Study Guide

Pharmacology for Nursing Care

Seventh Edition

RICHARD A. LEHNE, PhD

Prepared by

Sherry Neely, MSN, RN, CRNP
Associate Professor
Butler County Community College
Butler, Pennsylvania

Reviewed by

Shelia Bouie, RN, MSN
Assistant Professor
Richard J. Daley College
Chicago, Illinois

SAUNDERS

ELSEVIER

SAUNDERS
ELSEVIER

11830 Westline Industrial Drive
St. Louis, Missouri 63146

Notice

Knowledge and best practice in this field are constantly changing. As new research and experience broaden
our knowledge, changes in practice, treatment and drug therapy may become necessary or appropriate.
Readers are advised to check the most current information provided (i) on procedures featured or (ii) by the
manufacturer of each product to be administered, to verify the recommended dose or formula, the method
and duration of administration, and contraindications. It is the responsibility of the practitioner, relying on
their own experience and knowledge of the patient, to make diagnoses, to determine dosages and the best
treatment for each individual patient, and to take all appropriate safety precautions. To the fullest extent of
the law, neither the Publisher nor the Authors assumes any liability for any injury and/or damage to persons
or property arising out of or related to any use of the material contained in this book.

The Publisher

Acquisitions Editor: Kristin Geen
Senior Developmental Editor: Lauren Lake
Publishing Services Manager: Jeff Patterson
Senior Project Manager: Anne Konopka

Printed in the United States of America

Working together to grow
libraries in developing countries

www.elsevier.com | www.bookaid.org | www.sabre.org

ELSEVIER   BOOK AID
International   Sabre Foundation

Last digit is the print number: 9   8   7   6   5   4   3   2   1

Introduction

The critical thinking and study questions in this study guide include review of knowledge, application of knowledge to nursing care, and analysis of nursing situations that require clinical decision-making, and prioritization of nursing actions. When using this book as a study guide, the questions that do not have a ▶ or ✳ are excellent tools to augment the initial reading of the textbook before attending class and for review following classroom activities. Knowledge of the action, interactions, administration directives, and adverse effects is required before the nurse can engage in clinical decision-making.

The questions that have a ▶ or ✳ before their number require more than repetition of the information in the textbook. Questions preceded by ▶ require application and analysis of information while those preceded by ✳ require prioritization including selecting the most important information or action. Identifying the correct answer to these questions requires careful examination of the data and reflection on the patient in a holistic manner. The student will have to integrate other nursing knowledge such as developmental considerations, and laboratory values, as well as timing and prioritization of actions. These ▶ and ✳ critical thinking questions reflect the reasoning that students and new graduate nurses need to be able to perform in order to safely administer pharmacotherapy. They are an excellent source of review when preparing for the NCLEX® examination.

A useful strategy when presented with long situation questions in this workbook is to read the last sentence first. Knowing the question that is being asked guides identification of pertinent information in the case. When reading the rest of the information in the case, identify key words and data. Identify assessment findings and laboratory values that are normal or abnormal. Think about the situation to identify if it is a normal part of nursing care or if it requires collaboration with the prescriber.

Some of the questions and case studies require short answers. Some of these answers are knowledge based and some are questions for which there is not one correct answer or strategy. For the second type of question, the author has provided possible solutions and strategies that have been effective in her practice. Discuss these situations and challenges with faculty and peers. Develop new approaches and don't be afraid to "think outside the box."

Critical thinking by the nursing student requires assimilating classroom learning and clinical experience. No two experiences are the same. Be careful not to add additional information into the question based on your experience with patients when answering questions in this workbook. But DO engage in discussion about similar patient experiences with faculty and peers. Be prepared to explain your thinking. It will enrich your learning experience.

The author and Elsevier welcome any feedback you have about the content of the study guide.

Answers can be reviewed online http://evolve.elsevier.com/Lehne/.

Contents

Answers can be reviewed online http://evolve.elsevier.com/Lehne/.

Neurologic Drugs

Drugs for Pain

Psychotherapeutic Drugs

Drug Abuse

VI. DRUGS THAT AFFECT FLUID AND ELECTROLYTE BALANCE

VII. DRUGS THAT AFFECT THE HEART, BLOOD VESSELS, AND BLOOD

VIII. DRUGS FOR ENDOCRINE DISORDERS

1

Orientation to Pharmacology

OBJECTIVES

After reading and studying the corresponding chapter and completing the critical thinking and study questions, the student will be able to:

1. Analyze the significance of drug characteristics.
2. Describe nursing actions that assist nursing clinical decision making regarding administration of a prescribed drug.
3. Evaluate nursing situations that involve administration of drugs.
4. Identify nursing interventions that address barriers to adherence to the prescribed drug regimen.

CRITICAL THINKING AND STUDY QUESTIONS

✳ 1. Several nursing students are debating whether ease of administration, effectiveness, minimal adverse effects, and safety are the most important characteristics of a drug. Prioritize these from most to least important and describe the reason for your prioritization.

2. The following questions must be considered when the nurse administers medications. Describe the actions the nurse must take to answer each question relating to the properties of an ideal drug.
    a. Effectiveness—Is the drug doing what it is supposed to do?

b. Safety—Is there any reason why this drug should not be administered?

c. Selectivity—What effects in addition to the intended effect is the drug producing?

d. Reversible action—When will the effects of the drug start, peak, and stop?

e. Predictability—What individual factors will affect how this patient will respond to this drug?

f. Ease of administration—What characteristics of the medication will promote or hinder the patient taking the medication as prescribed? What can the nurse do to make it easier for the patient to take the medication as prescribed?

g. Freedoms from drug interactions—What possible interactions with the combination of drugs that the patient is taking are likely to occur?

h. Low cost—Can the patient afford this drug? What can the nurse do if the patient states that he or she cannot afford the prescribed medication?

i. Chemical stability—What can the nurse teach to ensure that the patient stores a medication so that it does not lose potency or become toxic?

j. Possession of simple generic name—What should the nurse do to ensure that the patient knows the name and desired action of the drug?

▸ 3. A patient returned to the nursing unit after an esophagogastroduodenoscopy (EGD). She did not receive her 0900 oral drugs before the procedure because of an order for nothing by mouth (NPO). What factors must the nurse consider when deciding which of the 0900 oral drugs should be administered at this time?

2

Application of Pharmacology in Nursing Practice

Answers can be reviewed online at http://evolve.elsevier.com/Lehne/.

OBJECTIVES

After reading and studying the corresponding chapter and completing the critical thinking and study questions, the student will be able to:

1. Explain how the nurse fulfills the responsibility for the six rights of drug administration.
2. Develop a teaching plan for a newly prescribed drug.
3. Describe the use of the nursing process in drug administration.
4. List the data that should be obtained in a preadministration assessment.
5. Recognize the importance of the liver and kidneys in pharmacokinetics.
6. Differentiate nursing actions for drug contraindications versus drug precautions.
7. Develop interventions to overcome self-care obstacles for drug therapy adherence.

CRITICAL THINKING AND STUDY QUESTIONS

▶ 1. The nurse is preparing to administer prescribed drugs to a patient in a hospital. Describe how the nurse ensures that these rights occur.
   a. Right drug

   b. Right route

   c. Right dose

   d. Right time

   e. Right patient

   f. Right assessment

   g. Right education

   h. Right documentation

   i. Right to refuse

   j. Right evaluation

▶ 2. The nurse is preparing to administer desloratidine (Clarinex). The medication administration record lists the patient's dose as 15 mg (3 tablets) once a day. The nursing drug handbook lists the normal dose as 5 mg. Why should the nurse check the original prescriber's order before contacting the pharmacy or prescriber?

▶ 3. Why does the nurse need to know the mechanism of action of an antihypertensive drug before administering the medication?

4. Research the drug furosemide (Lasix). Use the following chart to create a patient teaching handout using wording that the average adult patient could understand.

Furosemide (Lasix, Apo-furosemide)	
Therapeutic category and action	
Dosage, route, and time schedule	
Expected therapeutic response	
Nondrug measures to enhance therapeutic response	
Duration of treatment	
Method of drug storage	
Symptoms of common adverse effects	
Early toxicity symptoms	
Measures to minimize harm	
Major adverse drug-drug and drug-food interactions	
When to contact the prescriber	

5. Describe the needed nursing actions for each step of the nursing process for administering a medication for pain (analgesic) to a patient who is postoperative following gallbladder removal (cholecystectomy) and who does not want to cough and deep breathe because of the pain.
   a. Assessment

   b. Analysis: nursing diagnosis

   c. Planning

   d. Implementation

   e. Evaluation

6. List the data that should be obtained in a preadministration assessment.

▶ 7. The nurse is preparing to administer an anti-hypertensive drug (medication that lowers the blood pressure). The nurse assesses the patient's blood pressure, and it is 110/70 mm Hg, which is within normal limits. What action should the nurse take to determine if it is safe to administer the drug?

a. Call the prescriber, report the current blood pressure, and ask if the medication should be administered.

b. Hold the medication because the patient's blood pressure is too low to administer an antihypertensive drug.

c. Administer the medication because the antihypertensive medication is prescribed.

d. Assess the patient's baseline blood pressure and the blood pressure before and after the last dose of this medication to determine if the medication should be administered.

8. Why are liver and kidney function so important to assess before administering any drug?

9. The nurse is administering medications. The medication administration record (MAR) has cefazolin sodium (Ancef) prescribed for two different patients. One patient's chart states that the patient is allergic to cephalosporin. The other states that the patient is allergic to penicillin. Allergy to cephalosporin is a contraindication for cefazolin. Allergy to penicillin is a precaution for cefazolin. The nurse should assess both patients for their allergic symptoms and

a. hold both medications and notify the prescriber.

b. administer the medication to the patient who is allergic to penicillin because cefazolin is not a penicillin.

c. notify the prescriber of the allergy and administer the cefazolin cautiously to the patient who is allergic to penicillin because there is sometimes a cross allergy between penicillins and first-generation cephalosporins.

d. administer both medications if the patient did not have a life-threatening reaction with the previous drug reaction.

10. State interventions to overcome these factors that may interfere with a patient's ability to perform self-care with a medication regimen.

a. Unable to remember what they are supposed to do.

b. Lack money to pay for medications.

c. Believe drug is not needed.

3

Drug Regulation, Development, Names, and Information

Answers can be reviewed online at http://evolve.elsevier.com/Lehne/.

OBJECTIVES

After reading and studying the corresponding chapter and completing the critical thinking and study questions, the student will be able to:

1. Discuss the characteristics of reliable research studies.
2. Describe the role of the nurse in clinical testing of a new drug.
3. Apply information about new drugs to a patient's situation.
4. Describe the three types of names of drugs.
5. Recognize the benefit of knowing the generic name of drugs.
6. Explain the problems with use of trade names to identify drugs.
7. Recognize the characteristics of generic drugs.

CRITICAL THINKING AND STUDY QUESTIONS

1. The nurse is caring for a patient who has high blood cholesterol (hyperlipidemia). The patient states that she became worried about her high cholesterol when her sister had a "heart attack." She went to a health food store to see if they had any natural product that could help lower her cholesterol. She noticed a sign on the counter asking for volunteers to enter a study. Volunteers are to submit a copy of their blood cholesterol results and again at the end of a year after taking the product as directed for a full year. Explain why the results of this study may not be reliable based on these factors.
   a. Control
   b. Randomization

   c. Blinding

2. What new power was given to the FDA by the PREA (2003)?
   a. Testing of new drugs for dose content
   b. Testing of new drugs for additional ingredients
   c. Testing of new drugs on children
   d. Testing of new drugs on women

3. What role can the nurse fill to assist the FDA with the goals of FDA Amendment Act (2007)?
   a. Encourage patients to always take the full course of prescribed drugs
   b. Explain the importance of disposing of drugs that are older than 12 months.
   c. Report unusual effects of drugs.
   d. Teach patients how to read drug labels.

4. Angiotensin converting enzyme inhibitor (ACEI) drugs are used for high blood pressure (hypertension). These drugs can cause a dry cough in approximately 40% of patients. Newer, more expensive angiotensin II receptor blocker (ARB) drugs have been developed that produce essentially the same therapeutic effect but do not the cause the same cough.

A patient who is receiving an ACEI explains to the nurse that her friend is getting a new drug (ARB) and that she is sure it is better because it is new. Discuss how the nurse should respond.

5. Describe the three types of names of drugs.
   a. Chemical name

   b. Generic name

   c. Trade name

6. Why is it important for the nurse to learn the generic names of drugs? (Select all that apply.)
   a. The same generic name is never used for more than one medication.
   b. Generic names tell the nurse the chemical ingredients of the drug.
   c. The generic name of a drug will be the same no matter which company produces the drug.
   d. Generic names are easy to recall and pronounce.

   e. Generic names often suggest the action of the drug.
   f. Generic names of drugs in the same therapeutic class often have a similar suffix making them easy to identify.

7. When preparing discharge instructions for a patient the nurse should
   a. review the prescriptions written for discharge and include the stated trade name and generic name in discharge teaching.
   b. write and explain the generic name so the patient does not become confused.
   c. write and explain the trade name because it is easier for the patient to remember.
   d. ask the patient which name he or she uses for the drug and only use that name in discharge teaching.

8. A patient has been taking a brand-name drug for a chronic condition for several years. Recent changes in his insurance plan require the use of generic drugs whenever they are available. The patient asks the nurse if he should pay out of his pocket to continue receiving the brand-name drug. The nurse's response should be based on the fact that
   a. trade name drugs contain different active ingredients than generic drugs.
   b. generic drugs are equal in their therapeutic equivalency to their brand-name counterparts.
   c. generic drugs usually are not absorbed at the same rate as brand-name drugs.
   d. continuing to use the brand-name drug will prevent confusion.

9. The nurse is providing discharge teaching for a patient who has had outpatient surgery and who has been prescribed Percocet 2 tablets every 4 to 6 hours as needed for pain. Percocet is a combination of oxycodone, a narcotic, and acetaminophen, an over-the-counter (OTC) analgesic found in Tylenol and other OTC products. What should the nurse include in the teaching to avoid liver damage from excessive acetaminophen ingestion?

10. The nurse is teaching a patient about tamsulosin (Flomax), which has been prescribed for difficulty voiding due to an enlarged prostate. Because this person travels extensively and not all countries require prescriptions to get drugs, it is important for the nurse to teach the patient that
    a. a drug labeled Flomax may have different active ingredients in different countries.
    b. drugs purchased in countries other than the United States and Canada are usually unsafe.
    c. Flomax is not available anywhere except the United States and Canada.
    d. the doses of Flomax in countries that use the metric system are different than doses of drugs in the United States.

4

Pharmacokinetics

Answers can be reviewed online at http://evolve.elsevier.com/Lehne/.

OBJECTIVES

After reading and studying the corresponding chapter and completing the critical thinking and study questions, the student will be able to:

1. Define pharmacokinetics.
2. Identify nursing responsibilities when administering drugs.
3. Employ knowledge of factors that affect drug movement when administering drugs.
4. Use critical thinking to develop measures that prevent drug administration errors.
5. Identify nursing considerations for timing and routes of drug administration.
6. Research the metabolism and excretion of a drug and apply the information to nursing care.
7. Apply the principles of narrow therapeutic range, half-life, peak, and trough to nursing responsibilities when administering drugs.
8. Explain the clinical significance between a narrow and wide therapeutic range.

CRITICAL THINKING AND STUDY QUESTIONS

1. Describe the four processes of pharmacokinetics.
   a. Absorption

   b. Distribution

   c. Metabolism (biotransformation)

   d. Excretion

2. Drugs can cross cell membranes in three ways. Match the method of movement with characteristics for that method of movement.

   _____ a. Passage through channels   1. May require energy or pores

   _____ b. Direct penetration of the membrane   2. Requires small size

   3. Requires lipid solubility

   _____ c. Passage with the aid of a transport system

3. The four processes of pharmacokinetics have which of the following characteristics in common?
   a. Stimulation of receptors
   b. Blocking of processes
   c. Dose-response relationship
   d. Movement

4. Insulin is a hormone that is available as a drug. It combines with receptors on cardiac and skeletal muscle and fat cells to facilitate the transport mechanism that allows the glucose ($C_6H_{12}O_6$) molecule to enter the cell. Why does glucose require a transport mechanism to enter these cells? (Select all that apply.)
   a. Glucose is water soluble.
   b. Glucose is fat soluble.
   c. Glucose is too large to cross the cell membrane through a channel.
   d. Glucose is an ion.
   e. Glucose is a quaternary ammonium compound.

5. The nurse is caring for a patient who has recently been diagnosed with asthma and is prescribed an inhaled bronchodilator drug that is a quaternary ammonium compound. The patient does not like using the inhaler and asks the nurse why the prescriber did not just prescribe a pill. The nurse's response would be based on knowledge that the
   a. oral drug would not produce the desired effect.
   b. oral drug would be absorbed too quickly.
   c. inhaled drug and oral drug produce different therapeutic effects.
   d. inhaled drug has very limited absorption into the bloodstream and should cause less adverse effects.

6. Which of the following changes in pain medication orders for a second-day postoperative patient whose pain has decreased from 8 of 10 to 7 of 10 should the nurse question?
   a. Discontinue morphine sulfate 2 mg intravenous (IV) every 3 hours as needed and start morphine sulfate 2 mg tablets by mouth every 4 hours as needed.
   b. Discontinue morphine sulfate 2 mg IV every 3 hours as needed and start morphine sulfate 10 mg tablets by mouth every 4 hours as needed.

▶ 7. The nurse has a heavy assignment, including caring for a hospitalized patient who has been prescribed the following medications: 0800 glyburide (DiaBeta) 10 mg; 0900 quinapril HCl (Accupril) 20 mg. Breakfast is served at 0810. Hospital policy states that medications may be administered 30 minutes before and after the designated time. To save time, the nurse plans to administer both of these medications at 0830. Research these medications and describe why this is not a good plan.

8. Explain if the following factors would increase or decrease the absorption of an oral medication.
   a. Administer a chewable aspirin (acetylsalicylic acid) instead of an enteric-coated aspirin.

   b. The patient has an ileostomy.

   c. Take a medication immediately before or after vigorous exercise.

9. Describe why chemotherapy for cancer is administered through a central IV line instead of a peripherally inserted IV line.

10. Heparin sodium is available on the nursing unit in two concentrations. Heparin sodium 100 units/mL is for flushing IV lines, and heparin sodium 5000 units/mL is for subcutaneous administration. Identify measures that prevent accidental administration of the wrong concentration of this drug.

11. What steps does the nurse need to take before administering any IV medication?

12. Describe administration techniques for IV drugs that can decrease the chance of adverse reactions.

13. A 15-year-old young woman comes to a family planning clinic and is diagnosed with primary syphilis. Based on knowledge that developmentally this patient is not likely to adhere to a lengthy treatment plan, the best route for administering an antibiotic to this patient is
   a. a once-a-day oral pill.
   b. a depot intramuscular (IM) injection.
   c. an IV infusion.
   d. a topical cream.

▶ 14. The nurse would consult the prescriber regarding IM administration of any drug if the patient's laboratory test results include
   a. AST: 72 international units/L.
   b. Creatinine: 2.4 mg/dL.
   c. INR: 3.2.
   d. Potassium: 3.2 mEq/L.
   e. WBC: 13,000/mm.^{3}

15. Developmentally, which of the following routes is the least desirable for a hospitalized school-aged child who is receiving frequent doses of pain medication?
   a. Intramuscular
   b. Intravenous
   c. Oral
   d. Topical

16. The home health nurse notes that a family member has been crushing all of the patient's medications, including enteric-coated preparations and mixing them in pudding so that they are easier to swallow. The nurse should explain that enteric-coated drugs should not be crushed because
   a. they must be taken on an empty stomach.
   b. crushing these preparations destroys the medication.
   c. crushing these preparations can cause stomach distress or cause the acid in the stomach to alter the drug.
   d. crushing these preparations can delay medication absorption.

17. The nurse is teaching a patient how to take the medication nitroglycerin for anginal chest pain. Teaching on the route of administration should be based on the fact that nitroglycerin has an extensive first-pass effect, which means (Select all that apply.)
   a. most of the drug is inactivated by the liver before it reaches circulation when administered orally.
   b. most of the drug is activated by the liver, so it must be administered orally.
   c. once absorbed, the drug stays in systemic circulation for a long time because it is not metabolized by the liver.
   d. administration by dissolving under the tongue (sublingually) allows the drug to be absorbed directly into systemic circulation bypassing first pass in the liver.
   e. the drug can only be administered as a topical patch.

18. The nurse would expect that an IV antibiotic prescribed for bacterial meningitis would most likely get to the site of infection if the patient is
    a. an infant.
    b. a child.
    c. an adolescent.
    d. an adult.

✳ 19. The most effective way for the nurse to promote excretion of most anesthetics is to
    a. encourage deep breathing.
    b. maintain a patent IV line.
    c. monitor urine output.
    d. prevent constipation.

20. The nurse is preparing to administer the medication digoxin (Lanoxin) to a patient who has been receiving the drug for chronic heart failure (HF) and who recently went into renal failure. Research the metabolism and excretion of this drug and explain why the nurse needs to be cautious when administering digoxin to this patient.

21. Digoxin (Lanoxin) is a drug that has a narrow therapeutic range. When administering this drug the nurse needs to (Select all that apply.)
    a. administer the medication only on an as needed (PRN) basis.
    b. carefully monitor the patient for therapeutic and toxic effects.
    c. be diligent about administering the medication exactly as prescribed.
    d. monitor blood levels of the drugs to assess if they are in the therapeutic range.

22. Research the drugs heparin sodium and warfarin (Coumadin). Based on the action and half-life of these drugs, explain why heparin sodium administered subcutaneously (SC) can be administered the day before elective surgery, but the surgeon may delay elective surgery for several days to a week if a patient is receiving warfarin.

23. A patient stopped taking levothyroxine (Synthroid) 3 days ago. This drug has a half-life of 9 to 10 days. He tells the nurse that the drug must not have been necessary because he does not feel any different. The basis of the nurse's explanation on why the patient has not noticed any change in how he feels is the
    a. drug's previous doses have not been completely eliminated from the body.
    b. drug probably was not needed if the patient has not experienced any symptoms.
    c. patient's dose was probably too high, so the drug is still working.
    d. patient could not have been taking the drug as prescribed before stopping the drug 3 days ago.

24. Grapefruit juice inhibits the cytochrome P450 CYP3A4 drug metabolizing enzyme and inhibits p-glycoprotein in the intestines for weeks after ingestion. This especially affects calcium channel blockers, benzodiazepines, cyclosporine, and "statin" drugs. The nurse should teach a patient who is prescribed any of these drugs that drinking grapefruit juice can cause
    a. excessive first pass effect.
    b. excess levels of drug in the blood.
    c. lack of therapeutic effect of the drug.
    d. rapid excretion of the drug.

25. A patient is receiving vancomycin 500 mg every 6 hours IV for a serious infection. Vancomycin IV has an immediate onset and can be neurotoxic, but adequate levels of the drug are needed to treat the infection. The prescriber has ordered peak and trough levels to be drawn. When would the nurse expect the peak and trough levels to be drawn?
    a. Peak level 1.5 hours before infusion started and trough level immediately after infusion of the drug is complete.
    b. Peak level 1.5 hours after infusion and trough level 30 minutes before next dose.
    c. Peak level while the drug is infusing and trough level immediately after infusion of the drug is complete.
    d. Peak level while the drug is infusing and trough level 30 minutes before next dose.

26. Phenytoin (Dilantin) is a drug that has a narrow therapeutic range. Serum levels of these drugs are monitored periodically because the
    a. drug is very potent.
    b. drug is used for patients who have critical illnesses.
    c. dose of the drug that is needed to produce the desired effect is very high.
    d. difference between the dose that produces the desired effect and the dose that is toxic to the patient is very small.

5

Pharmacodynamics

Answers can be reviewed online at http://evolve.elsevier.com/Lehne/.

OBJECTIVES

After reading and studying the corresponding chapter and completing the critical thinking and study questions, the student will be able to:

1. Explain why knowledge of pharmacodynamics is needed for drug administration.
2. Describe the three phases of the dose-response relationship.
3. Recognize the significance of potency and drug-receptor interactions.
4. Identify the relationship of the type of receptor to onset of therapeutic effect.
5. Differentiate between appropriate and inappropriate nursing actions based on expected effects of a drug.
6. Compare the intrinsic activity and affinity of selected drugs.
7. Anticipate possible adverse effects of a drug based on excessive individual response.
8. Apply pharmacodynamic principles to nursing clinical decision making.

CRITICAL THINKING AND STUDY QUESTIONS

▶ 1. Increasing urinary fluid excretion, vasodilation, and decreasing heart rate are different mechanisms of action of drugs used to treat hypertension. Why does the nurse need to know the mechanism of action of an antihypertensive drug?

2. Describe the three phases of the dose-response relationship.
   a. Phase 1

   b. Phase 2

   c. Phase 3

3. The nurse is reading research about a drug. The literature states that the drug is potent. This means the drug
   a. produces its effects at low doses.
   b. produces strong effects at any dose.
   c. requires high doses to produce its effects.
   d. is very likely to cause adverse effects.

4. Except for gene therapy, which of the following statements are true about drug-receptor interactions? (Select all that apply.)
   a. Drugs can mimic the actions of endogenous molecules.
   b. Receptors for drugs do not respond to hormones and neurotransmitters produced by the body.
   c. The binding of a drug to its receptor is usually irreversible.
   d. Drugs can block the actions of endogenous molecules.
   e. Drugs can give the cell new functions.

5. A patient has been diagnosed with hypothyroidism and has been prescribed levothyroxine (Synthroid), a synthetic thyroid hormone replacement. An explanation of why the drug does not reach a peak therapeutic effect until taken regularly for 3 to 4 weeks is that thyroid hormone stimulates the family of receptors that are
   a. located on the cell surface (cell membrane–embedded enzymes).
   b. located on the cell surface and regulates the flow of ions in and out of the cell (ligand-gated channels).
   c. found within the cell and function to regulate protein synthesis (transcription factors).
   d. folded receptors that activate a G protein that then activates the effector (G protein–coupled receptor systems).

6. The nurse is administering morphine sulfate for moderate to severe postoperative pain. Based on the effect of modulating processes that are affected by morphine, the nurse should (Select all that apply.)
   a. assess respirations and hold the medication if adventitious breath sounds are present.
   b. assess respiratory rate and hold the medication if respirations are weak or less than 12/min.
   c. maintain the patient on complete bed rest with all four side rails elevated to prevent injury.
   d. assist the patient when ambulating to prevent injury.
   e. not administer the medication if the patient's behavior does not suggest that he is having moderate to severe pain.
   f. restrict fluids to prevent nausea.
   g. encourage ambulation if not contraindicated to promote bowel motility.

7. A patient has been receiving intravenous hydromorphone HCl (Dilaudid) 1 mg every 4 hours as needed for severe pain. The patient has been progressing and is experiencing less pain. The prescriber has discontinued the hydromorphone and prescribed intravenous pentazocine (Talwin) 30 mg every 4 hours as needed for moderate pain. This suggests that hydromorphone
   a. and pentazocine are agonists and have equally high affinity and intrinsic activity.
   b. and pentazocine are agonist-antagonist and have equally moderate affinity and intrinsic activity.
   c. is an agonist with a higher affinity and intrinsic activity than the agonist-antagonist pentazocine.
   d. is an agonist-antagonist with a lower affinity and intrinsic activity than the agonist pentazocine.

8. Metoprolol (Lopressor, Betaloc) is a drug that is a selective antagonist for $beta_1$-adrenergic receptors. When stimulated, $beta_1$-receptors of the heart increase the heart rate. The nurse should assess the patient receiving metoprolol for excessive response, which would be seen as
   a. hypertension and tachycardia.
   b. hypertension and bradycardia.
   c. hypotension and tachycardia.
   d. hypotension and bradycardia.

✳ 9. Research the pharmacokinetics of methadone HCl (Metadol), an opiate, and naloxone HCl (Narcan), a narcotic antagonist. A patient who has overdosed on methadone HCl is brought into the emergency department unresponsive with severely depressed respirations. The patient receives intravenous naloxone HCl with a dramatic improvement in the level of consciousness and respiratory rate and effort within minutes. What must the nurse be prepared to do 45 to 60 minutes after the naloxone HCl is administered?
   a. Assess for return of pain because the effect of the naloxone HCl should be peaking.
   b. Assess for the need to administer another dose of naloxone HCl because respiratory and CNS depression might occur as the naloxone HCl effect is ending.
   c. Prepare to administer the drug intramuscularly if the drug has not taken effect.
   d. Counteract effects of opiate withdrawal.

10. Ibuprofen is a nonsteroidal anti-inflammatory drug (NSAID) that is available over-the-counter. Based on the dose instructions on the label (or a drug handbook), what is the ED_{50} for mild to moderate pain relief?

▸ 11. The pediatrician has prescribed amoxicillin suspension 100 mg every 8 hours for a child who weighs 22 lb (10 kg). The nurse's drug handbook states that the recommended dosage of amoxicillin for a child weighing less than 20 kg is 20 to 40 mg/kg/day divided into three equal doses. The nurse should
    a. hold the medication and notify the pediatrician that the dose is more than the recommended dose.
    b. hold the medication and notify the pediatrician that the dose is less than the recommended dose.
    c. administer the medication and continue to assess the child.
    d. administer no more than 133 mg per dose.

12. When the therapeutic index of a drug is narrow, the nurse would expect
    a. the drug would produce the desired effect at low doses.
    b. blood levels of the drug to be monitored throughout therapy.
    c. the drug would produce many adverse effects at low doses.
    d. the drug should only be used in an emergency.

6

Drug Interactions

Answers can be reviewed online at http://evolve.elsevier.com/Lehne/.

OBJECTIVES

After reading and studying the corresponding chapter and completing the critical thinking and study questions, the student will be able to:

1. Identify common substances that can alter the effect, metabolism, and/or excretion of other drugs.
2. Describe the purpose of additive ingredients in drugs.
3. Explain the disulfiram (Antabuse) reaction.
4. Evaluate the process of drug administration and order transcription for common errors that can cause drug interactions.
5. Apply knowledge of pH-dependent ionization and partitioning to therapeutic uses.
6. Use knowledge of the effects of the hepatic microsomal enzyme system and P-glycoprotein on drug levels.
7. Research situations that can cause altered drug absorption, metabolism, and excretion.
8. Identify assessment data that suggest drug accumulation.
9. Solve drug administration problems that relate to interactions.

CRITICAL THINKING AND STUDY QUESTIONS

1. Identify which of the following substances can cause drug interactions. (Select all that apply.)
    a. Beer
    b. Chocolate
    c. Garlic
    d. Over-the-counter drugs
    e. Potassium
    f. Prescription drugs
    g. Tea
    h. Tobacco

2. A mother asks the nurse why her son was prescribed amoxicillin and potassium clavulanate (Augmentin) for otitis media if amoxicillin has not worked in the past. What should the nurse's response be based on?

3. The nurse is providing discharge teaching for a patient who will be taking metronidazole (Flagyl) after discharge. The drug information states to caution the patient that a disulfiram (Antabuse) reaction can occur. This means
   a. adverse reactions can occur if the patient takes metronidazole and the drug disulfiram.
   b. adverse reactions can occur if the patient ingests or absorbs alcohol while taking metronidazole.
   c. metronidazole must be taken with disulfiram to prevent adverse reactions.
   d. disulfiram is frequently prescribed for patients who are receiving metronidazole.

▶ 4. List some examples of how the nurse can inadvertently mix two drugs together during medication administration and possibly produce adverse effects.

▶ 5. It is the nurse's responsibility at this institution to decide what time a drug will be administered. Cholestyramine (Questran) has been prescribed for a patient who takes many drugs for diabetes and hypertension. The patient takes the other drugs at 0900 and 1700. At this institution, drugs can be given up to 1 hour before or after the assigned time. When should the cholestyramine be administered?

6. A patient has toxic levels of an alkaline drug in his blood. The drug is excreted unchanged in the urine. The nurse anticipates administration of which of the following substances to increase excretion of the alkaline substance?
   a. Sodium bicarbonate (baking soda)
   b. Antacids (TUMS)
   c. Acetylsalicylic acid (aspirin)
   d. Ascorbic acid (Vitamin C)

7. Patients receiving certain drugs that are metabolized by the CYP3A4 enzyme should not drink grapefruit juice because grapefruit juice inhibits the CYP3A4 enzyme and the drug transporter P-glycoprotein. The patient asks what might happen if she drinks grapefruit juice and takes the medication. The nurse's response is based on knowledge that the effect could be
   a. a lack of response to the drug because it does not get to the site of action.
   b. possible toxicity because metabolism and excretion of the drug can be impaired, and absorption may be increased.
   c. a lack of response because the drug will not be absorbed.
   d. liver damage because the CYP3A4 enzyme destroys the liver.

8. Smoking induces the CYP1A2 liver enzyme. Coumadin (warfarin), an anticoagulant blood thinner, is metabolized by the CYP1A2 enzyme. Because of this interaction, the nurse needs to be alert for what response in the patient receiving warfarin who also smokes tobacco?
   a. Excessively elevated INR
   b. Gums that bleed when teeth are brushed
   c. Sudden shortness of breath, change in mental status, or chest pain
   d. Unexplained bruising

9. A patient is taking digoxin (Lanoxin), a drug that is excreted by the kidneys in the active state. The nurse notes that the patient's laboratory values include significantly elevated creatinine levels, suggesting renal failure. Research digoxin and identify symptoms of digitalis toxicity for which the nurse should assess this patient.

10. The nurse is caring for a 92-year-old female who was admitted yesterday with pneumonia. Past history includes hypertension and heart failure. The patient is exhibiting signs that she is experiencing hallucinations. What information does the nurse need to provide to the prescriber to help determine if the behavior is related to a drug interaction?

11. A patient has been having severe diarrhea for the past 5 days after receiving a new antibiotic. He takes an anticonvulsant orally. What is the possible effect on the blood level of the anticonvulsant?

12. The nurse is getting ready to give two IV antibiotics. Both are scheduled at 0900. The nurse cannot find any information about the compatibility of these two drugs, but knows that it is important to stay on schedule to keep plasma levels stable. One drug (drug X) can be given over 20 minutes, and the other (drug Y) requires 1 hour to infuse. Describe what the nurse can do to safely administer these drugs if compatibility is unknown.

13. Describe how the nurse should respond to these possible drug-food interactions.
    a. The patient wants to take tetracycline with milk because it upsets his stomach.

b. The patient takes digoxin (Lanoxin) in the morning with breakfast.

c. A patient who is HIV positive has a poor appetite and is prescribed saquinavir (Invirase).

d. A patient who is taking a calcium channel blocker states that he does not drink grapefruit juice with his medication, only later in the day.

e. The patient has been prescribed tranylcypromine (Parnate), an MAO inhibitor for depression.

f. The patient has started taking warfarin (Coumadin) and only eats green vegetables occasionally.

7
Adverse Drug Reactions and Medication Errors

Answers can be reviewed online at http://evolve.elsevier.com/Lehne/.

OBJECTIVES

After reading and studying the corresponding chapter and completing the critical thinking and study questions, the student will be able to:

1. Identify patients who are at risk for drug reactions.
2. Assess the necessary nursing response when an adverse drug reaction occurs.
3. Anticipate the effect of sudden withdrawal from a drug for which the patient has developed a physical dependence.
4. Describe common symptoms of nephrotoxicity, neurotoxicity, and ototoxicity.
5. Research drugs for potential adverse effects.
6. Incorporate laboratory test analysis in nursing decision making relating to drug administration.
7. Apply knowledge of drug-induced long QT-syndrome to nursing care.
8. Determine appropriate nursing actions when adverse effects are probable.
9. Recognize the importance of correct dose calculation.
10. Apply the appropriate scope of nursing practice to medication administration situations.
11. Develop strategies that reduce the incidence of medication errors.
12. Summarize nursing responsibilities when a medication error occurs.

CRITICAL THINKING AND STUDY QUESTIONS

1. Which of the following is not an adverse effect of a drug as defined by the World Health Organization (WHO)?
   a. Constipation from codeine for pain
   b. Nausea and vomiting from chemotherapy
   c. Reflex tachycardia from calcium channel blocker vasodilators to lower blood pressure
   d. Respiratory depression from overdose on benzodiazepine sleeping pills

2. The nurse would contact the prescriber before administering a drug that depresses respirations if the adult patient's respiratory rate is less than how many breaths per minute?

3. Adverse drug reactions occur more often in (Select all that apply.)
   a. patients taking multiple drugs.
   b. patients taking potent drugs.
   c. situations where a drug error occurs.
   d. patients over 60 years of age.
   e. patients younger than 1 year of age.
   f. malnourished patients.
   g. accidental poisonings.

✳ 4. The nurse has administered quinapril (Accupril). One hour after administration, the patient reports a tingling sensation of the lips. The nurse notes that the patient's lips are "puffy" (perioral edema). The nursing action with the highest priority is to
   a. hold the next dose of the medication.
   b. document the finding and continue to assess the patient.
   c. notify the prescriber STAT.
   d. withhold all food and water.

5. Match the symptoms to the adverse effects.

   _____ a. Anaphylaxis
   _____ b. Hemorrhage
   _____ c. Neutropenia

   1. Bleeding with minor trauma such as brushing teeth
   2. Frequent or unusual infections
   3. Numbness and tingling around the mouth
   4. Platelet count less than 100,000/mm^3
   5. Unexplained bruising
   6. WBC count less than 5,000/mm^3

6. The nurse is administering metoprolol tartrate (Lopressor, Toprol), a beta$_1$-adrenergic receptor blocking drug that slows the heart rate and lowers the blood pressure. The nurse must teach the patient not to stop taking the drug suddenly because this could cause
   a. bradycardia and hypotension.
   b. bradycardia and hypertension.
   c. tachycardia and hypotension.
   d. tachycardia and hypertension.

7. Because the drug handbook lists gentamicin sulfate (Garamycin) as being ototoxic, the nurse should teach the patient to report
   a. dizziness.
   b. tinnitus.
   c. palpitations.
   d. rash.

8. Before administering lovastatin (Mevacor), a "statin" drug known to be toxic to the liver, the nurse reviews the patient's laboratory tests. Test results include alanine aminotransferase (ALT) 234 international units/L and aspartate aminotransferase (AST) 197 units/L. The nurse should
   a. administer the drug.
   b. assess the vital signs, and if stable, administer the drug.
   c. hold the drug medication and report the results to the prescriber within 24 hours.
   d. notify the prescriber STAT.

9. The nurse is teaching a patient who has been prescribed terbinafine HCl (Lamisil) tablets 250 mg once a day for 12 weeks for toenail onychomycosis. Because the drug can be hepatotoxic, the nurse teaches the patient to report (Select all that apply.)
   a. constipation.
   b. light-colored stool.
   c. rash.
   d. yellow-colored skin.
   e. pale conjunctiva.
   f. anorexia.
   g. angioedema.
   h. nausea and vomiting.
   i. tarry stool.

10. The nurse is administering a drug that has been known to cause long-QT syndrome to a female patient. Assessment findings that would warrant consultation with the prescriber include (Select all that apply.)
    a. lightheadedness or dizziness.

b. palpitations.
c. serum magnesium 1.9 mEq/L.
d. serum potassium 4.7 mEq/L.
e. medication regimen includes three drugs known to prolong QT interval.
f. nausea and vomiting.
g. constipation.
h. heart rate 58 beats/min.
i. heart rate 122 beats/min and BP 80/46 mm Hg.

11. What role does the nurse have on admission and discharge of a patient that is designed to significantly prevent adverse effects of drugs, especially due to polypharmacy and drug interactions?

12. A patient calls the telephone triage nurse at her doctor's office to report experiencing ankle edema and shortness of breath within 24 hours after starting a newly prescribed drug. The symptoms resolve when the drug is stopped but return when it is restarted. Drug information does not include peripheral edema and shortness of breath as adverse effects of this drug. Which of the following would not be an appropriate action by this nurse?
    a. Advise the patient to seek emergency care (call 911) if she experiences throat tightness.
    b. Consult with the prescriber regarding reporting these symptoms to www.fda.gov/medwatch.
    c. Explain that she needs to stop taking the drug and come in to be seen as soon as possible.
    d. Tell the patient to withhold taking all prescribed drugs until she can come in and be seen by the prescriber.

13. The nurse is caring for a 57-year-old black man who has been prescribed sulfamethoxazole and trimethoprim (Septra IV) and whose history includes a G-6-PD deficiency. Because this enzyme deficiency can cause hemolytic anemia in patients receiving sulfonamide, penicillin, and cephalosporin antibiotics, the nurse will monitor the patient for which of the following symptoms?
    a. Decreased urine output
    b. Fatigue and pale gums

c. Nausea and vomiting

d. Rubor and pruritis

14. The nurse is mentoring a student nurse. The student complains that it is unfair that the nursing program requires 100% proficiency in dose calculation on a dose calculation examination during the last semester. The student complains that students may be stressed by test taking and should not be expected to meet that level of proficiency. The basis of the nurse's response to the student is to

   a. support the student's efforts to overturn the policy because it is unrealistic.

   b. share with the student the policy that existed when the nurse was in school.

   c. support the school policy because 100% proficiency on dose calculations is required on the state board National Council Licensure Examination (NCLEX) examination.

   d. explain to the student that students must be able to calculate drug doses under stress because emergency situations are very stressful and that drug dose errors in these situations can be fatal.

15. The nurse is caring for a patient who is experiencing severe pain. Morphine sulfate 10 mg intramuscular (IM) is ordered every 4 hours as needed. The patient asks the nurse to administer the medication via an existing intravenous (IV) cap because he hates the pain of an IM injection. The nurse should

   a. explain to the patient that the nurse cannot change the route of a medication and that the patient can receive the medication IM as prescribed now or wait until the nurse pages the prescriber for the patient's request.

   b. administer the medication IM because that is the way that it is ordered.

   c. administer the medication via the intravenous cap.

   d. determine if the dose is safe for IV administration and administer it via the IV cap if it is safe.

▶ 16. The nurse is preparing to administer 0900 medications on an assigned patient. The medication administration record states Celebrex 20 mg

once a day. The medication supplied is Celexa 20-mg tablets. What should the nurse do?

17. A nurse has administered an incorrect dose (too high) of a prescribed drug to a patient. Which of the following interventions would be least likely to be beneficial in this situation?

   a. Assess the patient for effects of the drug.

   b. Place the nurse on unpaid leave.

   c. Report the error to the institution's safety coordinator.

   d. Require the nurse to identify possible strategies to prevent this type of error in the future.

18. Describe measures that the nurse can take to prevent medication errors including specific actions for the three most common types of fatal medication errors.

   a. Measures that apply to all types of errors

   b. Giving an overdose

   c. Giving the wrong drug

   d. Using the wrong route

19. Document the following information clearly and concisely using safe abbreviations and eliminating unsafe abbreviations.

"I went to give a dose of 200 milligrams of Celebrex and the patient wouldn't take it. She told me that she does not take any capsules, especially not funny looking ones that have those lines on them. I explained that the medication is a nonsteroidal anti-inflammatory drug for pain and swelling. She still insisted that she does not take this capsule. She told me that while I was at it I should ask that doctor where my pill is that I take to feel better. It looks like a little pink football. She said that she feels less depressed since she started taking it a few months ago but she didn't get any last night. Maybe it is OK because she still feels OK. I got her chart out and read the admission orders and medication list. Celebrex was on the order but it was not listed on the medication reconciliation list from admission. The selective serotonin receptor antagonist Celexa is on the list. I called the attending doctor who told me to consult her primary care practitioner, which I did. He D/C the Celebrex 200 milligrams qd and ordered Celexa 20 milligrams gd at hs.

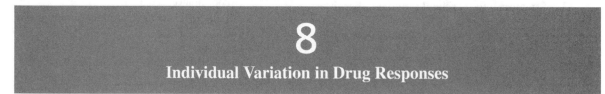

8

Individual Variation in Drug Responses

Answers can be reviewed online at http://evolve.elsevier.com/Lehne/.

OBJECTIVES

After reading and studying the corresponding chapter and completing the critical thinking and study questions, the student will be able to:

1. Identify the most accurate method for determining appropriate drug doses.
2. Evaluate nursing assessments and laboratory test results that reflect renal functioning.
3. Describe the effect of alterations in acid-base balance on drug distribution.
4. Examine the relationship of serum potassium levels and digoxin toxicity.
5. Compare pharmacodynamic and metabolic (pharmacokinetic) tolerance.
6. Determine the best nursing action when tachyphylaxis occurs.
7. Develop a teaching plan for a drug with a narrow therapeutic index and factors that can vary drug absorption and concentration.
8. Recognize appropriate nursing actions when adverse effects are probably caused by genetic variations.
9. Contrast differences in select drug metabolism between the sexes.
10. Predict the effect of nutritional status on drugs that are highly protein bound.

CRITICAL THINKING AND STUDY QUESTIONS

1. Dose requirements for drugs with a narrow therapeutic range are most accurately calculated based on
   a. age.
   b. body surface area.
   c. sex.
   d. weight.

▶ 2. Aminoglycoside antibiotics are potentially nephrotoxic antibiotics. What assessments and laboratory tests should the nurse monitor when a patient is receiving aminoglycoside antibiotics?

3. A patient is totally dependent on a respirator to initiate respirations. Recent laboratory values include pH 7.48, pCO_2 32 mm Hg, and

HCO$_3$ 20 mEq/L, indicating respiratory alkalosis. The effect of this acid-base imbalance on acidic drugs would be

a. ionization of the drug in the blood, increasing the blood level of the drug.

b. trapping of the drug in the cells, decreasing the blood level of the drug.

4. A terminal cancer patient has been receiving narcotic analgesics for severe pain for more than 6 months. The prescriber has increased the dose of the long-acting opiate and added an "as needed" opiate for breakthrough pain. The nurse should

a. recognize that the higher dose is needed because the patient would have undergone down-regulation of opiate receptors.

b. recognize that the additional medication is needed because cancer causes an up-regulation of opiate receptors.

c. question the higher dose of medication because the patient is at risk for narcotic addiction.

d. question why the medication is being prescribed on a regular and an as needed basis.

5. The difference between pharmacodynamic and metabolic (pharmacokinetic) tolerance is that there is a decreased response to the drug in tolerance and

a. both involve high levels of the drug in the blood, but pharmacodynamic tolerance involves lack of response, and metabolic tolerance involves normal response.

b. both involve high levels of the drug in the blood, but metabolic tolerance involves lack of response, and pharmacodynamic tolerance involves excessive response.

c. pharmacodynamic tolerance is lack of response to high levels of the drug in the blood, and metabolic tolerance is lack of response because of low levels of the drug in the blood.

d. pharmacodynamic tolerance is excessive response to low levels of the drug in the blood, and metabolic tolerance is lack of response to high levels of the drug in the blood.

6. A nitroglycerin transdermal patch is ordered to be applied at 0900 and removed at 2100. The patch from the previous day is still in place when the nurse is preparing to administer the 0900 patch. The best action by the nurse is:

a. leave the old patch on and apply the new one in a different site.

b. remove the old patch and apply the new one in a different site.

c. remove the old patch and do not apply a new patch until tomorrow.

d. remove the old patch and consult with the prescriber for further directions.

7. Research the drug lithium carbonate (Eskalith) and identify important teaching points about fluid, electrolyte, and food considerations when administering the drug.

8. The nurse is caring for a 57-year-old black man who has been prescribed sulfamethoxazole and trimethoprim (Septra IV) and whose history includes a G-6-PD deficiency. Because this enzyme deficiency can cause hemolytic anemia in patients receiving sulfonamide, penicillin, and cephalosporin antibiotics, the nurse will monitor which laboratory tests?

a. BUN and creatinine

b. Hematocrit and hemoglobin

c. AST and ALT

d. PT and INR

9. Based on differences in metabolism of alcohol between the sexes, if both a man and woman consume the same amount of alcohol (on a weight-adjusted basis) and take the drug metronidazole (Flagyl), the disulfiram reaction between alcohol and the drug in the woman should (Select all that apply.)

a. last longer than in the man.

b. abate sooner than in the man.

c. be more intense than in the man.

d. be less intense than in the man.

10. Warfarin sodium (Coumadin) is a drug that slows the formation of clots. It is highly protein bound. Only the unbound fraction of the drug is active. If the nurse is administering warfarin to a malnourished patient with a serum protein level of 4.9 gm/dL, the nurse would expect the patient's response to the drug to be

a. more intense with a greater risk for bleeding.

b. less intense with a greater risk for bleeding.

c. more intense with a lesser risk for bleeding.

d. less intense with a lesser risk for bleeding.

9

Drug Therapy During Pregnancy and Breast-Feeding

Answers can be reviewed online at http://evolve.elsevier.com/Lehne/.

OBJECTIVES

After reading and studying the corresponding chapter and completing the critical thinking and study questions, the student will be able to:

1. Apply knowledge of drug safety during pregnancy and lactation to clinical cases.
2. State principles that guide prescribing of drugs during pregnancy.
3. Employ principles of pharmacokinetics to drug transfer to a fetus.
4. Recognize symptoms of opiate addiction in a neonate.
5. Formulate nursing interventions that can decrease the incidence of exposure of pregnant women to teratogenic substances.
6. Identify factors that make it difficult to detect teratogens.
7. Use the FDA pregnancy category of drugs in nursing practice.
8. Discuss benefit versus risk of pharmacotherapy during pregnancy.
9. Recognize the role of the nurse in situations where exposure to a teratogen has occurred.
10. Teach interventions to decrease the risk of adverse effects from maternally administered drugs to the fetus and breast-fed neonate.

CRITICAL THINKING AND STUDY QUESTIONS

1. The nurse is working in an obstetric office. A pregnant patient states that she has stopped taking all of her medications because she has heard that medications are harmful to the developing baby. The nurse's response should be based on
   a. pregnant women should not take any drugs.
   b. the health of the fetus depends on the health of the mother.
   c. all drugs have been tested and the prescriber will know which drugs are harmful to the fetus.
   d. the health of the fetus is always the first consideration when drugs are prescribed to pregnant women.

2. Identify the principles to be considered when a drug is prescribed for a pregnant woman.

3. Based on pharmacokinetics, drugs are most likely to pass into fetal circulation if they are
   a. highly polar.
   b. ionized.
   c. protein bound.
   d. lipid soluble.

4. A mother with a history of heroin addiction has delivered a full-term infant. Which signs and symptoms suggest the infant is experiencing withdrawal symptoms?
   a. Shrill cry and irritability
   b. Respiratory depression and lethargy
   c. Peripheral cyanosis and hypotension
   d. APGAR score of 3 at 1 minute and 4 at 5 minutes

5. A mother with a history of heroin addiction has delivered a full-term infant. What should be included in the nursing care of this neonate to address possible drug withdrawal in the neonate?

6. Exposure to teratogens during the embryonic period can produce gross malformation in the fetus. What are nursing actions that can decrease teratogenesis during this period?

7. A mother is grieving because her newborn has an anatomic defect. She asks why scientists have not been able to identify all substances that cause birth defects. When the mother is truly ready to discuss this question, what explanation should the nurse provide?

8. A pregnant woman with a history of controlled hypertension asks the nurse why the prescriber changed her high blood pressure medication from quinapril (Accupril) to methyldopa (Aldomet). The nurse's response should be based on the knowledge that
   a. methyldopa is more effective for treating hypertension during pregnancy.
   b. methyldopa is pregnancy category B and quinapril is pregnancy category C in the first trimester and category D in the second and third trimesters.
   c. the dose of quinapril is more potent than the dose of methyldopa.
   d. quinapril crosses the placenta, but methyldopa does not.

9. Recommendations for levothyroxine state that the drug should be continued and increased during pregnancy. Research the drug and explain why this is recommended.

10. An important role of the nurse when a pregnant woman has a known exposure to a known teratogen during week 4 of the pregnancy would be
   a. ordering an ultrasound.
   b. providing the diagnosis from the ultrasound to the parents.
   c. recommending termination of pregnancy if a severe malformation is detected.
   d. providing information and emotional support.

11. The nurse is providing discharge teaching to a postpartum mother who is breast-feeding her neonate. The mother has a chronic condition that requires drug therapy. What should the nurse include in teaching regarding breast-feeding and drug therapy?

10

Drug Therapy in Pediatric Patients

Answers can be reviewed online at http://evolve.elsevier.com/Lehne/.

OBJECTIVES

After reading and studying the corresponding chapter and completing the questions and the case studies, the student will be able to:

1. Identify the effects of organ system immaturity on drug doses and responses.
2. Apply knowledge of pharmacokinetics to pediatric cases.
3. Determine needed assessments relating to potential adverse effects.
4. Recognize drugs that are uniquely contraindicated for pediatric patients.
5. Use body surface area to calculate safe drug doses.
6. Employ knowledge of developmental characteristics of pediatric development and family centered care to increase adherence to the drug therapy regimen.

7. Accurately measure pediatric doses.
8. Compare differences in infant and adult blood-brain barriers.

CRITICAL THINKING AND STUDY QUESTIONS

1. Premature infants are at risk for
   a. inadequate and short-lived response to drugs.
   b. intense and prolonged response to drugs.
   c. inadequate but prolonged response to drugs.
   d. intense but short-lived response to drugs.

2. An infant is diagnosed with scurvy caused by vitamin C deficiency. Based on the principles of pH-dependent ionization and ion trapping and the differences in gastrointestinal physiology in the infant, the nurse would expect that the prescribed dose of vitamin C (ascorbic acid) adjusted for weight would be
   a. less than an adult dose.
   b. equal to an adult dose.
   c. more than an adult dose.

▶ 3. A pregnant patient received morphine sulfate late in labor. The neonate was born 22 minutes later. Because the drug crosses the placenta and the characteristics of the blood-brain barrier of the neonate, it is important to assess the neonate for
   a. vomiting.
   b. irritability.
   c. tachycardia.
   d. respiratory depression.

4. In general terms, describe the capacity of the liver to metabolize drugs from birth through puberty.

5. The nurse is administering a drug that is excreted primarily unchanged in the urine to a 15-month-old child. The nurse would expect the dose of this drug, adjusted for weight, to be
   a. less than an adult dose.
   b. equal to an adult dose.
   c. more than an adult dose.

6. Which over-the-counter (OTC) drugs should not be administered to children younger than 19 years of age, especially during or after a viral illness, because of the danger of Reye's syndrome? (Select all that apply.)
   a. Acne cleansers
   b. Alka-Seltzer
   c. Anacin
   d. Ascriptin
   e. Astringents
   f. Kaopectate
   g. Dristan
   h. Pepto-Bismol
   i. Robitussin
   j. Sudafed
   k. St Joseph's baby aspirin
   l. TUMs
   m. Tylenol
   n. Vitamin C

7. Which of the following is the recommendation by the CDC for OTC cough and cold drug use in children younger than 2 years of age?
   a. Do not give any OTC drugs to a child younger than 2 years of age.
   b. Do not give any OTC cough and cold preparations to a child younger than 2 years of age.
   c. OTC cough and cold drugs are safe and effective if the preparation are specifically made for children and are properly measured.
   d. Use accurate measuring devices specifically designed for pediatric use when administering OTC cough and cold drugs to children younger than 2 years of age.

8. Which of the following are recommended by the American Academy of Pediatrics (AAP) as safe and effective for relieving cold symptoms in children? (Select all that apply).
   a. Acetaminophen (Tylenol)
   b. Diphenhydramine (Benadryl)
   c. Dexomethorphan ("DM" cough suppressants)
   d. Ibuprofen (Motrin)
   e. Suction nasal secretions with a bulb syringe
   f. Use a humidifier

▶ 9. The nurse is preparing to administer 10 mL of medication to a shy 4-year-old child. Which of the following nursing interventions is most likely to gain cooperation from the child with taking the drug?
   a. Mix the medication in a 6-ounce glass of juice to mask the taste.

b. Use a syringe to accurately measure the medication and squirt the medication into the child's mouth.

c. Place the medication in a large empty glass so that the child can see that there is only a small amount of medication.

d. Ask the parents if they have any special technique for administering medication that has been effective with this child.

10. Drugs do not readily cross into an adult's central nervous system (CNS). This is not true in neonates. What difference between the adult and the neonate makes what drug characteristics more of a concern in neonates than in adults?

11. A new mother says it is impossible to get her infant to take an oral suspension of an antibiotic. She tells you that she has been putting the medicine in the baby's formula. What can the nurse do to increase adherence to the drug regimen?

CASE STUDIES AND PATIENT TEACHING

(Use a separate piece of paper for your responses.)

Case Study 1

The recommended adult dose of a drug is 500 mg twice a day.

1. Based on body surface area, what is the recommended dose for a child who is 43 inches tall and 48 lbs in weight?

2. The prescriber has prescribed 225 mg of the drug above twice a day for this child. Is this a safe dose for this child?

3. The drug is available in an elixir of 250 mg/5 mL. How much medication will the nurse administer?

Case Study 2

1. Carbamazepine (Tegretol) 15 mg three times a day has been prescribed for a 4-year-old child who has a seizure disorder. It is recommended that the dose not exceed 35 mg/kg in children younger than 6 years of age. What is the maximum recommended dose for a child who weighs 40 pounds? Is the prescribed dose safe?

2. Carbazepine is available as a suspension containing 100 mg/5 mL. How much drug should be administered at each dose?

3. The nurse will administer the carbamazepine using a
   a. 1-cc syringe.
   b. 3-cc syringe.
   c. calibrated plastic medicine cup.
   d. measuring spoon.

4. Before administering the drug, the nurse notes a recent lab carbamazepine level. The level is 4 mcg/L. The nurse should
   a. administer the drug and continue nursing care.
   b. administer the drug and notify the prescriber of the lab results.
   c. withhold the drug and page the prescriber STAT.
   d. withhold the drug and monitor for symptoms of toxicity.

Answers can be reviewed online at http://evolve.elsevier.com/Lehne/.

OBJECTIVES

After reading and studying the corresponding chapter and completing the critical thinking and study questions, the student will be able to:

1. Identify factors that increase the risk of adverse effects from drugs in the older adult.
2. Develop nursing interventions that can decrease the incidence of adverse drug reactions and drug-drug interactions in the older adult.
3. Incorporate anticipated changes that occur with aging when interpreting laboratory test results relating to drug therapy for the older adult.
4. Assist the older adult with overcoming obstacles to adherence to the prescribed drug regimen.
5. Respond to symptoms that require consultation with the prescriber when caring for the aging adult.

CRITICAL THINKING AND STUDY QUESTIONS

1. Which statements about older adults and pharmacotherapy are generally true? (Select all that apply.)
   a. The goal of therapy for the older adult is to cure the disease.
   b. There is a wider individual variation in drug response in the older adult.
   c. Older adults are less sensitive to drugs.
   d. Older adults absorb less of the dose of medication than younger individuals.
   e. Absorption of many drugs slows with aging.
   f. Changes in body fat and lean body mass that occur with aging can cause lipid-soluble drugs to decrease in effect and water-soluble drugs to have a more intense effect.
   g. Liver enzyme activity may be increased in the older adult.
   h. Drug accumulation secondary to decreased renal excretion is the most common cause of adverse reactions in older adults.

   i. A reduction in the number of receptors and/or decreased affinity for receptors in the older adult may decrease the response to drugs that work by receptor interactions.

2. When evaluating kidney function in the older, debilitated adult, it is most important for the nurse to review the results of the
   a. serum blood urea nitrogen (BUN).
   b. serum creatinine.
   c. creatinine clearance.
   d. renal ultrasound.

3. How can the nurse decrease the incidence of adverse drug reactions and drug-drug interactions in the older adult based on the following factors?
   a. Altered pharmacokinetics

   b. Multiple severe illnesses and multiple-drug therapy

   c. Poor adherence

4. An older adult with liver disease is receiving several drugs that are normally highly protein bound. The patient's serum albumin is 2.8 mg/dL (normal 3.5 to 5 mg/dL). The nurse needs to assess the patient for symptoms of
   a. excessive action of the drugs.
   b. inadequate action of the drugs.

▶ 5. The nurse is preparing to administer ketorolac (Toradol) to an 83-year-old female who has joint pain and resides in an extended-care facility. Of the following symptoms, which would warrant withholding the drug and contacting the prescriber?
   a. Difficulty waking up in the morning
   b. Dizziness when changing from a prone to upright position
   c. Fecal impaction
   d. Tarry stools

6. A 76-year-old patient, who has mild arthritis and a cataract of the left eye, has been prescribed four medications with varied time intervals. Identify the steps that the nurse could use to promote adherence to a prescribed drug regimen.

▶ 7. The nurse is aware that anticholinergic adverse effects of drugs can be more common and a greater problem in the elderly than in the younger adult. Which of the following anticholinergic effects would warrant prompt consultation with the prescriber?
   a. Blurred vision
   b. Dry mouth
   c. Has not voided in 16 hours
   d. No BM for 48 hours

OBJECTIVES
(CHAPTERS 12-109)

The following are the overall objectives for this workbook. After reading and studying the corresponding chapters and completing the questions and the case studies, the student will be able to:

- Recognize common suffixes of generic names of drugs.
- Apply knowledge of pathophysiology of diseases and chronic conditions to nursing clinical decision making for teaching and safe administration of prescribed drug therapy.
- Use the nursing process to develop a plan of nursing care for patients receiving drug therapy.
- Incorporate knowledge of pharmacokinetics and pharmacodynamics when planning, providing, and evaluating nursing care.
- Recognize situations that can cause altered drug absorption, metabolism, and excretion.
- Calculate safe and therapeutic drug doses.
- Use critical thinking to develop measures that prevent drug administration errors.
- Safely administer prescribed drugs.
- Identify patients who are at risk for drug reactions.
- Assess for adverse effects of drug therapy.
- Differentiate between medically acceptable and significant adverse effects.
- Develop interventions to minimize adverse effects.
- Apply knowledge of routes of administration to clinical cases.

- Develop a teaching plan for a prescribed drug.
- Evaluate the factors that the nurse, patient, or caregiver must consider when deciding whether to administer or withhold a prescribed drug.
- Review the patient history for significant data relating to drug therapy.
- Incorporate developmental, genetic, gender, economic, and other issues that affect drug therapy in nursing care.
- Evaluate laboratory test results for needed nursing responses.
- Differentiate among normal, abnormal, and critical assessment findings and test results.
- Interpret the significance of laboratory values as they relate to drug therapy and nursing care.
- Respond appropriately when abnormal data is identified.
- Differentiate between critical and noncritical situations.
- Communicate pertinent data to the prescriber in an appropriate time frame.
- Document nursing care relating to drug administration.
- Recognize common factors at different developmental stages that affect adherence to prescribed drug regimen.
- Work with patients to develop realistic goals for drug therapy.
- Prioritize nursing actions relating to drug therapy.

Answers can be reviewed online at http://evolve.elsevier.com/Lehne/.

OBJECTIVES

See page 28 for the Objectives.

CRITICAL THINKING AND STUDY QUESTIONS

1. Two drugs that alter synaptic transmission are in the same therapeutic class. Which would the nurse expect to have more adverse effects?
   a. Selective drug
   b. Nonselective drug

2. The nurse can identify possible adverse effects of drugs that alter synaptic transmission by identifying (Select all that apply.)
   a. normal responses to receptor activation.
   b. whether the drug increases or decreases receptor activation.
   c. the dose of the drug.
   d. the target cell.
   e. whether the drug is selective or nonselective for specific receptors.
   f. the axon that is affected.
   g. the body cells that have receptors for the drug.

3. Selective serotonin reuptake inhibitors are a class of antidepressant drugs. Their mechanism of action is to
   a. increase the release of serotonin from the vesicles into the synapse.
   b. decrease the synthesis of serotonin in the axon.
   c. decrease the pumping of serotonin back into the axon from which it was released.
   d. stimulate receptors for serotonin.

4. A cholinergic (mimics the action of acetylcholine) drug would cause the heart rate to slow because the drug
   a. stimulates cardiac receptors for acetylcholine.
   b. causes an increased release of acetylcholine.
   c. causes a decreased release of acetylcholine.
   d. blocks receptors for acetylcholine.

5. What characteristics allow naloxone (Narcan) to take the place of the opiate at opiate receptors and reverse respiratory depression caused by an opiate (narcotic) analgesic? (Select all that apply.)
   a. Binding of naloxone and opiates to opiate receptors is reversible.
   b. Naloxone has a longer half-life than opiates.
   c. Naloxone has a stronger affinity for the receptor.
   d. Naloxone is selective for opiate receptors.
   e. The dose of naloxone is larger than the dose of the opiate.

6. What would be the possible adverse effects on these organs and/or processes of a nonselective drug that is administered to slow the heart rate that acts by blocking stimulation of beta$_1$ and beta$_2$ sympathetic nervous system receptors? (Think of the opposite of "fight or flight.")
   a. Eyes

   b. Respiratory rate

   c. Airway

d. GI motility

▸ 7. Based on the adverse effects that are possible in question 6, the nurse would be especially cautious when administering a nonselective blocker of beta$_1$ and beta$_2$ receptors to patients with which chronic disorders?

e. Production of glucose by the liver and release into the blood

13

Physiology of the Peripheral Nervous System

Answers can be reviewed online at http://evolve.elsevier.com/Lehne/.

OBJECTIVES

See page 28 for the Objectives.

b. Lungs

CRITICAL THINKING AND STUDY QUESTIONS

1. Match the divisions of the nervous system to functions that can be influenced by drugs.

_____ a. Autonomic   1. Involuntary process and
_____ b. Central   skeletal muscle
_____ c. Parasympa-   2. Thinking, emotion, and
        thetic   processing data
_____ d. Peripheral   3. Skeletal muscle and
_____ e. Somatic   parasympathetic
                                  4. Heart, secretory glands,
                                  and smooth muscle
                                  5. Involuntary processes

c. Heart

2. List the effects on these body parts that are relevant to drug therapy that occur when the parasympathetic nervous system is stimulated.
   a. Eye

d. Gastrointestinal tract

e. Urinary bladder

3. A nurse receives a soldier from a combat zone who is experiencing sudden intense vomiting. What symptoms, if present, suggest that he might have been exposed to nerve gas? (Select all that apply.)
   a. Diminished bowel sounds
   b. Diarrhea
   c. Rapid pulse and elevated blood pressure
   d. Sensitivity to bright light (photophobia)
   e. Squinting
   f. Urinary frequency

4. Sympathetic nervous stimulation ("fight or flight") can cause which of the following? (Select all that apply.)
   a. Increase heart rate
   b. Dilate bronchi
   c. Constrict pupils
   d. Inhibit the release of epinephrine from the adrenal gland
   e. Maintain blood flow to the brain
   f. Compensate for blood loss by vasodilation
   g. Constrict surface blood vessels
   h. Dilate surface blood vessels
   i. Stimulate sweating
   j. Shunt blood from muscles to vital organs during exercise
   k. Decrease blood pressure
   l. Increase blood glucose

5. The nurse is caring for a patient whose temperature is 102.4° F. The nurse notes that the patient's skin is flushed and sweaty. Vital signs include pulse of 96 beats/min and respirations of 25 breaths per minute. Describe why stimulation of the sympathetic nervous system would respond to fever in this way.
   a. Dilate surface vessels and sweating

6. A patient asks the nurse why so many drugs have the adverse effect of impairing male sexual functioning. The nurse's response is based on what knowledge?

7. A patient with a blood pressure (BP) of 188/104 mm Hg takes a potent vasodilating drug to lower the blood pressure. One hour after administration, the BP has dropped to 135/78 mm Hg in response to the drug. The patient's pulse is 124 BPM. The nurse interprets this pulse as the body's baroreceptors response to a rapid drop in blood pressure causing
   a. diuresis.
   b. reflex tachycardia.
   c. orthostatic hypotension.
   d. vasodilation.

8. Most drugs that affect muscarinic receptors of the parasympathetic nervous system produce adverse effects because
   a. high doses are needed to get therapeutic effects.
   b. muscarinic receptors are present on all postganglionic neurons.
   c. most drugs that affect muscarinic receptors are nonselective.
   d. muscarinic receptors are stimulated by epinephrine, which is secreted by the adrenal gland.

9. Why would stimulation of nicotinic$_N$ (N_n) receptors cause widespread effects?

b. Increase heart and respiratory rates

10. Complete this chart.

Effects of parasympathetic muscarinic receptor stimulation and blocking		
Location	Cholinergic (Muscarinic)—Substances that stimulate muscarinc receptors	Anticholinergic (Antimuscarinic)—Substances that block muscarinic receptors
Eye		
Heart		
Lungs		
Bladder		
Gastrointestinal (GI) tract		
Sweat glands		
Sex organs		
Blood vessels (not caused by nervous system activation)		

11. Based on the chart that you created, what would be logical therapeutic uses for
    a. cholinergic (muscarinic) drugs?

    b. anticholinergic (antimuscarinic) drugs?

12. What are reasons why scientistists might not have developed cholinergic or anticholinergic drugs for conditions that you listed in question 11?

13. Complete this chart.

Effects of sympathetic (adrenergic) receptor stimulation and blocking			
Receptor	*Location*	*Adrenergic—Substances that stimulate adrenergic receptors*	*Adrenergic blocker— Substances that block adrenergic receptors*
Alpha$_1$ (α_1)	Eye		
	Arterioles of skin, organs, and mucous membranes		
	Veins		
	Male sex organs		
	Prostate capsule		
	Bladder		
Alpha$_2$ (α_2)	Presynaptic nerve terminals		
Beta$_1$ (β_1)	Heart		
	Kidney		
Beta$_2$ (β_2)	Arterioles of heart, lungs, and skeletal muscle		
	Bronchi		
	Uterus		
	Liver		
	Skeletal muscle		

14. Based on the chart that you created, what would be logical therapeutic uses for
    a. alpha$_1$-adrenergic drugs?

    b. alpha$_1$-adrenergic blocking drugs?

    c. beta$_1$-adrenergic drugs?

    d. beta$_1$-adrenergic blocking drugs?

    e. beta$_2$-adrenergic drugs?

    f. beta$_2$-adrenergic blocking drugs?

15. Which adrenergic receptor is the "brakes" of the system that prevents excessive sympathetic effects?

16. What would be the possible adverse effects of a nonselective drug that acts by blocking stimulation of beta$_1$ and beta$_2$ sympathetic nervous system receptors on these organs and/or processes?

    a. Eyes

    b. Respiratory rate

    c. Airway

    d. GI motility

    e. Production of glucose by the liver and release into the blood

▶ 17. Based on the possible adverse effects, the nurse would be especially cautious when administering a nonselective blocker of beta$_1$ and beta$_2$ receptors to patients with which chronic disorders?

18. Despite the fact that no nerves terminate at muscarinic receptors on blood vessels, what is the effect of muscarinic drugs on the blood pressure?

19. What three factors determine adrenergic receptor stimulation by a drug?

20. The only neurotransmitter that activates beta$_2$ adrenergic receptors is
    a. acetylcholine.
    b. dopamine.
    c. epinephrine.
    d. norepinephrine.

21. Nerve gas is deadly because it can be absorbed through the skin and has an irreversible effect on cholinesterase. The victim experiences increased bronchial secretions, tight chest, dimming of vision, drooling, involuntary defecation and urination, muscle tremors, convulsions, coma, and death. Based on these symptoms, does nerve gas induce or inhibit cholinesterase?

▶ 22. Monoamine oxidase (MAO) inhibitors are a class of antidepressants that inhibit the breakdown of norepinephrine by MAO. The nurse is caring for a patient who has been taking an MAO inhibitor and consumed large amounts of foods containing tyramine. What symptoms would the nurse expect and why? (See Fig. 13-8 in the textbook.)

23. What three factors must be considered when studying drugs that work by receptor interaction?

Answers can be reviewed online at http://evolve.elsevier.com/Lehne/.

OBJECTIVES

See page 28 for the Objectives.

CRITICAL THINKING AND STUDY QUESTIONS

1. Define these terms.
   a. Agonist

   b. Antagonist

▶ 2. The nurse is preparing to administer bethane-chol (Urecholine). Which of the following findings would warrant the nurse holding the medication and contacting the prescriber? (Select all that apply.)
   a. Pulse 110 beats/min
   b. BP 100/60
   c. Wheezing
   d. Drooling
   e. Postoperative abdominal distention
   f. Recent bowel resection
   g. Recent vaginal delivery of a 7-lb neonate
   h. Postvoid residual of 350 mL of urine
   i. Positive hemoccult of stool
   j. TSH 0.2 microunits/mL; T_4 18 mcg/dL

3. A 48-year-old woman with a history of rheumatoid arthritis has been diagnosed with Sjögren's syndrome. Cevimeline (Evoxac) 30-mg capsule, three times daily has been prescribed. Why is it important to assess this patient for electrolyte imbalances?

4. A camper finds some wild mushrooms and eats them. Which of the following symptoms would the camp nurse expect if he is experiencing muscarinic poisoning? (Select all that apply.)
   a. Tachycardia
   b. Hypertension
   c. Profuse salivation and lacrimation
   d. Constipation
   e. Dilated pupils that do not respond to light
   f. Wheezing

✳ 5. The emergency department nurse receives a patient brought in by an ambulance with suspected poisoning from exposure to muscarinic insecticide. A priority nursing action is to prepare
   a. to relieve the pain of muscle spasms.
   b. for possible respiratory arrest.
   c. to place the patient in a side-lying position because the patient is likely to vomit.
   d. to administer intravenous fluids.

6. Why is "antimuscarinic drug" a better term than "anticholinergic drug"?

7. Why might excessive doses of atropine cause sympathetic nervous system stimulation symptoms?

▶ 8. The nurse has administered atropine as a preoperative medication. The patient complains of a sudden feeling of warmth. Her skin is warm and dry, and her face is flushed. The nurse should
   a. notify the surgeon STAT.
   b. asses the patient's vital signs and notify the surgeon.
   c. assess the patient's vital signs and mental status and notify the OR that surgery must be postponed.
   d. assess the patient's vital signs and mental status and, if within normal limits, document the findings and continue the preoperative protocol.

9. What form of atropine would be prescribed for a person who is at risk to be exposed to toxic levels of insecticide or nerve gas?
   a. Extended-release tablet
   b. Enteric-coated tablet
   c. Self-injectable pen
   d. Intravenous solution

10. Oxybutynin (Ditropan) is a prescribed anticholinergic drug that is available in four formulations. A patient has experienced many adverse effects when taking oxybutynin immediate-release tablets (Ditropan IR) for overactive bladder (OAB). She asks the nurse how the transdermal patch could cause less adverse effects if it is essentially the same drug. The nurse's response should be based on the knowledge that
   a. transdermal absorption bypasses metabolism in the intestinal wall.
   b. the transdermal form is water soluble and poorly absorbed.
   c. the transdermal form is a different drug than oral oxybutynin.
   d. the transdermal form is less effective than the extended release (ER) oral form.

11. The nurse is teaching a patient about darifenacin (Enablex), a newly prescribed drug for OAB that selectively blocks muscarinic$_3$ (M$_3$) receptors. The nurse should teach the patient that likely adverse effects include (Select all that apply.)
   a. blurred vision.
   b. confusion.
   c. diarrhea.
   d. dry eyes.
   e. photophobia.
   f. sleepiness.
   g. tachycardia.

12. The nurse is administering trospium (Sanctura XR) to a 78-year-old woman who has a history of overactive bladder (OAB), hypertension, diabetes, osteoarthritis, and osteoporosis. As the nurse explains the drug action, the patient asks how this drug is different from oxybutynin (Detrol LA), which is cheaper. The basis of the nurse's response is that trospium (Sanctura) should not cause
   a. constipation.
   b. dizziness.
   c. dry mouth.
   d. interactions with other drugs.

13. Why is lack of the adverse effect in the situation in the previous question so important for the patient described?

14. Emergency department prescriber's orders for a patient with advanced HIV admitted with a mycobacterium infection include clarithromycin (Biaxin) 500 mg PO twice a day and continue with all home medications. The patient's regimen includes darifenacin (Enablex) ER 15 mg once a day, delavirdine 400 mg, three times daily, nevirapine 200 mg twice a day, and ritonavir 600 mg twice a day. Based on possible drug interactions with darifenacin, the nurse should
   a. give the medications with food to prevent GI distress.
   b. administer the medications so that there is at least 1 hour between each medication.
   c. review the home medications and the medication order with the prescriber.
   d. hold all of the medications.

15. The nurse should review the results of the echocardiogram (ECG) and the history for unexplained fainting or long-QT syndrome before administering
    a. darifenacin (Enablex).
    b. oxybutynin (Ditropan, Oxytrol).
    c. solifenacin (VESIcare).
    d. tolterodine (Detrol).
    e. trospium (Sanctura).

16. What response to tolterodine (Detrol) would the nurse expect if a patient lacks the P450 cytochrome CYP2D6 isoenzyme?
    a. More adverse effects
    b. Lack of therapeutic response
    c. Prolonged drug action
    d. Need to take the drug on an empty stomach

17. Trospium (Sanctura) 20 mg once a day is prescribed for an older adult patient with OAB. The nurse instructs the patient to take the medication
    a. one hour before breakfast.
    b. one hour after breakfast.
    c. with the first bite of breakfast.
    d. anytime during the day as long as it is at the same time each day.

18. The nurse is caring for a patient who has taken an overdose of a tricyclic antidepressant drug that has pronounced antimuscarinic properties. The nurse should prepare to (Select all that apply.)
    a. support breathing.
    b. administer atropine.
    c. administer drugs for hypotension.
    d. administer phenothiazine antipsychotic drugs to treat delirium.
    e. administer physostigmine.

▶ 19. A patient has received a mydriatic medication as part of an eye examination. Before leaving the office, what instructions would be most useful for the patient's comfort and safety?

CASE STUDIES AND PATIENT TEACHING

(Use a separate piece of paper for your responses.)

Case Study 1

A frail-appearing, 66-year-old female with a history of type 2 diabetes mellitus, hypertension, depression, and OAB is admitted to a medical unit with the diagnosis of altered mental status. Assessment findings include BP 182/110 mm Hg, P 118, R 14, and T 102.4 °F. The patient is becoming confused and is exhibiting symptoms that suggest she is hallucinating. The patient resists efforts to open her eyes for pupil assessment. Skin is flushed and warm; mucous membranes are dry. Bowel sounds are hypoactive, and there are multiple areas of dullness when percussing the abdomen. The bladder is palpable above the pubic symphysis, with bladder scan reading 350 mL. Admission laboratory test results include BUN 32 mg/dL; creatinine 2.3 mg/dL; glucose 178 mg/dL; WBC 12,400/mm³. Creatinine clearance has been ordered, and the collection was started at 0600. The nurse is preparing the patient's 0900 medications including tolterodine (Detrol).

1. What do laboratory test results suggest?

2. What concern does the nurse have about administering tolterodine?

3. What symptoms suggest antimuscarinic toxicity?

4. What should the nurse do?

5. The prescriber discontinues the tolterodine. The patient's condition improves. The patient is concerned about bladder control. What teaching can the nurse provide to assist a patient with OAB to attain bladder control?

Case Study 2

The recommended subcutaneous dose of atropine for a child is 0.01 mg/kg, not to exceed 0.4 mg.

1. What is the recommended dose for a child who is 32 inches long and weighs 24 lb?

2. Based on the recommended dose, how much medication will the nurse draw into the syringe if atropine is available as 0.5 mg/mL?

Case Study 3

Create a patient teaching handout for cevimeline (Evoxac) using this format.

cevimeline (Evoxac)	
Reason for taking this drug	
Dose and administration directions	
Teaching relating to possible adverse effects	
Things to report to your prescriber	
Drug interactions	

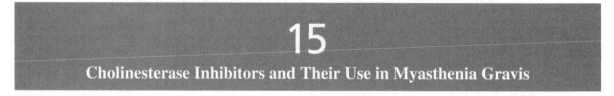

15

Cholinesterase Inhibitors and Their Use in Myasthenia Gravis

Answers can be reviewed online at http://evolve.elsevier.com/Lehne/.

OBJECTIVES

See page 28 for the Objectives.

CRITICAL THINKING AND STUDY QUESTIONS

1. Cholinesterase inhibitors can
   a. intensify transmission at neuromuscular junctions.
   b. intensify transmission at muscarinic, ganglionic, and neuromuscular junctions.
   c. prevent transmission at neuromuscular junctions.
   d. prevent transmission at muscarinic, ganglionic, and neuromuscular junctions.

2. The principle reason why physostigmine is preferred over neostigmine for reversing muscarinic toxicity is related to the
   a. ability of the drug to cross the blood-brain barrier.
   b. absence of significant adverse effects.
   c. mechanism of action.
   d. rate of onset of action.

▸ 3. A 66-year-old male has been taking ambenonium (Mytelase) for myasthenia gravis for 4 years. He is admitted to the hospital for a prostate biopsy after his PSA laboratory test was elevated. The ambenonium is scheduled to be administered. The nurse should
   a. administer the drug.
   b. hold the drug.

c. assess for urine retention before and after administering the drug.

d. consult with the urologist before administering the drug.

▸ ■ 4. The nurse is caring for a patient who is prescribed pyridostigmine (Mestinon) 240 mg, three times daily for myasthenia gravis. The patient states that he is experiencing an extreme increase in muscle weakness and that he needs the nurse to administer 300-mg doses. The nurse should

a. administer 240 mg because that is the dose ordered by the prescriber.

b. administer 300-mg doses because myasthenia gravis patients often need to adjust their dose of medication according to symptoms.

c. call the prescriber and request an order for the increased dose.

d. immediately assess the patient for other symptoms including excessive muscarinic stimulation, such as increased secretion, increased bowel sounds, bradycardia, and wheezing, and contact prescriber with patient's request and assessment findings.

5. Match the medication to its use.

_____ a. Atropine
_____ b. Echothiophate
_____ c. Edrophonium
_____ d. Malathion
_____ e. Neostigmine
_____ f. Physostigmine
_____ g. Pralidoxime
_____ h. Tabun

1. Used to diagnose myasthenia gravis
2. Antidote for poisoning by organophosphate insecticides
3. Used to treat drug-induced muscarinic blockade
4. Irreversible cholinesterase inhibitor used to treat glaucoma
5. Irreversible cholinesterase inhibitor nerve gas that can be used in bioterrorism
6. Antidote for cholinergic crisis
7. Short-acting reversible cholinesterase inhibitor that does not cross blood-brain barrier
8. Organophosphate insecticide

CASE STUDIES AND PATIENT TEACHING

(Use a separate piece of paper for your responses.)

Case Study 1

A patient who is receiving a reversible cholinesterase inhibitor for myasthenia gravis is brought into the emergency department by his family because of extreme muscle weakness and difficulty breathing.

1. In this situation, why is it important to determine if the cause of the weakness is myasthenic crisis versus cholinergic crisis?

2. What assessments should the nurse perform? What questions should the nurse ask the patient and family? Why?

3. The prescriber is unsure, by history, if the patient is experiencing myasthenic crisis or cholinergic crisis. He orders administration of edrophonium to differentiate. What should the nurse do along with preparing to administer the edrophonium?

4. The nurse is doing discharge teaching for this patient. What teaching should the nurse do to help the patient monitor the response to medication for his myasthenia gravis?

Case Study 2

The nurse has been asked to speak to a 4-H group in a farming community on preventing poisoning by organophosphate insecticides. The nurse has stressed the importance of following all directions provided and seeking clarification if any directions are unclear.

1. What information should the nurse include to prevent
   a. exposure when using insecticides through the skin or eyes?
   b. exposure when using insecticides through the respiratory tract?
   c. oral exposure?

2. What symptoms warrant seeking immediate medical attention when using pesticides?

3. What is the treatment for pesticide poisoning?

16

Drugs That Block Nicotinic Cholinergic Transmission: Neuromuscular Blocking Agents and Ganglionic Blocking Agents

Answers can be reviewed online at http://evolve.elsevier.com/Lehne/.

OBJECTIVES

See page 28 for the Objectives.

CRITICAL THINKING AND STUDY QUESTIONS

1. A woman who is 8 weeks pregnant must have surgery. The anesthesiologist administers vecuronium (Norcuron), a quaternary ammonium compound, to achieve muscle relaxation. The most likely effect of this medication on the developing fetus is
   a. no detectable effect.
   b. respiratory depression.
   c. bradycardia.
   d. teratogenesis.

2. Neuromuscular blocking agents (Select all that apply.)
   a. block nicotinic$_M$ (N$_M$) receptors on the motor end-plate.
   b. block the sensation of pain.
   c. can be administered orally, intramuscularly, and intravenously.
   d. can cause respiratory arrest.
   e. cross the blood-brain barrier.
   f. do not cause loss of consciousness.
   g. may lower BP by vasodilation.
   h. have a primary effect of spastic paralysis.

3. The nurse is aware that neuromuscular blocking agents do not alter consciousness or pain perception. The nurse instructs a patient who has received tubocurarine to blink her eyes to indicate if she is e`xperiencing pain. Is this an appropriate assessment technique? Why?

4. Preoperative laboratory test results include potassium 3.1 mg/dL. It is important for the nurse to inform the anesthesiologist of this result because it can cause normal doses of tubocurarine to cause
   a. tachycardia.
   b. inability to reverse the blockade.
   c. respiratory arrest.
   d. the patient to sense pain during the procedure.

5. The nurse should assess for and plan interventions to relieve muscle pain 12 to 24 hours after surgery for patients who have received
   a. succinylcholine.
   b. atracurium.
   c. pancuronium.
   d. tubocurarine.

6. An anesthesia resident is supervising the reversal of the neuromuscular blockade for a patient who has received succinylcholine. She asks the nurse to administer 0.5 mg of neostigmine (Prostigmin) intravenously. The nurse should
   a. administer the medication slowly to prevent respiratory depression.
   b. question the resident because neostigmine intensifies the neuromuscular blockade caused by succinylcholine, a depolarizing neuromuscular blocker.
   c. only administer the medication if mechanical assistance for ventilation is available.
   d. question the resident as to whether atropine also should be administered to prevent respiratory depression.

7. A patient will be receiving succinylcholine before electroconvulsive therapy. A nursing priority is
   a. administering the succinylcholine.
   b. administering atropine if toxicity occurs.
   c. performing the electroconvulsive therapy.
   d. preparing for possible respiratory arrest.

8. Succinylcholine is routinely administered to patients during certain endoscopic procedures. The endoscopy nurse reviews each patient history before the procedure. What information should the nurse look for because it would be a

40

concern and should be reported to the anesthesiologist relating to succinylcholine use?

CASE STUDIES AND PATIENT TEACHING

(Use a separate piece of paper for your responses.)

Case Study 1

The postanesthesia care unit (PACU) nurse is caring for a patient who received tubocurarine during surgery to remove a cancerous section of the bowel. The patient is admitted to the PACU with mechanical ventilation and a nasogastric (NG) tube to low-intermittent suction.

1. What are priority assessments that the PACU nurse must monitor while the patient is still under the effects of tubocurarine?

2. The NG tube is draining a large amount of bile-colored liquid. How does this affect potassium levels and nursing care?

3. As the patient regains neuromuscular functioning, the nurse instructs the patient to take deep breaths. How does deep breathing counteract the adverse effects of histamine release stimulated by the tubocurarine?

Case Study 2

A patient is receiving a neuromuscular blocker for prolonged paralysis during mechanical ventilation.

1. Describe measures that should be included in nursing care and their rationale.

2. The patient spikes a temperature of 102° F within an hour after the neuromuscular agent infusion is begun. The infusion of the neuromuscular blocking agent is stopped, and the patient receives a dose of dantrolene (Dantrium), and the patient's temperature begins to drop. Why was dantrolene administered to lower this patient's temperature instead of an antipyretic such as acetaminophen?

17
Adrenergic Agonists

Answers can be reviewed online at http://evolve.elsevier.com/Lehne/.

OBJECTIVES

See page 28 for the Objectives.

CRITICAL THINKING AND STUDY QUESTIONS

1. What common term for adrenergic agonists reflects that their effects mimic sympathetic nervous system stimulation?

2. Direct-acting adrenergic drugs mimic the action of (Select all that apply.)
   a. acetylcholine (ACh).
   b. dopamine.
   c. epinephrine (epi).
   d. norepinephrine (NE).

3. Match the medication to its mechanism of action. (Some will have more than one answer.)

_____ a. Amphetamines
_____ b. Cocaine
_____ c. Ephedrine
_____ d. MAO inhibitors
_____ e. Most sympa-
        thomimetics
_____ f. Tricyclic
        antidepressants

1. Promotion of NE release
2. Inhibition of NE reuptake
3. Inhibition of NE inactivation
4. Direct receptor activation

4. Catecholamines (Select all that apply.)
   a. are inactivated before reaching systemic circulation if administered orally.
   b. cross the blood-brain barrier activating the central nervous system (CNS).
   c. include the drugs epinephrine, norepinephrine, isoproterenol, dopamine, and dobutamine.
   d. are effective when administered by any parenteral route.
   e. have a long half-life.
   f. are polar molecules.
   g. are destroyed by monoamine oxidase (MAO) and catechol-O-methyltransferase (COMT) enzymes in the liver and intestinal wall.
   h. usually have a duration of 3 to 6 hours.

▶ 5. The nurse is caring for a patient who is receiving a dopamine intravenous (IV) drip. The nurse has been assessing her patient every 15 minutes. The nurse notes that since the last assessment the IV dopamine solution has turned pink. The nurse should
   a. stop the IV infusion, assess the patient for adverse effects, and notify the prescriber.
   b. stop the infusion, notify the pharmacy for an immediate replacement, and assess the patient.
   c. continue to assess the patient and infuse the solution as prescribed.
   d. continue to assess the patient and infuse the solution as prescribed for up to 24 hours after being hung.

6. Based on Table 17-2, which catecholamine would stimulate the heart while producing the least unintended effects?

7. A woman who is pregnant at 30 weeks of gestation is receiving terbutaline. The drug book states that it is a drug used to bronchodilate. The patient does not have a history of asthma and denies any problems with bronchoconstriction. What would be a logical problem for which she is receiving the terbutaline?

8. Based on the general principles of pharmacokinetics and relative specificity, patients with what chronic diseases would be at most risk for adverse effects from adrenergic agonists? (Select all that apply.)
   a. Chronic obstructive pulmonary disease (COPD)
   b. Cirrhosis of the liver
   c. Hypertension
   d. End-stage renal disease
   e. Osteoarthritis

9. A patient experiences sudden AV block. IV epinephrine is ordered STAT. What should nursing care related to administration of this drug include?

▶ 10. The nurse is working in the emergency department. A local anesthetic combined with epinephrine is often used when performing procedures on extremities that need a small area of anesthesia and are likely to bleed. Assessment findings that would warrant caution before administering a drug containing epinephrine include (Select all that apply.)
   a. blood pressure 86/50 mm Hg.
   b. blood pressure 175/90 mm Hg.
   c. history of angina pectoris.
   d. history of AV heart block.
   e. poor capillary refill.

f. palpitations.

g. pulse 50 beats/min.

h. pulse 110 beats/min.

i. weak peripheral pulse.

11. The nurse is administering terbutaline to a patient in preterm labor who has a history of asthma and gestational diabetes. It is important to assess this patient for which possible adverse effect of terbutaline?

a. Hot, dry, flushed skin

b. Hypotension

c. Sensitivity to light

d. Urinary urgency

12. A patient has a history of depression. Treatment by which of the following antidepressants is most likely to decrease the inactivation of dopamine and increase the risk of toxicity?

a. Bupropion (Wellbutrin)

b. Nortriptyline (Pamelor)

c. Sertraline (Zoloft)

d. Tranylcypromine (Parnate)

13. Dobutamine HCl (Dobutrex) is available in a vial of 250 mg/20 mL. The prescribed dose for a patient weighing 110 lb is 250 mcg/min. To administer this medication the nurse must

a. administer it by IV push over 5 minutes.

b. infuse the vial by IV piggyback over 20 minutes.

c. dilute the vial in at least 50 mL of diluent and infuse at a rate of 30 mL/hr.

d. dilute the vial in 250 mL and infuse at a rate of 150 mL/hr.

14. Phenylephrine (NeoSynephrine) is available over the counter (OTC) as a nasal decongestant. A patient states that he understands why the label says it should not be used if he has high blood pressure, but he does not understand why it should not be used by diabetics. The nurse's response is based on knowledge that phenylephrine can cause (Select all that apply.)

a. anorexia.

b. hypoglycemia in the diabetic patient.

c. hyperglycemia in the diabetic patient.

d. a tremor, which the patient may interpret as hypoglycemia.

15. The nurse is performing discharge teaching for a patient who was hospitalized with newly diagnosed hyperthyroidism. What teaching should the nurse include regarding commonly used OTC medications?

CASE STUDIES AND PATIENT TEACHING

(Use a separate piece of paper for your responses.)

Case Study 1

A female in cardiogenic shock is ordered an IV infusion of dopamine at a rate of 400 mcg/min. The patient weighs 154 lb.

1. What does the nurse need to do before beginning the infusion?

2. The prescriber decreases the prescribed dose to 300 mcg/min. The dopamine infusion is available in a dilution of 100 mg/250 mL. The infusion pump is calculated in mL/hr. What is the flow rate that the nurse will program into the infusion pump?

3. The nurse is administering the IV dopamine infusion. The nurse assesses the large antecubital vein and notes the site is swollen, cold, and extremely pale. The basis of the nurse's response is

a. dopamine can only be infused through a central vein.

b. a clot has formed and can break off and become an embolus.

c. the IV infusion must continue at this site until another IV is successfully started.

d. vasoconstriction can cause tissue necrosis at the site of extravasation.

4. What treatment can prevent necrosis if dopamine extravasation occurs? How is it administered? How does it work?

Case Study 2

A 4-year-old child comes to the emergency department with angioedema, wheezing, and hypotension after eating a peanut butter cookie. Epinephrine is administered.

1. Describe how it treats the symptoms of anaphylactic shock.

2. The child is prescribed an epinephrine auto-injector (EpiPen Jr). What should the nurse teach the parents and child about administering the medication?

3. How can the parents ensure that the child of this age has his pen available at all times?

18

Adrenergic Antagonists

Answers can be reviewed online at http://evolve.elsevier.com/Lehne/.

OBJECTIVES

See page 28 for the Objectives.

CRITICAL THINKING AND STUDY QUESTIONS

1. An advantage of alpha antagonists is that they
   a. are more potent.
   b. work on specific receptors.
   c. have irreversible action.
   d. are capable of treating a wide variety of illnesses.

2. Match the disorder with the desired outcome. (Answers may be used more than once.)

   _____ a. Alpha$_1$ agonist toxicity
   _____ b. Benign prostatic hyperplasia (BPH)
   _____ c. Essential hypertension (HTN)
   _____ d. Pheochromocytoma
   _____ e. Raynaud's disease

   1. Blood pressure (BP) 90/60 mm Hg to120/80 mm Hg
   2. Warm, pink tissue
   3. Pain less than 2 on a scale of 1 to 10 in toes and fingers
   4. Brisk capillary refill
   5. Post-void residual less than 75 mL

3. The generic name of alpha$_1$ receptor antagonists shares the common suffix
   a. (-azole).
   b. (-lol).
   c. (-osin).
   d. (-sartan).

4. Before administering alfuzosin (Uroxatral) to a patient, it is most important for the nurse to evaluate which of the following laboratory test results?
   a. AST/ALT
   b. BUN/Creatinine
   c. FBS/HbA$_{1C}$
   d. Na$^+$K$^+$

5. A patient has just been prescribed prazosin (Minipress). Which of the following statements would indicate a need for further teaching?
   a. "I should avoid driving and other hazardous activities for 12 to 24 hours after I first take this medication or have a dose increase."
   b. "I should take the medication first thing in the morning."
   c. "I should sit on the edge of the bed for a few minutes before standing up when I get up in the morning."
   d. "I should be sitting or lying 30 to 60 minutes after I take the first dose of this medication."

6. A patient is receiving terazosin (Hytrin) for hypertension. An adverse effect that may warrant the prescriber changing to another drug in the same class is
   a. hypotension.
   b. nasal congestion.
   c. headache.
   d. reflex tachycardia.

7. A patient asks why his prescriber told him he should not take sildenafil (Viagra) for erectile dysfunction when he is taking an alpha$_1$-adrenergic antagonist for his high blood pressure.

The basis of the nurse's response is the concern that this combination of drugs can cause
a. atrial fibrillation.
b. migraine headache.
c. prolonged erection.
d. severe hypotension and vascular collapse.

8. When administering tamsulosin (Flomax), which of the following assessments would indicate that therapy has achieved the desired effect?
a. Post-void residual less than 250 mL
b. Voiding 250 mL every 2 to 3 hours while awake
c. Position changes without dizziness
d. Absence of dysuria when voiding

9. Tamsulosin (Flomax) should be administered
a. with food.
b. 30 minutes after the same meal each day.
c. 1 hour before or 2 hours after the same meal each day.
d. with a full glass of water and remain upright for 30 minutes.

10. Which of these factors, if identified in the history of a patient who has just been prescribed alfuzosin (Uroxatral), would be a concern to the nurse? (Select all that apply.)
a. Angina pectoris
b. Advanced HIV infection
c. Diabetes mellitus type 2
d. Erectile dysfunction
e. Frequent urinary tract infections
f. Hepatitis B
g. Hypertension
h. Ventricular dysrhythmia

11. A patient who is receiving phenoxybenzamine (Dibenzyline) to treat pheochromocytoma faints. BP is 75/40 mm Hg, P 135 beats/min. The nurse contacts the prescriber and plans to administer:
a. epinephrine.
b. norepinephrine.
c. intravenous fluids.
d. metoprolol.

12. The generic name of beta$_1$ and beta$_2$ receptor antagonists shares the common suffix
a. (-azole).
b. (-lol).
c. (-zosin).
d. (-sartan).

13. An assessment finding that would warrant holding a beta blocker and consulting the prescriber is?
a. Apical pulse 48 beats/min
b. BP 110/70 mm Hg
c. 2+ ankle edema
d. Capillary blood sugar 90 mg/dL

14. Which of these assessment findings, if identified 1 hour after administering metoprolol (Lopressor), should the nurse report to the prescriber immediately?
a. Drop in apical pulse from 80 to 65 beats/min
b. Warm, flushed, dry skin
c. Crackles throughout lung fields
d. Headache

15. Which of these conditions, if identified in the history of a patient receiving a drug that blocks beta$_1$-adrenergic receptors, would be a concern to the nurse? (Select all that apply.)
a. Anxiety
b. AV heart block
c. Benign prostatic hyperplasia (BPH)
d. Chronic obstructive pulmonary disease (COPD)
e. Depression
f. Diabetes insipidus
g. Diabetes mellitus
h. Hypertension
i. Hypothyroidism
j. Migraine headaches
k. Severe allergic reaction to bee stings

16. Which of these laboratory findings, if identified in a patient who is prescribed metoprolol (Lopressor), should the nurse report to the prescriber immediately?
a. Creatinine 1.2 mg/dL
b. Ejection fraction on echocardiogram of 20%
c. Hemoglobin A$_{1C}$ (glycosylated hemoglobin) 5.5%
d. Sinus rhythm on electrocardiogram (ECG)

17. Which of these findings would be most significant if a patient was prescribed propranolol (Inderal)?
a. Apical pulse 100 beats/min
b. Expiratory wheezing
c. BP 160/90 mm Hg
d. Urinary urgency

18. Which adrenergic antagonists block alpha$_1$, beta$_1$, and beta$_2$ receptors?
    a. Atenolol and bisoprolol
    b. Acebutolol and pindolol
    c. Carvedilol and labetalol
    d. Propranolol and timolol

19. The nurse should be especially vigilant to monitor for excessive cardiosuppression in a patient who is receiving metoprolol and
    a. atorvastatin (Lipitor).
    b. hydrochlorothiazide (HydroDIURIL).
    c. terazosin (Hytrin).
    d. verapamil (Calan).

CASE STUDIES AND PATIENT TEACHING

(Use a separate piece of paper for your responses.)

Case Study 1

A 58-year-old male has just been prescribed prazosin (Minipress) for hypertension.

1. Explain the common adverse effects and nursing teaching needed to provide both comfort and safety for this patient.

2. What assessments should be performed before the nurse administers an alpha$_1$-adrenergic antagonist for hypertension, and what assessment findings would warrant not administering the medication and notifying the prescriber?

3. The patient's BP is not controlled by his prescribed alpha$_1$ antagonist. The prescriber has added a loop diuretic and a beta$_1$ blocker. The patient asks, "Why do I have to take three different medications for my blood pressure? Can't I just have a higher dose of one medication?" How should the nurse explain the rationale for this drug regimen?

4. Why is it important to address ejaculation problems and other adverse effects with this patient?

Case Study 2

A 45-year-old male is being treated for hypertension. Several types of antihypertensive medications have been tried without success. He also has been taking glargine insulin (Lantus) 22 units every morning and aspart insulin (NovoLog) on a sliding scale according to blood sugar for diabetes. His prescriber orders metoprolol 50 mg once a day. When the patient tries to fill the prescription using his insurance, the pharmacist notifies him that his insurance only covers the less expensive beta blocker, propranolol, unless the patient experiences adverse effects or has an absolute contraindication for the use of propranolol. The prescriber can appeal to the insurance company and justify the use of the more expensive decision. The prescriber asks the office nurse to initiate the insurance appeal form.

1. Describe and explain the adverse effects that this patient might experience relating to his diabetes diagnosis and propranolol.

2. The insurance appeal is approved, and the patient receives metoprolol, a beta$_1$-selective adrenergic antagonist. The patient states "I'm glad I do not have to take propranolol. I have had frequent episodes of hypoglycemia because with my job I cannot always eat when I should." What should the nurse do and why?

3. The nurse discovers that this patient has a history of poor adherence to medication regimens. Why are beta-adrenergic blockers poor choices for this patient?

Answers can be reviewed online at http://evolve.elsevier.com/Lehne/.

OBJECTIVES

See page 28 for the Objectives.

CRITICAL THINKING AND STUDY QUESTIONS

1. Match the medication to its effect. Select all that apply.

   _____ a. Clonidine
   _____ b. Guanethidine
   _____ c. Methyldopa
   _____ d. Reserpine

   1. Depletes norepinephrine (NE) from adrenergic neurons
   2. Activates alpha$_2$ receptors
   3. Blocks NE release and depletes NE storage
   4. Adverse effects of orthostatic hypotension and diarrhea
   5. Adverse effects of hemolytic anemia and liver damage
   6. Adverse effects of drowsiness and dry mouth
   7. Less likely to cause orthostatic hypotension
   8. Rebound hypertension if stopped abruptly

✳ 2. Depletion of neurotransmitters norepinephrine and serotonin by reserpine makes it a priority for the nurse to assess the patient's
   a. blood count.
   b. bowel sounds.
   c. mental status.
   d. stool for blood.

3. Which of these factors would be most significant if a patient was prescribed clonidine?
   a. Also taking a tricyclic antidepressant
   b. Need to operate complex machinery
   c. Positive Coombs' test
   d. Woman of child-bearing age

▸ 4. The nurse is caring for a patient who is receiving reserpine for hypertension. The patient is passive, has poor eye contact and appetite, and is difficult to engage in conversation. The nurse is concerned that the patient is experiencing a drug-induced depression. The nurse should share her concern with the
   a. patient.
   b. patient and the prescriber.
   c. prescriber and the family.
   d. patient, the prescriber, and the family.

5. A patient was started on reserpine 0.5 mg once a day 4 days ago for hypertension unresponsive to other antihypertensive agents. The nurse assesses the patient's blood pressure, which is 155/72 mm Hg. The patient is discouraged. The nurse's response should be based on which of the following?
   a. It takes 1 to 2 weeks for NE depletion to occur.
   b. At first reserpine promotes NE release, which can elevate BP temporarily.
   c. Ensure that the medication is being taken on an empty stomach.
   d. Reserpine primarily affects systolic blood pressure.

✳ 6. A patient is receiving guanethidine for uncontrolled hypertension. Which of the following laboratory test results should be reported to the prescriber immediately?
   a. ALT 35 units/L
   b. BUN 20 mg/dL
   c. Creatinine clearance 100 mL/min (eGFR)
   d. Urine catecholamines 870 mcg/24 hr

▸ 7. A patient is receiving methyldopa. Which of the following laboratory tests should be monitored throughout therapy? (Select all that apply.)
   a. Albumin
   b. ALT
   c. Bilirubin
   d. Coombs' test
   e. Glucose
   f. Hematocrit
   g. Hemoglobin
   h. LDH
   i. Potassium
   j. Sodium
   k. Troponin T

8. The nurse is teaching a 56-year-old truck driver about taking clonidine. It is very important to explain that he should take the
   a. two doses 12 hours apart.
   b. larger dose at bedtime.
   c. medication with food.
   d. medication on an empty stomach.

9. Match the drug with the contraindications and/or precautions. (Answers may be used more than once.)

   _____ a. Clonidine
   _____ b. Guanethidine
   _____ c. Methyldopa
   _____ d. Reserpine

   1. Active peptic ulcer disease
   2. Tricyclic antidepressants
   3. Pregnancy
   4. Pheochromocytoma
   5. History of depression
   6. Hepatitis

▶ 10. A patient is receiving methyldopa 250 mg twice a day. Vital signs are 170/90 mm Hg, P 92, and R 20. The nurse is reviewing new laboratory test results, which include ALT 35 international units/L, creatinine 0.8 mg/dL, BUN 20 mg/dL, Coombs' test positive, sodium 145 mEq/L, and potassium 4.8 mEq/L. The nurse should
   a. administer the medication and continue to assess the patient.
   b. administer the medication and notify the prescriber of the vital signs and laboratory results.
   c. hold the medication and notify the prescriber of the vital signs and laboratory results.
   d. hold the medication and page the prescriber STAT.

CASE STUDIES AND PATIENT TEACHING

(Use a separate piece of paper for your responses.)

Case Study 1

A 68-year-old active retired woman who plays tennis has been prescribed guanethidine 10 mg once a day for hypertension not controlled by other agents. The prescriber asks the office nurse to provide teaching regarding this medication.

1. What teaching should the nurse present?

2. The patient returns to the office 1 week after initiation of therapy. Her pulse has increased to 88 beats/min, up from a baseline of 80 beats/min and BP 170/78 mm Hg, up from a baseline of 165/70 mm Hg. What could be causing this elevation?

3. Why are anticholinergic antidiarrheal agents appropriate for diarrhea caused by this medication, and when would the patient expect to experience diarrhea as an adverse effect?

OBJECTIVES

See page 28 for the Objectives.

CRITICAL THINKING AND STUDY QUESTIONS

1. Which of the following are characteristics of drugs that can affect the brain? (Select all that apply.)
   a. Lipid soluble
   b. Highly ionized
   c. Move via transport systems
   d. Protein bound
   e. Water soluble

2. A 3-month-old infant is infected with meningitis. Why would the nurse expect an infant to be more responsive to the prescribed antibiotic than a college student?

3. A patient who has been taking a medication at the same dose for a period of time for a seizure disorder experiences an increase in seizure activity. The prescriber increases the dose of the medication. This may be an example of
   a. addiction.
   b. physical dependence.
   c. tolerance.

CASE STUDIES AND PATIENT TEACHING

(Use a separate piece of paper for your responses.)

Case Study 1

A patient has recently been diagnosed with major depression. Medication has just been prescribed that alters CNS neurotransmission. The patient verbalizes concerns to the nurse because the medication "is not working." She is also experiencing some daytime sedation.

1. How should the nurse respond?

2. The patient asks why drug companies have not been able to develop new psychotherapeutic drugs that do not have adverse effects. What would be the basis of the nurse's response?

3. There are many psychotherapeutic drugs that are effective in treating patient symptoms. What factors decrease patient adherence with these medications?

Answers can be reviewed online at http://evolve.elsevier.com/Lehne/.

OBJECTIVES

See page 28 for the Objectives.

CRITICAL THINKING AND STUDY QUESTIONS

1. Select all of the following that apply to Parkinson's disease (PD).
   a. The cause of symptoms is degeneration of neurons that supply dopamine to the striatum.
   b. PD causes a slowing of movement.
   c. Current drug treatment prevents further neuronal degeneration and controls symptoms.
   d. PD is hereditary in some cases.
   e. Drug therapy can prolong life.
   f. Excess dopamine inhibits muscle movement.
   g. Findings on autopsy include neurotoxic fibrin strands (Lewy bodies).
   h. Symptoms are called extrapyramidal adverse effects when they are drug induced.
   i. Symptoms include tremor when attempting movement.
   j. Symptoms may include depression, dementia, and memory loss.
   k. The symptoms of tremor and rigidity are most disabling.

2. Match the following drugs and descriptors:

   _____ a. Amantadine (Symmetrel)
   _____ b. Apomorphine (Apokyn)
   _____ c. Bromocriptine (Parlodel)
   _____ d. Entacapone (Comtan)
   _____ e. Levodopa (L-Dopa)
   _____ f. Levodopa/ Carbidopa

   1. Is not dependent on enzyme conversion to become active
   2. Inhibits catechol-*O*-methyltransferase (COMT) degradation of dopamine
   3. Inhibits dopamine breakdown by MAO-B
   4. Promotes dopamine release

   _____ g. Pergolide (Permax)
   _____ h. Pramipexole (Mirapex)
   _____ i. Ropinirole (Requip)
   _____ j. Selegiline (Eldepryl)
   _____ k. Tolcapone (Tasmar)

   5. Promotes dopamine synthesis
   6. Stimulates dopamine receptors (Sinemet/ Parcopa)

3. A realistic outcome for a patient receiving drug therapy for PD is
   a. absence of tremor.
   b. to attain a normal gait.
   c. to improve ability to perform activities of daily living.
   d. to reverse neurodegeneration.

4. Expected beneficial effects of levodopa on PD usually are
   a. dramatic relief of symptoms that stay suppressed with continued use.
   b. gradual relief of symptoms, peaking in approximately 5 years.
   c. relief of symptoms that increase over 1 to 2 years then decline as tolerance develops.
   d. relief of symptoms that steadily increase over months but decline to pretreatment state within 5 years.

5. Selegiline (Eldepryl, Zelapar) and rasagiline (Azilect) improve mild PD symptoms by
   a. blocking acetylcholine stimulation of GABA release.
   b. inhibiting the enzyme that breaks down dopamine.
   c. blocking the effect of GABA on skeletal muscles.
   d. increasing dopamine secretion.

6. The nurse has explained the medication levodopa to a patient who was recently diagnosed
   with PD. The patient has researched the
   disease and asks why dopamine is not prescribed. The nurse's response is based on the
   knowledge that
   a. dopamine cannot cross the blood-brain
      barrier.
   b. dopamine has significant adverse effects.
   c. dopamine requires decarboxylase to be
      absorbed and levels of this enzyme are
      depleted as a person ages.
   d. drug manufacturers have not been able to
      develop dopamine as a drug.

7. A PD patient who is receiving levodopa dis-
   plays violent, twisting, jerking movements of
   the extremities. The nurse holds the medications, notifies the prescriber, and documents
   this adverse effect as
   a. ballismus.
   b. choreoathetosis.
   c. fasciculation.
   d. tremor.

✳ 8. Which of these findings would be of most
   concern if the nurse is preparing to administer levodopa?
   a. Blood pressure 140/85 mm Hg
   b. Dark-colored urine
   c. Pulse 110 beats/min
   d. Tics

9. A PD patient complains that he has episodes
   of intense PD symptoms that last from 10
   minutes to 2 or 3 hours. These occur at any
   time and are different from the feeling that
   he gets when the drug is losing effectiveness
   before the next dose is due. Dietary teaching that may help this "on-off" phenomenon
   includes avoiding which of the following near
   the time of medication administration?
   a. Foods with a high glycemic index
   b. High-fat meals
   c. High-protein foods
   d. Refined carbohydrates

10. Psychotic symptoms caused by treatment
    with levodopa are often treated with
    a. chlorpromazine (Thorazine).
    b. clozapine (Clozaril).
    c. haloperidol (Haldol).
    d. risperidone (Risperdal).

11. The nurse should instruct patients who are pre-
    scribed levodopa to avoid dietary supplemen-
    tation of
    a. ascorbic acid (vitamin C).
    b. biotin.
    c. niacin.
    d. pyroxidine (vitamin B_6).

▶ 12. The nurse is bathing a patient who is receiv-
    ing levodopa for PD and notes an asymmet-
    ric, irregular darkly pigmented mole on the
    patient's back. The nurse should
    a. continue to assess the patient.
    b. notify the prescriber immediately.
    c. tell the patient that he should consult a
       dermatologist.
    d. stop administering the levodopa until the
       prescriber can be contacted.

13. Sinemet and Parcopa are levodopa-carbidopa
    combinations used when a patient has
    decreased responsiveness to levodopa. Addi-
    tion of carbidopa to the regimen (Select all
    that apply.)
    a. adds to the therapeutic effect because carbi-
       dopa more readily crosses the blood-brain
       barrier than levodopa.
    b. allows for an increase in levodopa dosage
       without significant adverse effects.
    c. decreases adverse effects, such as nausea
       and vomiting.
    d. decreases the risk of adverse effects of
       abnormal movements and psychiatric
       symptoms.
    e. inhibits decarboxylation of levodopa in the
       central nervous system (CNS).
    f. inhibits the conversion of levodopa to
       dopamine in the intestines and in tissue out-
       side the CNS.
    g. stimulates decarboxylation of levodopa by
       pyroxidine (vitamin B_6).

✳ 14. A hospitalized patient is prescribed Parcopa
    (25 mg levodopa/100 mg carbidopa). The hos-
    pital pharmacy substitutes the equivalent
    Sinemet product. A priority nursing assess-
    ment that would warrant further investigation
    before administering the Sinemet is
    a. anorexia.
    b. drooling.
    c. hypertension.
    d. tremor.

15. A patient is being switched from levodopa to a levodopa-carbidopa preparation. The nurse instructs the patient to
    a. allow at least 8 hours to pass after the last dose of levodopa before starting the new medication.
    b. start taking the new medications when symptoms of the old drug wearing off begin.
    c. take the new medication on an empty stomach.
    d. take the new medication within 3 hours after the last dose of the levodopa to prevent return of PD symptoms.

16. It is important for the nurse to teach the patient who is prescribed pramipexole (Mirapex) to avoid use of which OTC medication for heartburn?
    a. nizatidine (Axid)
    b. famotidine (Pepcid)
    c. cimetidine (Tagamet)
    d. ranitidine (Zantac)

▶ 17. A patient who has been taking pramipexole (Mirapex) for years is prescribed pramipexole (Mirapex) 1.5 mg. The hospital pharmacy stocks pramipexole 0.25 mg. How many tablets should the nurse administer?
    a. $^1/_2$ tablet
    b. 2 tablets
    c. 4 tablets
    d. 6 tablets

✳ 18. Which of these laboratory test findings would be most significant when a patient is receiving ropinirole (Requip)?
    a. ALT 285 international units/L
    b. BUN 22 mg/dL
    c. e GFR 55 mL/min
    d. Hb 11.8 g/dL

19. The medication administration record (MAR) for a patient with PD lists apomorphine (Apokyn) 1 mg subcutaneous with trimethobenzamide (Tigan) 300 mg, up to three doses per day as needed. The nurse should administer these medications if the patient experiences
    a. a sleep attack.
    b. an "off" episode.
    c. nausea.
    d. psychotic symptoms.

20. A common early complication of most drugs prescribed for PD that the nurse should consider when developing a plan of care for a PD patient is
    a. confusion.
    b. hypertension.
    c. nausea.
    d. somnolence.

✳ 21. Which of these assessment findings would be most significant if a patient was receiving bromocriptine (Parlodel)?
    a. Abnormal movements
    b. Confusion
    c. Red, swollen, hot hands
    d. S3 heart sound

✳ 22. A patient who is receiving tolcapone (Tasmar) complains of nausea and abdominal pain. His urine is dark amber. Which of the following laboratory test results would be most significant when the nurse reports these symptoms to the prescriber?
    a. ALT 175 international units/L; AST 159 international units/L
    b. BUN 22 mg/dL; Creatinine 1.1 mg/dL
    c. Hb 12 g/dL; Hct 39%
    d. Na⁺ 142 mEq/L; K⁺ 4.8 mEq/L

23. The nurse notes an orange color to the urine of a PD patient who is scheduled to receive a dose of entacapone (Comtan). The nurse should
    a. assess for symptoms of liver failure.
    b. consult with the prescriber.
    c. continue nursing care including administration of the medication.
    d. hold the medication and contact the prescriber immediately.

24. Selegiline (Eldepryl) should not be administered if a patient is receiving (Select all that apply.)
    a. butorphanol (Stadol).
    b. fluoxetine (Prozac).
    c. hydromorphone (Dilaudid).
    d. meperidine (Demerol).
    e. paroxetine (Paxil).
    f. sertraline (Zoloft).

CASE STUDIES AND PATIENT TEACHING

(Use a separate piece of paper for your responses.)

Case Study 1

A 54-year-old male welder who is married and has two adult children and one in college has recently been diagnosed with PD.

1. What assessments does the nurse need to make to aid in determining the needed therapy for this patient?

2. The patient is prescribed levodopa 0.5 gm twice daily and amantadine 100 mg twice daily. What teaching regarding administration of levodopa can the nurse provide that prevents or minimizes nausea and vomiting while maximizing drug absorption?

3. The nurse is teaching the patient and his wife about adverse effects of levodopa and amantadine. What teaching should be provided regarding possible postural hypotension, psychotic symptoms, and dermatologic changes?

4. Eighteen months after diagnosis the patient is admitted to a medical unit for a 10-day "drug holiday" because of significant adverse effects. It is anticipated that the patient will have a severe return of symptoms including rigidity and postural instability. What are probable nursing issues and what interventions will the nurse employ to address these problems?

5. The patient's major complaint is increased dyskinesias. The family provides the nurse with a history of progressive memory loss, increased tremors, mottled discoloration of the skin, and the inability to walk straight. He took his last dose of levodopa at 1200. The prescriber orders Sinemet (25 mg carbidopa with 100 mg levodopa) twice daily. What are the advantages of administering carbidopa to this patient?

6. Describe the precautions needed when switching a patient from levodopa to carbidopa with levodopa/carbidopa (Sinemet).

22

Alzheimer's Disease

Answers can be reviewed online at http://evolve.elsevier.com/Lehne/.

OBJECTIVES

See page 28 for the Objectives.

CRITICAL THINKING AND STUDY QUESTIONS

1. The daughter of a patient asks about the pathophysiology and pharmacologic treatment of Alzheimer's disease (AD). Which of the following information could be included in the nurse's explanation? (Select all that apply.)
   a. An early symptom of AD is loss of appetite.
   b. Current drug therapy for AD is not highly effective for relieving symptoms.
   c. High levels of the neurotransmitter acetylcholine are found in patients with AD.
   d. Neuritic plaques composed of a core beta-amyloid are found in the hippocampus and cerebral cortex of patients with AD.
   e. In AD, the orderly arrangement of microtubules is disrupted forming neurofibrillar tangles.
   f. Neurotoxic effects of beta-amyloid can be blocked by blocking the action of endoplasmic reticulum-associated binding protein (ERAB), which is found in high levels in patients with AD.
   g. Research suggests that individuals with copies of the gene that codes for apolipoprotein E2 (apoE2) are at increased risk for AD.

h. The American College of Physicians recommends trying a cholinesterase inhibitor in all patients with mild to moderate AD.
i. The neuronal damage occurring with AD is reversible if diagnosed early in the disease.
j. A blood test can confirm the diagnosis of AD.
k. Effects of drugs are long lasting.

2. High levels of homocysteine are associated with an increased risk of AD and other disorders. The nurse can teach patients to lower their homocysteine levels by eating a diet high in vitamins B_6 and folate found in
a. citrus fruits and meat.
b. fruits and vegetables.
c. dairy products and eggs.
d. green leafy vegetables and legumes.

3. Research suggests that some patients with AD regularly display more intense symptoms
a. in the morning.
b. before meals.
c. in the evening.
d. during the night.

＊ 4. The nurse is caring for a patient who is receiving rivastigmine (Exelon) for AD. Because of common adverse effects, a nursing priority would be
a. orthostatic BP precautions.
b. ensuring adequate fluids and nutrition.
c. assessing for unusual bruising or bleeding.
d. reviewing other prescribed drugs for drug interactions.

5. Research suggests cholinesterase inhibitors
a. enhance transmission by central cholinergic neurons.
b. decrease the formation of neuritic plaque.
c. maintain the orderly arrangement of microtubules.
d. prevent the degeneration of cortical neurons.

6. Adverse effects of cholinesterase inhibitors come from parasympathetic stimulation. Common adverse effects include
a. blurred vision.
b. diarrhea.

c. fatigue.
d. tachycardia.

▸ 7. The nurse should be particularly cautious when administering a cholinesterase inhibitor drug to any patient with a history of (Select all that apply.)
a. asthma.
b. chronic obstructive pulmonary disease (COPD).
c. heart failure (HF).
d. hypertension.
e. peptic ulcer disease.
f. peripheral vascular disease.

8. Which of the following treatments for dyspepsia could potentially decrease the renal excretion of memantine (Namenda) and cause toxicity?
a. Calcium carbonate (TUMS)
b. Lansoprazole (Prevacid)
c. Ranitidine (Zantac)
d. Sodium bicarbonate (baking soda)

▸ 9. Which of the following laboratory results would warrant withholding administration of memantine (Namenda) and notifying the prescriber?
a. ALT 112 international units/L
b. BUN 18 mg/dL
c. eGFR 45 mL/min
d. Potassium 4.7 mEq/L

▸ 10. The nurse is assigned an 87-year-old woman who was admitted from an extended-care facility with pneumonia. The nursing report reveals that the patient is extremely confused and combative. Why is it important for the nurse to not assume that the patient has AD?

CASE STUDIES AND PATIENT TEACHING

(Use a separate piece of paper for your responses.)

Case Study 1

A 77-year-old male who has a history of AD, diabetes mellitus (DM), hypertension, and seasonal allergies has been admitted with a hip fracture that occurred when wandering around the house at night. He is scheduled for an open reduction and internal fixation of the fracture the next morning. On admission the nurse discovers that the patient's wife had been administering Ginkgo biloba for the past 8 months in hope that it would improve his memory.

1. Why is it important for the nurse to report this to the orthopedic surgeon?

2. The patient's wife is concerned that his confusion, memory loss, and wandering has not improved much and that he seems to have gotten worse since the weather got warm. The wife provided a list of all of the patient's prescribed medications, which include hydrochlorothiazide (HydroDIURIL), metformin (Glucophage), and tacrine (Cognex). Based on the patient history, what class of over-the-counter (OTC) medication does the nurse need report to the prescriber because it could be contributing to the patient's sudden decline in functioning?

3. What assessments (including reviewing laboratory tests) should the nurse perform before administering the tacrine (Cognex), and what findings would warrant consulting the prescriber?

4. The patient's ALT is 178 international units/L, and his bilirubin is 3.2 mg/mL. The prescriber instructs the wife and patient to discontinue the tacrine (Cognex), not take any OTC antihistamines, and to start donepezil (Aricept). The wife asks the nurse why the prescriber changed the medication to a medication in the same class if the tacrine is not working well and is hurting her husband's liver.

5. The wife asks why the prescriber is giving her husband less medication (5 mg once a day versus 40 mg, four times a day). The nurse's response should include what information?

6. The nurse should teach the wife what information regarding adverse effects of donepezil (Aricept)?

7. The patient's wife heard from friends of something sold in the health food store to cure AD. The friend said that the store provided results of research that states that the supplement is effective in improving memory in AD patients. She is on a limited budget and asks the opinion of the nurse. How should the nurse respond?

23
Drugs for Multiple Sclerosis

Answers can be reviewed online at http://evolve.elsevier.com/Lehne/.

OBJECTIVES

See page 28 for the Objectives.

CRITICAL THINKING AND STUDY QUESTIONS

1. A 26-year-old woman seeks medical care for blurred vision and severe muscle weakness. Which of the following from her history are possible risk factors for multiple sclerosis (MS)? (Select all that apply.)
   a. She smokes.
   b. She is overweight.
   c. She lives in North Carolina.
   d. She has had mononucleosis twice while in college.

e. Her father has had a cerebral vascular accident ([CVA], stroke).

f. Her maternal and paternal grandparents were Norwegian immigrants.

2. Match the diagnostic test with its function.

_____ a. CSF analysis   1. Detects areas of demyelination

_____ b. MRI

_____ c. VEP   2. Measures how quickly the brain responds to visual stimuli

     3. Assesses immune activity in CNS

3. Current drug therapy for MS can (Select all that apply.)
   a. cure the disease.
   b. decrease the formation of lesions.
   c. decrease symptoms during a relapse.
   d. improve mobility and safety.
   e. produce remissions in all types of MS.
   f. slow the disease process.

4. Treatment with immunomodulators for relapsing-remitting MS should (Select all that apply.)
   a. always include a drug classified as an immunosuppressant.
   b. begin as soon as possible after MS is diagnosed.
   c. only be used if attacks last more than 1 week.
   d. only be used during periods of relapse.
   e. continue indefinitely unless it is totally ineffective or toxic.

▶ 5. The nurse is administering high-dose intravenous (IV) methylprednisolone to a patient who is experiencing an acute relapse of MS. The nurse would need to be especially careful of monitoring the patient who has the chronic condition of
   a. asthma.
   b. diabetes mellitus (DM).
   c. hypertension.
   d. rheumatoid arthritis.

▶ 6. A patient with MS who is hospitalized with pneumonia is receiving the immunomodulator interferon beta-1a (Avonex) IM 30 mcg once a week. It would be most important for the nurse to report which of the following laboratory test results to the prescriber?
   a. ALT 45 international units/L
   b. Hemoglobin A$_{1C}$ 5.2%

c. RBC 4.9 million cells per microliter
d. WBC 12,000/mm^3

▶ 7. A patient is prescribed an initial subcutaneous dose of 8.8 mcg of interferon 1a (Refib) for the first 2 weeks of therapy. The drug is supplied as 22 mcg/0.5 mL. How much drug should the patient administer with each dose?

8. Assessing for symptoms of progressive multifocal leukoencephalopathy before infusing natalizumab (Tysabri) must focus on recent changes because many symptoms of this adverse effect
   a. are similar to symptoms of MS.
   b. can be prevented.
   c. occur in hours.
   d. predict if the drug will not be effective.

9. A patient reports perioral paresthesias and wheezing after the last dose of natalizumab (Tysabri). The infusion nurse should
   a. administer diphenhydramine before starting the infusion.
   b. administer the drug over 2 hours.
   c. administer the drug in at least 100 mL of diluent.
   d. consult the prescriber.

▶ 10. The nurse is administering mitoxantrone (Novantrone) to a patient who was unresponsive to other immunomodulating drugs for MS. The nurse should hold the medication and contact the prescriber if the patient exhibits
   a. diaphoresis and low blood sugar.
   b. dizziness and orthostatic hypotension.
   c. headache and elevated blood pressure.
   d. weight gain of 3 lb in 24 hours and shortness of breath.

11. When a patient is receiving mitoxantrone (Novantrone), liver function tests (LFT) should be assessed once
   a. a month.
   b. every 3 months.
   c. every 6 months.
   d. a year.

▶ 12. A patient is scheduled to receive mitoxantrone (Novantrone). Which of the following would be definite reasons to withhold the medication and contact the prescriber? (Select all that apply.)
   a. ALT 100 international units/L
   b. Amenorrhea
   c. Blue-green colored urine
   d. LVEF 60%
   e. hCG 35 international units/L
   f. Neutrophils 1000 cells/mm³
   g. Yellow-tinged skin

▶ 13. A patient who is receiving mitoxantrone (Novantrone) should not receive which of the following immunizations? (Select all that apply.)
   a. Hepatitis A vaccine
   b. Hepatitis B vaccine
   c. Influenza vaccine
   d. Measles, mumps, and rubella (MMR)
   e. Pneumococcal polysaccharide vaccine (Pneumovax)
   f. Tetanus plus diphtheria toxoids for adults (Td)
   g. Varicella virus vaccine

▶ 14. A patient with MS experiences nausea, vomiting, tea-colored urine, clay-colored stool, and right upper quadrant (RUQ) tenderness. ALT results are 200 international units/L. The nurse would consult with the prescriber if the patient was prescribed
   a. betaseron.
   b. copaxone.
   c. mitoxantrone.

15. Match the symptoms of MS to the drugs used to manage them. (You may use more than one answer.)

_____ a. Amantadine (Symmetrel)
_____ b. Baclofen (Lioresal)
_____ c. Bethanechol (Urecholine)
_____ d. Botulinum toxin
_____ e. Docusate sodium
_____ f. Donepezil (Aricept)
_____ g. Enemeez
_____ h. Fluoxetine (Prozac)
_____ i. Gabapentin (Neurontin)
_____ j. Hyoscyamine
_____ k. K-Y jelly
_____ l. Meclizine (Antivert)
_____ m. Modafinil (Provigil)
_____ n. Nortriptyline (Pamelor)
_____ o. Primidone (Mysoline)
_____ p. Psyllium (Metamucil)
_____ q. Terazosin (Hytrin)
_____ r. Tolterodine (Detrol)
_____ s. Vardenafil (Levitra)

1. Ataxia and tremor
2. Constipation
3. Depression
4. Difficulty starting or stopping urination and incomplete bladder emptying
5. Dizziness and vertigo
6. Fatigue
7. Fecal incontinence
8. Impaired bladder emptying
9. Memory impairment
10. Neuropathic pain
11. Sexual dysfunction
12. Sleep disturbances
13. Spasticity
14. Urinary frequency, urgency, and incontinence

CASE STUDIES AND PATIENT TEACHING

(Use a separate piece of paper for your responses.)

Case Study 1

A 32-year-old college professor has been diagnosed with relapsing-remitting MS after the birth of her first child.

1. What assessments are important for the nurse to include when caring for this patient?

2. Her symptoms have significantly resolved. What are the primary factors of the pathophysiologic process of MS that explain how the symptoms can abate but the disease is still present?

3. What are some possible nursing diagnoses for this patient throughout the disease process?

4. When the nurse is administering medications, the patient refuses the drug stating "What's the use? My mom had MS and the drugs didn't help. She died in 1990. She was only 57 years old." What should be the basis of the nurse's response?

5. The patient with MS is started on the immunomodulator interferon beta-1a (Avonex) IM 30 mcg once a week. What should the nurse include in teaching regarding this drug?

6. The patient and the prescriber have tried treatment with the immunomodulators without success. They have agreed to try the immunosuppressant mitoxantrone (Novantrone). What teaching should the nurse provide this patient?

7. What steps does the nurse need to take before administering the mitoxantrone (Novantrone) by IV infusion?

8. The patient is experiencing fecal incontinence. What pharmacologic and nonpharmacologic measures can be employed to prevent this problem?

24
Drugs for Epilepsy

Answers can be reviewed online at http://evolve.elsevier.com/Lehne/.

OBJECTIVES

See page 28 for the Objectives.

CRITICAL THINKING AND STUDY QUESTIONS

1. Convulsions
   a. always occur as a symptom of epilepsy.
   b. are the same as seizures.
   c. may involve brief periods of unconsciousness.
   d. only refer to abnormal movements.

2. The experimental procedure called kindling suggests that
   a. children may outgrow seizure disorders.
   b. early treatment may prevent more serious seizure disorders.
   c. seizures caused by trauma will occur within 24 hours of the trauma.
   d. seizure disorders rarely can be controlled by drugs.

3. Antiepileptic drugs can exert their effect by increasing the effect of which of the following?
   a. Calcium
   b. Gamma-aminobutyric acid
   c. Glutamate
   d. Sodium

4. Complex partial seizures differ from simple partial seizures in that they involve
   a. fear and depression.
   b. hearing, seeing, or tasting things that are not present.
   c. lack of response to the environment.
   d. motor twitching.

5. Which of the following is restricted by some state laws for individuals who have had a seizure in the past 1 to 2 years?
   a. Certification to teach preschool through high school
   b. Licensure as a nurse
   c. Licensure as a pharmacist
   d. Licensure to drive

6. The nurse can assist the prescriber with obtaining the effective dose of ethosuximide (Zarontin) for absence seizures by teaching the patient and/or family to
   a. comply with scheduled lab tests for drug levels.
   b. increase doses if seizure activity increases.
   c. note adverse effects.
   d. observe and record seizure activity.

7. A patient who has been taking valproic acid (Depakene) and carbamazepine (Tegretol) is to begin attempting drug withdrawal. To prevent adverse effects, the nurse reinforces teaching that the
   a. dose of both drugs should both be gradually decreased.
   b. dose of one drug should be gradually decreased while maintaining the usual dose of the second drug.
   c. carbamazepine should be stopped and the valproic acid continued for at least a week.
   d. valproic acid should be stopped and the carbamazepine continued for at least a week.

8. When caring for a patient who is receiving phenytoin (Dilantin), which of the following assessments require immediate nursing intervention?
   a. Continuous back and forth movements of the eyes
   b. Drowsiness
   c. Excessive growth of gum tissue
   d. Inadequate consumption of products rich in calcium and vitamin D

9. When administering phenytoin (Dilantin), at what serum level should the nurse consider therapy to be potentially toxic?
   a. Greater than 1 mcg/L
   b. Greater than 5 mcg/mL
   c. Greater than 10 mcg/mL
   d. Greater than 15 mcg/mL

✳▸ 10. A 47-year-old patient has been taking phenytoin (Dilantin) for years without significant adverse effects or seizures. Serum levels usually are 12 to 16 mcg/mL. The patient is admitted with sudden onset of multiple seizures. Serum phenytoin levels now are 7 mcg/mL. What question is most important for the nurse to ask?
   a. "Have you changed from brand name to generic phenytoin?"
   b. "Have you noticed a rash anywhere on your body?"
   c. "Have you had any change in or addition of any other medications?"
   d. "Have you been diagnosed with any liver disease?"

11. A parent has received instructions regarding administration of 5 mL twice a day of phenytoin (Dilantin suspension) to their child.

Which of these statements made by the parent suggests a need for further teaching?
   a. "I must be sure to shake the medication thoroughly before measuring the dose."
   b. "I should give him a teaspoonful of the drug at each dose."
   c. "I should give him the medication with breakfast and with a snack before bedtime."
   d. "It is important that I space the drug doses as I have been instructed."

✳▸ 12. When a patient who is receiving carbamazepine (Tegretol) complains of vertigo, which action should the nurse take first?
   a. Ensure patient safety.
   b. Page the prescriber STAT.
   c. Review most recent lab results of CBC, BUN, and electrolytes.
   d. Withhold the medication.

13. The nurse is teaching a patient about adverse effects that occur with carbamazepine (Tegretol). Which of the following would not be included in this teaching?
   a. Avoid situations where you are likely to be exposed to people with contagious infections.
   b. Contact the prescriber if you experience double vision.
   c. Plan your day to allow for rest periods.
   d. Use an electric razor because you may bleed easily.

14. The nurse is administering carbamazepine (Tegretol) to a patient of Asian descent. In order to reduce the risk of life-threatening skin reactions, it would be important for the nurse to verify that the patient had a laboratory test result done that showed
   a. absence of the human leukocyte antigen b*1502 (HLA-B*1502).
   b. absence of inflammation.
   c. adequate hydration.
   d. adequate RBCs.

15. The nurse instructs patients who have just received a prescription for carbamazepine (Tegretol) to avoid consuming grapefruit juice for which of the following periods?
   a. Four hours after taking the medication
   b. No more than twice a week when taking the medication
   c. Not at all when taking the medication
   d. Two hours before taking the medication

16. When teaching about adverse effects of valproic acid, the nurse should emphasize the importance of reporting which of the following adverse effects that suggest the possibility of a life-threatening reaction?
    a. Abdominal pain and lack of appetite
    b. Heartburn and belching
    c. Rash and tremor
    d. Weight gain and hair loss

17. A woman who is of child-bearing age must take valproic acid to control seizures. Which of the following statements if made by the patient suggest a need for further teaching?
    a. "If I get pregnant, the baby should be okay as long as I stop taking the drug within 2 months of becoming pregnant."
    b. "I need to inform all of my healthcare providers that I am taking valproic acid."
    c. "I need to take folic acid supplements in case I accidentally get pregnant."
    d. "I need to use two reliable forms of birth control."

▶ 18. When administering valproic acid to an elderly patient, the nurse notes the patient chewing the tablet. The nurse should
    a. ask the pharmacy to send the divalproex sodium (Depakote) sprinkles form of the drug.
    b. contact the prescriber.
    c. crush subsequent doses and put them in applesauce or pudding.
    d. crush subsequent doses and mix them in 5 mL of warm water.

19. A patient with a history of hypertension and complex partial seizures has been prescribed oxcarbazepine (Trileptal) 100 mg twice a day and spironolactone (Aldactone). It is important for the nurse to assess which of the following symptoms of hyponatremia?
    a. Dry mucous membranes and flushed skin
    b. Hyperactive bowel sounds and tall tented T waves on electrocardiogram (ECG)
    c. Muscle spasms and paresthesias
    d. Weakness and nausea

▶ 20. If a patient who is receiving lamotrigine (Lamictal) develops a rash, the nurse should
    a. assess vital signs.
    b. continue nursing care.

c. review laboratory test results.
d. withhold the medication and contact the prescriber.

✳ ▶ 21. Which of the following data, if not known by the prescriber, would be most important for the nurse to communicate to the prescriber when a patient is receiving gabapentin (Neurontin)?
    a. Dizziness
    b. Fasting blood sugar 110 mg/dL
    c. Urine output of 200 mL in 8 hours
    d. Patient is also receiving phenytoin (Dilantin)

22. Levetiracetam (Keppra)
    a. can cause loss of muscle strength.
    b. can decrease the effectiveness of warfarin (Coumadin).
    c. mechanism of action is blockade of sodium channels.
    d. should be administered with food to decrease gastrointestinal (GI) adverse effects.

▶ 23. It is important for the nurse to monitor laboratory test results for which of the following findings if a female patient is prescribed topiramate (Topamax)?
    a. Creatinine 1.5 mg/dL
    b. HCO_3 20 mEq/L
    c. HCT 32%
    d. WBC 4600/mm^3

24. A patient is receiving topiramate (Topamax) in addition to carbamazepine (Tegretol) for tonic-clonic seizures. The nurse should teach the patient to observe for critical adverse effects of topiramate including
    a. ataxia.
    b. difficulty concentrating.
    c. sudden eye pain.
    d. weight loss.

▶ 25. The nurse notes that tiagabine (Gabitril) is ordered but no other antiepileptic drugs (AEDs) are prescribed for this patient. The nurse should:
    a. administer the medication.
    b. administer the medication and ask the patient why they are taking the medication.
    c. withhold the medication and institute seizure precautions.
    d. withhold the medication and consult the prescriber STAT.

26. The nurse teaches that which of the following AEDs can increase the liver metabolism of contraceptives and increase the risk of unintended pregnancy? (Select all that apply.)
    a. carbamazepine (Tegretol)
    b. gabapentin (Neurontin)
    c. lamotrigine (Lamictal)
    d. levetiracetam (Keppra)
    e. oxcarbazepine (Trileptal)
    f. phenobarbital (Luminal)
    g. primidone (Mysoline)
    h. phenytoin (Dilantin)
    i. topiramate (Topamax)
    j. valproic acid (Depakene)
    k. zonisamide (Zonegran)

27. The nurse would consult the prescriber before administering the drug if the nurse notes that a patient who was prescribed zonisamide (Zonegran) had a known anaphylactic reaction to
    a. acarbose (Precose).
    b. insulin aspart (Novolog).
    c. glipizide (Glucotrol).
    d. metformin (Glucophage).

CASE STUDIES AND PATIENT TEACHING

(Use a separate piece of paper for your responses.)

Case Study 1

A 26-year-old female, who is 8 months pregnant, is admitted to the neurologic intensive care unit with the diagnosis of head injury. An automobile accident has left the patient unconscious. On admission an intravenous (IV) line of $D_5 \frac{1}{2}$ NS at 50 mL/hr is started. Within the first 24 hours on the unit, the patient has several tonic-clonic seizures. Standing orders on the unit allow the nurse to administer diazepam (Valium) 5 mg IV push. The prescriber is notified of the seizure and orders an IV loading dose of phenytoin (Dilantin) 800 mg followed by 100 mg every 6 hours, a phenytoin level the next day, and IV cimetidine 300 mg twice a day.

1. What nursing precautions are needed when administering phenytoin and cimetidine intravenously?

2. The phenytoin is available for IV infusion in a concentration of 50 mg/mL. How long should the nurse take when administering the 800-mg loading dose?

3. What symptoms should the nurse be alert for because of the possible interaction of phenytoin and cimetidine?

4. The next day, the phenytoin level is 14 mcg/mL. Why is it critical for the nurse to closely monitor plasma drug levels of phenytoin?

5. One week later, the patient goes into labor. Based on initiation of phenytoin near the end of the pregnancy, what fetal effects are most likely to occur?

6. What precautions might be taken to protect the fetus during drug therapy, during delivery, and after delivery?

7. Two weeks later, the patient is stabilized and has been transferred to the neurologic progressive unit. On admission the nurse notes a fine maculopapular rash on the patient's trunk. What should the nurse do and why?

8. Phenytoin (Dilantin) is discontinued. Carbamazepine (Tegretol) is substituted as the patient's antiseizure drug. The patient is concerned about taking seizure medication because she wants to have more children. She has been advised about possible adverse effects to the fetus. In addition to referring concerns to the prescriber, what information could the nurse provide about seizures, AEDs, and pregnancy?

Case Study 2

The nurse is working in a neurologic clinic of a major pediatric hospital. One responsibility is obtaining a complete history at the initial visit.

1. What data would be important for the nurse to collect from the parents of a 3-year-old boy who was referred because of new-onset seizures?

2. The patient weighs 35 lbs and is prescribed phenytoin 20 mg every 12 hours. The suggested initial dose is 2.5 mg/kg/day in divided doses. Is this a safe and effective dose for this child?

3. Phenytoin is available as a suspension of 125 mg/mL. How much drug should be administered at each dose, and what measuring device should the nurse teach the parents to use?

4. What care can the nurse teach the parents to provide to minimize the adverse effect of gingival hyperplasia?

5. Despite increasing doses, the child continues to have tonic-clonic seizures. The pediatric neurologist discontinues the phenytoin and orders valproic acid. Based on mechanism of action, why might valproic acid alone be effective when phenytoin was not effective?

Case Study 3

A 19-year-old college student has been diagnosed with partial seizures and has been prescribed carbamazepine (Tegretol) 100 mg twice a day. The patient reports his new diagnosis and drug therapy to the nurse at the college health center.

1. What information would be important for the college health clinic to collect to assist the student with managing his health and illness?

2. What can the nurse teach that enables the patient to assist the prescriber with evaluating the effectiveness of the prescribed drug?

3. What should the nurse teach about adverse effects of carbamazepine (Tegretol) including when he should seek medical attention?

4. What adverse effect of all antiepileptic drugs would warrant the nurse carefully monitoring the student's mental status?

5. What should the nurse teach about AEDs and alcohol?

6. At a later visit, the student tells the college health center nurse that he is discouraged because he has been on medication for over a month and continues to have seizures. How should the nurse respond?

7. The student plans to visit home between the fall and spring semester, which is 3000 miles from the college. What teaching should the nurse provide relating to precautions that should be taken with travel?

8. Developmentally, what are common barriers to adherence to drug therapy for this patient, and what are possible nursing interventions to address these barriers?

9. What communication techniques would be most likely to influence this individual?

25

Drugs for Muscle Spasm and Spasticity

Answers can be reviewed online at http://evolve.elsevier.com/Lehne/.

OBJECTIVES

See page 28 for the Objectives.

CRITICAL THINKING AND STUDY QUESTIONS

1. A patient who has chronic back pain asks the nurse why ibuprofen was prescribed instead of a muscle relaxant for his muscle spasms. The basis of the nurse's response is based on what knowledge?

2. It is important for the nurse to assess for nausea, vomiting, tea-colored urine, clay-colored stool, right upper quadrant (RUQ) tenderness, yellowish discoloration to eyes or skin, and elevated alanine aminotranferase (ALT) in patients receiving which of the following drugs? (Select all that apply.)
   a. baclofen (Lioresal)
   b. carisoprodol (Soma)
   c. chlorzoxazone (Paraflex)
   d. cyclobenzaprine (Flexeril)
   e. dantrolene (Dantrium)
   f. diazepam (Valium)
   g. metaxalone (Skelaxin)
   h. methocarbamol (Robaxin)
   i. orphenadrine (Norflex)
   j. tizanidine (Zanaflex)

✳ 3. Priority nursing interventions and teaching for a patient receiving a central muscle relaxant are related to
   a. emotional support.
   b. nutrition.
   c. safety.
   d. skin integrity.

4. Which of the following statements, if made by a patient who has been taking methocarbamol (Robaxin) for 6 months after an accident, would be a concern for the nurse?
   a. "I plan to stop taking this medication on Monday because I have to go back to work."
   b. "My urine has been a funny dark green color."
   c. "I had hepatitis several years ago."
   d. "I have to be careful when I stand up because sometimes I get dizzy."

5. A resident is writing orders for hospitalized patients. The nurse would question an order written for baclofen (Lioresal) for a patient with
   a. cerebral palsy.
   b. a cerebral vascular accident (CVA).
   c. multiple sclerosis.
   d. a spinal cord injury.

CASE STUDIES AND PATIENT TEACHING

(Use a separate piece of paper for your responses.)

Case Study 1

A 19-year-old male is admitted to the neurologic intensive care unit after a motorcycle accident. He is paraplegic with severe lower extremity muscle spasms. He is receiving intrathecal baclofen. A pump is being used to infuse the drug because abrupt discontinuation can cause rhabdomyolysis and multiple organ system failure.

1. What is rhabdomyolysis, what organ is particularly sensitive to its effects, and what assessment findings would suggest that this is occurring?

2. The patient is transferred to a rehabilitation unit. Baclofen 20 mg is prescribed 4 times a day. What assessments should be included in the nurse's plan of care for this patient relating to drug therapy?

3. Developmentally, this patient is at risk for nonadherence to therapy. Why should the patient be discouraged from abrupt discontinuation of baclofen?

4. Dantrolene (Dantrium) would be more convenient for this patient because it only needs to be taken once a day. Why is it not a good choice for this patient?

Case Study 2

A patient with multiple sclerosis is admitted with pneumonia. She is receiving cyclobenzaprine (Flexeril) to relieve muscle spasms.

1. What are common anticholinergic adverse effects associated with this drug and nursing interventions relating to these effects?

2. What nonpharmacologic interventions and teaching could the nurse provide to help relieve the patient's discomfort and prevent complications?

Case Study 3

A patient returns to the recovery room after general anesthesia. The vital signs have increased from normal to a temperature of 103.6° F, pulse 116, respirations 22 breaths per minute, and BP 145/99 mm Hg. The patient is developing muscular rigidity.

1. Why are antipyretics not appropriate to treat this fever?

2. Dantrolene 150 mg IV push is prescribed. The recommended dose to treat malignant hyperthermia is initially 2 mg/kg to a maximum of 10 mg/kg. The patient weighs 185 lb, and the initial prescribed dose is 150 mg. Is this a safe and therapeutic dose?

3. Why is it important to position the patient on his side with the side rails up?

26
Local Anesthetics

Answers can be reviewed online at http://evolve.elsevier.com/Lehne/.

OBJECTIVES

See page 28 for the Objectives.

CRITICAL THINKING AND STUDY QUESTIONS

1. The nurse is caring for a patient who has just returned to the nursing unit after an endoscopic procedure involving topical anesthesia applied to the throat. What should be included in nursing care relating to this anesthesia?

✱ 2. The nurse is assisting the emergency department nurse practitioner with anesthetizing and suturing of multiple wounds on the extremities

of a man who was attacked by a dog. Which of these new developments would be of most concern to the nurse?
   a. Numbness and tingling around the mouth
   b. Rash
   c. Respirations 24 breaths per minute
   d. Restlessness

✱ 3. A mother received epidural anesthetic 10 minutes before delivering a 7-lb 10-ounce girl at 39 weeks of gestation. The neonate is brought to the nursery from the delivery room. Which of the following findings would be a concern to the nursery nurse?
   a. Apical pulse 160 beats/min
   b. Positive Babinski's
   c. Respirations 22 breaths per minute
   d. Temperature 36.8°C

✱ 4. A patient is admitted to a surgical floor at 10 AM (1000) after a total abdominal hysterectomy performed with spinal anesthetic. During

the assessment at 4 PM (1600) the nurse notes that the patient has not voided. The patient denies a need to void. The initial action by the nurse would be to
a. administer bethanechol 5 mg subcutaneously ordered as needed for urinary retention.
b. tell the patient that she needs to go to the bathroom to attempt to void.
c. sit the patient upright on a bedpan to attempt to void.
d. perform a bladder scan.

5. Topical local anesthetic should be applied
a. using the lowest effective dose.
b. gently to areas of skin that are abraded.
c. as a thick film over the entire affected area.
d. extending approximately ½ inch beyond the affected area.

6. In general, anesthetics that are small in the size of particles, highly lipid soluble, and do not readily ionize have a
a. fast onset and long duration.
b. slow onset and long duration.
c. fast onset and short duration.
d. slow onset and short duration.

7. Using a vasoconstrictor, such as epinephrine, with a local anesthetic (Select all that apply.)
a. allows for the use of less anesthetic.
b. causes local vasoconstriction.
c. can cause adverse effects from systemic absorption of the vasoconstrictor.
d. causes local vasodilation.
e. delays onset of anesthesia.
f. delays systemic absorption.
g. improves blood flow to the affected area.
h. increases the risk of toxicity.
i. reduces blood flow to the affected area.
j. reduces the risk of toxicity.
k. requires the use of a larger dose of anesthetic.

8. When a patient is receiving a local anesthetic with epinephrine, the nurse should carefully assess for which effects from the epinephrine?
a. Convulsions and respiratory depression
b. Headache and urinary retention
c. Rapid pulse and rising BP
d. Slowed pulse and dropping blood pressure (BP)

9. A patient who has a known allergy to chloroprocaine (Nesacaine) should not receive
a. articaine (Septocaine).
b. lidocaine (Xylocaine).
c. mepivacaine (Carbocaine).
d. tetracaine (Pontocaine).

10. Cocaine differs from other ester-type local anesthetics in that it
a. can be particularly dangerous if given to a patient with heart failure (HF).
b. causes intense vasoconstriction.
c. is known to cause physical dependence.
d. produces CNS excitement, then depression.

11. A patient received intravenous regional anesthetic containing lidocaine without epinephrine when he had ankle surgery. At what point would the patient be at greatest risk for bradycardia, hypotension, and respiratory depression from the lidocaine?
a. Immediately after injection of the lidocaine
b. When the surgeon makes the incision
c. When the patient is in the postanesthesia unit
d. When the patient is in his hospital room on the medical-surgical unit

CASE STUDIES AND PATIENT TEACHING

(Use a separate piece of paper for your responses.)

Case Study 1

An 8-year-old child, accompanied by both parents, comes to the emergency room with a scalp laceration sustained when he fell off of his bicycle. The plan includes administration of lidocaine with epinephrine to close the wound with 6 to 8 interrupted sutures. The child is tearful but cooperative.

1. What would be the nursing responsibilities for this procedure?

Case Study 2

A patient received lidocaine for the removal of an ingrown toenail. Seeping blood made it difficult to visualize the work area. Epinephrine is a vasoconstrictor that is often combined with lidocaine to delay systemic absorption of the lidocaine. As a vasoconstrictor, it would have decreased the blood seepage.

1. Why was it not used in this situation?

2. The patient has had this procedure before and is concerned about pain. She verbalizes a desire to use ice immediately to prevent pain. What precautions should the nurse provide regarding the use of cold?

3. The patient asks if she can use over-the-counter (OTC) topical lidocaine anesthetic on her toe when sensation returns to relieve discomfort. What teaching should the nurse provide?

27
General Anesthetics

Answers can be reviewed online at http://evolve.elsevier.com/Lehne/.

OBJECTIVES

See page 28 for the Objectives.

CRITICAL THINKING AND STUDY QUESTIONS

1. General anesthesia (aka, anaesthesia) involves the absence of
   a. sensibility to pain.
   b. consciousness and sensibility to pain.
   c. consciousness and sensibility to pain and temperature.
   d. consciousness and sensibility to pain, temperature, and taste.

2. Describe the ideal anesthetic.

3. What are the agents included in a balanced anesthetic?

4. Match the class of drugs to the properties of ideal anesthesia that they produce.
   _____ a. Neuromuscular blocking agents
   _____ b. Nitrous oxide
   _____ c. Opioids
   _____ d. Short-acting barbiturates

   1. Analgesia
   2. Produce state of unconsciousness
   3. Muscle relaxation

5. The primary goal of using multiple agents to achieve anesthesia is to
   a. decrease the pain after the procedure.
   b. make the patient unable to feel pain during the procedure.
   c. permit full anesthesia with less adverse effects.
   d. prevent the patient from remembering the experience.

6. Current data indicates that inhalation anesthetics (Select all that apply.)
   a. depress transmission at excitatory synapses.
   b. depress transmission at inhibitory synapses.
   c. enhance transmission at excitatory synapses.
   d. enhance transmission at inhibitory synapses.

7. Nitrous oxide has an extremely high minimum alveolar concentration (MAC). Because of this
   a. the drug can be administered at low doses and achieve adequate anesthesia.
   b. surgical anesthesia cannot be obtained with nitrous oxide.
   c. the drug can achieve adequate, safe anesthesia if a high enough dose is administered slowly.
   d. the drug will make the patient unresponsive to painful stimuli.

* 8. The nurse is caring for a patient in the postanesthesia care unit (PACU). The assessment that the nurse should give the highest priority is
   a. breathing.
   b. level of consciousness.
   c. pain.
   d. urinary output.

* 9. A patient has received succinylcholine during surgery. A priority nursing outcome during nursing care in the PACU is
   a. blood pressure will be 110/60 to 120/70 mm Hg.
   b. dressing will be dry and intact.
   c. patient will void at least 250 mL of clear yellow urine.
   d. temperature will be 36.5°C to 37°C.

10. The nurse should assess all postoperative patients who have received inhaled anesthesia for
    a. diarrhea.
    b. excessive salivation.
    c. urinary urgency.
    d. wheezing.

▶ 11. The nurse is completing the preoperative checklist for a same-day surgery patient who has been called to the operating room (OR). The patient makes a comment to the nurse that he hopes they really knock him out because he really needs a lot of a drug to get a good effect. On further discussion the patient reveals that he has been using oxycodone (OxyContin) illegally for 2 years and that his last dose was 6 hours ago. The nurse should
    a. call the OR and cancel the surgery.
    b. note the medication on the patient's chart and send the patient to the OR.
    c. notify anesthesia and the surgeon of the finding.
    d. nothing, the medication should be out of the patient's system.

▶ 12. A male patient who has received midazolam (Versed), a preoperative benzodiazepine, informs the nurse that he needs to "pass his water." The nurse should initially
    a. assist the patient to the bathroom, staying with the patient at all times.
    b. provide the patient a urinal and ask him to try to use it while still in bed.
    c. provide the patient with a urinal and assist him with standing.
    d. insert a Foley catheter.

▶ 13. The assessment finding that would warrant the nurse withholding morphine from a postoperative patient is
    a. blood pressure 160/92 mm Hg.
    b. pain 9 on a scale of 1 to 10.
    c. respirations 8 breaths per minute.
    d. temperature 38.2°C.

14. A patient has received halothane during surgery. The PACU nurse would be concerned if the patient was unable to be aroused how soon after the halothane inhalation ended?
    a. 10 to 15 minutes
    b. 15 to 30 minutes
    c. 30 to 60 minutes
    d. 60 to 90 minutes

▶ 15. A 14-month-old received halothane during surgery. Which of the following immediate postoperative assessment findings would be a concern?
    a. Blood pressure 86/54 mm Hg
    b. Pulse 68 beats/min
    c. Respirations 30 breaths per minute
    d. Temperature 39.8°C

16. The PACU nurse has received a patient who had emergency surgery including general anesthetic with isoflurane (Forane) from the operating room. The family has just arrived, and the nurse has learned that the patient has been taking the calcium channel blocker amlodipine (Norvasc). Because of the similarity in effects of isoflurane and amlodipine on the cardiovascular system, the nurse should assess carefully for early signs of
    a. bradycardia.
    b. hypertension.
    c. hypotension.
    d. tachycardia.

17. Match the drug to the adverse effect.

_____ a. Desflurane
_____ b. Enflurane
_____ c. Halothane
_____ d. Isofloflurane
_____ e. Ketamine
_____ f. Propofol
_____ g. Sevoflurane

1. High risk of bacterial infection
2. Hypotension can occur from vasodilation
3. Can induce seizures
4. Delirium and psychotic symptoms can occur post-operatively or days or weeks after surgery
5. Can produce heat and fire in administration apparatus
6. May prolong QT interval
7. Tachycardia and hyper-tension can occurs if blood levels drop suddenly

18. Nitrous oxide is widely used in surgery because
    a. it has significant analgesic effects with-out significant cardiac or respiratory depression.
    b. it can produce a state of unconsciousness at very low doses.
    c. full anesthesia can be achieved with nitrous oxide alone.
    d. postoperative nausea and vomiting are uncommon.

19. A cataract surgery patient receives midazolam and fentanyl. The nurse would expect these medications to produce (Select all that apply.)
    a. absence of anxiety.
    b. analgesia.
    c. balanced anesthesia.
    d. flaccid paralysis.
    e. sedation.
    f. unconsciousness.

CASE STUDIES AND PATIENT TEACHING

(Use a separate piece of paper for your responses.)

Case Study 1

A 65-year-old white male with a history of lung cancer has been admitted the evening before surgery and is scheduled for a thoracotomy at 8 AM under balanced general anesthetic. He is 5 feet 6 inches and weighs 210 lb. The patient has a productive cough and admits to tobacco use for the last 40 years, smoking one pack of cigarettes per day. He has hypertension and takes hydrochlorothiazide, which has been effective in keep-ing his blood pressure under control.

✳ 1. What would be priority concerns of the PACU nurse for this patient relating to general anesthetic?

2. What actions should the PACU nurse employ relating to this concern?

Case Study 2

The nurse is admitting a patient with a history of dia-betes mellitus type 2 and hypertension to the same-day surgery unit who is scheduled for an inguinal herniorrhaphy.

1. What data is important for the nurse to collect?

2. The patient is in the PACU and has just awakened, but is very drowsy. Describe nursing interventions relating to the effects of inhalation anesthetic that are needed when a patient first awakens.

3. The postoperative patient reports that he awoke during surgery and was in pain, but was unable to tell the surgeon. What should the nurse do?

28

Opioid (Narcotic) Analgesics, Opioid Antagonists, and Nonopioid Centrally Acting Analgesics

Answers can be reviewed online at http://evolve.elsevier.com/Lehne/.

OBJECTIVES

See page 28 for the Objectives.

CRITICAL THINKING AND STUDY QUESTIONS

1. A patient is admitted to the emergency department (ED) with chest pain. The electrocardiogram (ECG) indicates inferior wall myocardial infarction. A STAT dose of morphine sulfate is prescribed. What is the most important effect of the morphine in this situation?
   a. Decreases cardiac workload and oxygen consumption
   b. Sedates patient so the patient is not aware of danger of situation
   c. Slows respirations so the patient feels calm
   d. Suppresses awareness of body functioning

∗ 2. The nurse is ambulating a postoperative patient in the hall who is receiving an opioid analgesic for pain when the patient complains of severe nausea. What should the nurse do first if all options are possible?
   a. Administer the prescribed antiemetic.
   b. Assist the patient to sit down.
   c. Get an emesis basin.
   d. Walk the patient back to his room.

▶ 3. A patient who has received morphine becomes slightly disoriented. If this effect is due to the morphine, which intervention by the nurse might aid in reversing this adverse effect?
   a. Assist the patient to ambulate.
   b. Instruct the patient to change positions slowly.
   c. Instruct the patient to take slow, deep breaths.
   d. Keep the room well lit.

4. A 54-year-old cancer patient asks why his dose of oral morphine is so much higher than the intravenous (IV) dose he was receiving postoperatively. The basis of the nurse's response is
   a. hepatic first pass metabolizes some of the drug before it reaches the central nervous system.
   b. morphine is not lipid soluble and does not readily cross the blood-brain barrier.
   c. the kidneys excrete oral morphine faster than IV morphine.
   d. tolerance develops more rapidly if the patient has first received parenteral morphine.

5. The nurse would expect the dose of morphine for a postoperative patient to be higher than usual for the patient's size and age if prescribed for a patient who routinely uses
   a. alprazolam (Xanax).
   b. ethanol (Alcohol).
   c. oxycodone (OxyContin).
   d. temazepam (Restoril).

∗ 6. A neonate is born to a known heroin addict. The infant is exhibiting symptoms of opioid withdrawal. Which of these nursing issues is of the highest priority as the nurse cares for the neonate in the nursery?
   a. Altered nutrition
   b. Disturbed sleep
   c. Fluid deficit
   d. Parenting

7. A cancer patient who is receiving oxycodone (OxyContin) for pain relief develops a rash after being prescribed an antibiotic. The prescriber discontinues the antibiotic and prescribes diphenhydramine (Benadryl). The nurse would include in the plan of care assessment and interventions for which possible effects of this drug combination?
   a. Delirium
   b. Fever
   c. Hypotension
   d. Urinary retention

69

* 8. A patient who has overdosed on oxycodone (OxyContin), an opiate, is brought into the ED unresponsive with severely depressed respirations. The patient receives IV naloxone HCl (Narcan), a narcotic antagonist, with an improvement in level of consciousness and respiratory rate and effort within minutes. The nurse is scheduled to go to lunch in 15 minutes. A priority nursing concern for this patient is
   a. prevention of abstinence syndrome.
   b. short half-life of oxycodone.
   c. short half-life of naloxone.
   d. substance abuse.

9. A fentanyl (Duragesic) patch has been prescribed for a patient after multiple musculoskeletal injuries in a car accident. The most important reason why the nurse should teach the patient not to apply heat in the area of the patch is because doing so could cause
   a. inactivation of the drug.
   b. loosening of the patch from the skin.
   c. prolongation of the drug effect.
   d. respiratory depression.

10. Transmucosal fentanyl (Actiq) is not appropriate for acute pain relief in children because the
   a. digestive enzymes in a child's mouth inactivate the drug.
   b. dose is too high.
   c. onset of effect takes too long.
   d. taste is bitter.

11. The nurse should assess for respiratory depression for 24 hours after a patient has discontinued use of
   a. intrathecal morphine.
   b. intramuscular meperidine (Demerol).
   c. oral methadone (Dolophine).
   d. transmucosal fentanyl (Actiq).

12. An aphasic patient, who has been receiving meperidine 75 mg every 3 to 4 hours for pain for the past 36 hours, has suddenly become restless and irritable. The last dose of meperidine was 4 hours ago. It is important for the nurse to withhold the meperidine, do a complete assessment on the patient, and contact the prescriber with the findings because
   a. respiratory depression is imminent.
   b. the patient is becoming physiologically dependent on the meperidine.

   c. tolerance to the meperidine has developed.
   d. toxicity from a metabolite may be occurring.

13. A nurse is responsible for obtaining the history for patients undergoing colonoscopy and other procedures in an outpatient gastroenterology department. The most frequently used procedural medications are midazolam (Versed) and meperidine (Demerol). Which of the following antidepressant medications, if taken by a patient, is most critical for the nurse to communicate to the anesthesiologist who will be administering the conscious sedation?
   a. Bupropion (Wellbutrin)
   b. Nefazodone (Serzone)
   c. Phenelzine (Nardil)
   d. Venlafaxine (Effexor)

14. A cancer patient has been taking increasing doses of oxycodone (OxyContin) for pain relief. Which of the following adverse effects is most likely to persist with long-term use of this drug?
   a. Constipation
   b. Euphoria
   c. Respiratory depression
   d. Sedation

15. A cancer patient has received instructions regarding administration of oxycodone (OxyContin). Which of these statements made by the patient would indicate that the patient needs further teaching?
   a. "I need to inform my doctor if I experience episodes of pain between doses."
   b. "I should tell all of my healthcare providers that I am taking this drug regularly."
   c. "I should not take this drug if I am allergic to Percocet, but not Tylenol."
   d. "If I have difficulty swallowing the pill, I should crush it and take it with a small amount of applesauce."

* 16. Which of these findings would be most important for the nurse to report to the prescriber if a patient was receiving propoxyphene?
   a. Anorexia
   b. Drowsiness
   c. Dysphoria
   d. Headache

▶ 17. The nurse is caring for a patient who has just received the first IV dose of pentazocine (Talwin). Which of the following, if present within minutes of injecting the drug, would be a reason for the nurse to contact the prescriber immediately?
   a. Constricted pupils
   b. Diaphoresis
   c. Drowsiness
   d. Respirations 18 breaths per minute

18. Because it is an opioid agonist-antagonist, the nurse is less likely to have to administer an opioid antagonist, such as naloxone (Narcan), for respiratory depression when administering which of the following opioid analgesics?
   a. Buprenorphine (Buprenex)
   b. Fentanyl (Sublimaze)
   c. Meperidine (Demerol)
   d. Remifentanil (Ultiva)

✳ 19. A patient is admitted to the ED after a traumatic injury and is in severe pain from compound fractures. It is most critical that the nurse carefully assess the patient before administering an opioid for evidence of
   a. asthma.
   b. diabetes.
   c. head injury.
   d. hypertension.

20. The nurse would consult the prescriber if the nurse identified that a patient had which history and was prescribed tramadol (Ultram) for pain relief?
   a. Heart failure (HF)
   b. Chronic obstructive pulmonary disease (COPD)
   c. Dementia
   d. Seizure disorder

▶ 21. A cancer patient is prescribed clonidine (Duraclon) for burning pain. Before administering the drug, the nurse should carefully review the patient's history, laboratory results, and orders and assess for (Select all that apply.)
   a. abuse of opioids.
   b. anticoagulant therapy.
   c. bradypnea.
   d. elevated ALT and/or AST.

   e. elevated serum creatinine.
   f. fever.
   g. hypotension.
   h. tachycardia.

✳ 22. A nursing priority relating to the most common adverse effects for patients receiving intrathecal ziconotide (Prialt) is
   a. breathing.
   b. circulation.
   c. elimination.
   d. safety.

23. The nurse is working in an outpatient cancer center. When a patient is experiencing uncontrolled pain, it is important for the nurse to communicate the quality of pain (sharp, dull, etc.) to the prescriber because it influences analgesic
   a. dose.
   b. metabolism.
   c. route.
   d. timing.

CASE STUDIES AND PATIENT TEACHING

(Use a separate piece of paper for your responses.)

Case Study 1

A 67-year-old obese female who has a history of osteoarthritis, type 2 diabetes mellitus (DM), cholecystitis, and hypertension undergoes right knee replacement surgery. Postoperative orders include IV morphine 4 mg every 3 hours for pain relief, and continuous passive motion (CPM) apparatus is to be applied at 20° range of motion, 2 cycles per minute, for 10 hours per day, not exceeding 2 hours at a time.

1. Why is the pain medication ordered every 3 hours instead of every 3 hours as needed?

2. Physical therapy (PT) is prescribed twice a day. Why is it important for the nurse to communicate the timing of the last dose of morphine to the physical therapist when sending the patient for PT?

3. What assessments must the nurse make before administering the morphine and what would be assessment findings that warrant withholding the medication and consulting the prescriber?

4. The pharmacy supplies a morphine solution for injection in a tubex containing 10 mg/mL. The drug handbook recommends that morphine be injected in a dilution of 5 mL administered over 5 minutes. How much morphine will the nurse withdraw from the tubex before diluting with sterile water?

5. What must the nurse do with the additional morphine left in the tubex after the proper dose has been withdrawn?

6. At 2 PM (1400) the patient appears relaxed and is visiting with family. The patient is sitting in a chair, and CPM machine is off. The patient requests morphine for operative site pain (4 of 10). The last dose of morphine was administered at 10 AM (1000). What should the nurse do?

7. Why is it important for the nurse to assist the patient with returning to bed before administering the morphine?

8. What interventions can the nurse provide to a patient who is prescribed an opioid on an as needed basis to achieve the best control of pain?

9. What assessments and nursing interventions might the nurse employ to prevent, identify, and address the following adverse effects of morphine?
   a. Constipation
   b. Urinary retention
   c. Orthostatic hypotension
   d. Miosis
   e. Nausea and vomiting

10. The patient reports right upper quadrant pain that is worse 30 minutes after receiving a dose of morphine. What in the patient's history could be causing this effect, and what should the nurse do?

Case Study 2

The nurse is providing preoperative teaching to a 35-year-old female who has been admitted for an abdominal hysterectomy. Patient-controlled analgesia (PCA) is anticipated as the mechanism of postoperative pain relief.

1. What preoperative teaching should the nurse provide this patient to enhance pain relief and prevent adverse effects, including respiratory depression?

2. Postoperatively the patient is ordered morphine IV via PCA pump for her postoperative pain. The pump is set to deliver 1 mg of morphine per injection and up to a maximum of 5 mg per hour. What are the advantages and disadvantages of PCA?

3. The patient is resting quietly. The nurse check assesses her respiratory rate as 8 breaths per minute. What other assessments should be performed, and what actions should the nurse take?

4. What measures, other than drug therapy, can the nurse employ to reduce this patient's pain?

Case Study 3

A patient continues to require morphine long after the usual time frame for opioids after the type of surgery that was performed. She tells you that she has no tolerance for pain, but the prescriber has decided that she must stop the morphine. The nurse is concerned that the patient may have been dependent on drugs before coming to the hospital, and withdrawing the morphine may lead to abstinence syndrome.

1. How should the nurse address these concerns?

2. What are the symptoms of abstinence syndrome that the nurse should include in patient assessment?

3. Is it possible that the patient could be having uncontrolled pain, not be a substance abuser, and not have any other medical problems?

4. How does physical dependence on opioid analgesics differ from abuse and addiction?

5. Describe a situation where physical dependence on opioid analgesics is acceptable.

Case Study 4

An oncology patient is prescribed Avinza (morphine) for chronic pain.

1. Why does the nurse teach the patient to swallow the pill whole?

2. The patient's social history includes a small glass of wine with dinner each night. In addition to intensifying the CNS depression of any opiod drug, why is this a problem with Avinza?

3. The patient tells the nurse that he has difficulty swallowing the pill. What should the nurse do?

29

Pain Management in Patients with Cancer

Answers can be reviewed online at http://evolve.elsevier.com/Lehne/.

OBJECTIVES

See page 28 for the Objectives.

CRITICAL THINKING AND STUDY QUESTIONS

1. Match the following types of pain to cause, origin, or characteristics (Some may be used more than once.)

_____ a. Neuropathic
_____ b. Nociceptive
_____ c. Somatic
_____ d. Visceral

1. Adjunctive drugs most effective
2. Bone, joint, muscle
3. Burning, numb, cold
4. Diffuse, aching
5. Opioids most effective
6. Organ
7. Peripheral nerve injury
8. Sharp, localized
9. Tissue injury

▸ 2. An oncology patient with a history of hypertension and type 2 diabetes mellitus complains of burning pain in his feet. The pain is constant (4/10) but intensifies (7/10) when he tries to walk. The nurse reviews the patient's medication administration record (MAR) and notes that the patient is prescribed oral valsartan (Diovan) 80 mg once a day, oral metformin (Glucophage) 500 mg twice a day, and intravenous (IV) hydromorphone (Dilaudid) 2 mg every 3 hours as needed, oral acetaminophen 650 mg every 4 hours as needed for temperature greater than 102°F. The patient's last dose of hydromorphone was 6 hours ago and he has not received acetaminophen in the past 24 hours. Based on the patient's complaint, the nurse should

a. administer the acetaminophen.
b. administer the hydromorphone.
c. ask the patient if anything has relieved this pain in the past.
d. explain to the patient that the pain is not due to his cancer and that it will improve with increased ambulation.

3. The most reliable indicator of the need for pain relief is
   a. changes in vital signs that can occur with pain.
   b. extensiveness of the cancer involvement.
   c. patient's expressions and reluctance to move.
   d. patient's report of a need for pain relief.

✳ 4. When developing a plan of care for pain management for the cancer patient, it is most important for the nurse to identify outcomes based on achieving (Select all that apply.)
   a. a rating of pain less than 3 on a scale of 0 to 10.
   b. comfort that allows the patient to complete all activities of daily living (ADL).
   c. pain relief that is acceptable to the patient.
   d. total pain relief.

5. A cancer patient whose history includes type 2 diabetes mellitus informs the nurse that she is experiencing constant pain in her feet. Based on the type of foot pain commonly experienced by diabetics, the nurse would consult the prescriber regarding possibly ordering a/an
   a. analgesic, such as acetaminophen (Tylenol).
   b. neurologic-acting adjunct drug, such as gabapentin (Neurontin).
   c. nonsteroidal anti-inflammatory drug (NSAID), such as naproxen (Aleve).
   d. opioid agonist analgesic, such as morphine.

✳ 6. Which of these laboratory test results would be of most concern to the nurse when a cancer patient treated with chemotherapy is taking a pain reliever that contains ibuprofen?
   a. ALT 40 international units/L
   b. BUN 22 mg/dL
   c. Platelet count 80,000/m^3
   d. WBC 5500/m^3

7. A postoperative cancer patient was receiving morphine sulfate IV 10 mg every 4 hours for pain. The prescriber has discontinued the IV morphine and ordered morphine sulfate 20-mg tablet every 4 hours. The nurse recognizes that this is a/an
   a. dose that cannot be compared with the IV dose.
   b. equianalgesic dose.
   c. less potent dose than the IV dose.
   d. more potent dose than the IV dose.

▶ 8. The nurse knows that respiratory depression is most likely to occur with which of the following pain regimens?
   a. A loading dose of 10 mg of morphine before starting PCA.
   b. Increasing long-term IV dose of morphine from 5 mg to 7 mg.
   c. Patient-controlled analgesia (PCA) morphine at 1 mg of morphine per injection and up to a maximum of 5 mg per hour.
   d. 60 mg of IV morphine every hour to a patient who has been receiving steadily increasing doses of morphine.

9. Generally the best pain control regimen for a hospitalized patient who has been known to abuse opioids and who has severe pain is
   a. agonist-antagonist opioids.
   b. codeine administered orally.
   c. intermittent IV dosing of meperidine (Demerol).
   d. IV opioid agonist administered by PCA.

CASE STUDIES AND PATIENT TEACHING

(Use a separate piece of paper for your responses.)

Case Study 1

The nurse is caring for a 68-year-old retired steelworker who is postoperative a right lung lobectomy for lung cancer. The patient is ordered morphine IV via PCA pump for postoperative pain. The pump is set to deliver 1 mg of morphine per injection and up to a maximum of 5 mg per hour. Vital signs are BP 150/92 mm Hg, pulse 94, respirations 24. Chest tube is intact and draining. Other assessment findings are within expected limits except the patient is restless and grimaces with movement. He is reluctant to use the incentive spirometer. He has not complained of pain.

1. What actions should the nurse take?

2. What psychosocial issues might influence this patient to be reluctant to use prescribed opioid analgesia?

3. What nursing approaches might increase the chance that the patient will use all available resources to obtain pain relief and increase adherence to prescribed therapy?

4. What teaching can the nurse provide regarding benefits of controlled pain for this patient?

Case Study 2

A cancer patient is being discharged on oxycodone and acetaminophen (Percocet).

1. What teaching should the nurse provide regarding the opioid and nonopioid components of this drug?

The patient's pain is not relieved by 2 Percocet (oxycodone 10 mg and acetaminophen 325 mg) tablets taken every 4 hours. The prescriber has discontinued the Percocet and ordered oxycodone CR (OxyContin) 40 mg twice a day, oxycodone IR 5 mg every 6 hours as needed, and acetaminophen 650 mg every 6 hours. The patient is overwhelmed by the multiple medications and asks why he cannot just take 3 Percocet tablets every 4 hours.

2. How should the nurse respond?

3. What interventions can the nurse offer to help the patient understand his analgesic regimen?

4. What teaching should the nurse provide regarding the adverse effect of constipation?

5. What teaching can the nurse provide to enable the patient to assist the prescriber with decisions regarding analgesic prescription?

Case Study 3

A patient who is receiving radiation therapy for metastatic breast cancer complains of pain.

1. Describe the nurse's role in implementing the clinical approach to pain management recommended by the Agency for Health Care Policy and Research (AHCPR).
   a. Ask and assess
   b. Believe
   c. Choose
   d. Deliver
   e. Empower and enable

2. Describe what the nurse should include when assessing and documenting the patient's pain.

Case Study 4

Developmental Considerations

1. Identify the pain scale that would be most effective in evaluating pain for these cancer patients. Explain how it is used and why you think it would be the best method of evaluating this patient's pain.
   a. A 3-month-old infant
   b. A 3-year-old who is shy
   c. A 15-year-old with osteosarcoma
   d. An adult who is nonverbal because of a laryngectomy
   e. An elderly patient with dementia

2. Describe physiologic differences in the infant, child, and elderly that must be considered when pain medication is prescribed.

Answers can be reviewed online at http://evolve.elsevier.com/Lehne/.

OBJECTIVES

See page 28 for the Objectives.

CRITICAL THINKING AND STUDY QUESTIONS

1. Migraine headaches (Select all that apply.)
   a. always start with an abnormal sensation (aura).
   b. cannot be treated effectively after the pain starts.
   c. involve inflammation of intracranial blood vessels.
   d. involve vasoconstriction of intracranial blood vessels.
   e. therapy includes drugs and nonpharmacologic measures to prevent attacks.
   f. therapy should start at the earliest sign of attack.

2. A patient who experiences migraine headaches including severe gastrointestinal (GI) distress asks why pills do not help her headaches. Which of the following statements suggest that the patient did not understand the nurse's explanation?
   a. "If I vomit, the pills may be expelled."
   b. "Pills are only effective if taken before a migraine starts."
   c. "Taking a drug for the nausea, vomiting and gastroparesis might help."
   d. "The pills may not be absorbed fast enough to help."

3. The primary reason why abortive medication for migraine headaches should not be used more than 1 or 2 days a week is
   a. abuse potential.
   b. development of chest pain.
   c. development of tolerance, and medication is not effective.
   d. medication overuse headache.

▶ 4. Which of these patient assessment findings would be most significant if the nurse was preparing to administer ergotamine to a patient who is experiencing the start of a migraine headache?
   a. ALT 30 international units/L
   b. Blood pressure 90/58 mm Hg
   c. Capillary refill 8 seconds
   d. Flashes of light in visual fields

5. A rationale for administering both ergotamine and metoclopramide (Reglan) to a patient to abort a migraine headache includes that the metoclopramide
   a. minimizes sensitivity to light.
   b. prevents adverse effects of weakness and myalgia from ergotamine.
   c. provides additional vasoconstriction to relieve cranial vessel vasodilation.
   d. reverses gastric stasis, which improves absorption of the ergotamine.

6. Which of the following over-the-counter medications has not demonstrated effectiveness in relieving mild to moderate migraine headache pain?
   a. Aspirin
   b. Acetaminophen
   c. Acetaminophen, aspirin, and caffeine
   d. Ibuprofen

▶ 7. The nurse would consult the prescriber before administering ergotamine or triptan drugs for migraine headache to a patient with (Select all that apply.)
   a. cardiovascular disease.
   b. diabetes mellitus.
   c. hypertension.
   d. infection.
   e. peptic ulcer disease.
   f. possible pregnancy.

8. Which of the following are true about triptan therapy for migraine headaches?
   a. Administering an oral dose of the drug after subcutaneous administration will prevent recurrence of the headache.
   b. One dose provides long-lasting relief for 80% of patients.
   c. It relieves headache, nausea, and sensitivity to sound and light.
   d. Peripheral vasoconstriction is the primary concern with adverse effects.

＊▶ 9. The nurse has administered sumatriptan (Imitrex) subcutaneously to a 35-year-old smoker who was admitted for depression and is experiencing a migraine headache. One hour after administration the patient complains of heavy arms and chest pressure. The nurse should
   a. assess vital signs and PQRST the chest pain.
   b. continue care; this is a normal adverse effect.
   c. notify the prescriber STAT.

10. Which of the following nursing problems would be a risk when administering haloperidol (Haldol) for migraine headache?
    a. Altered tissue perfusion
    b. Fluid volume deficit
    c. Safety
    d. Skin integrity

11. A college student has been prescribed propranolol to prevent migraine headaches and frovatriptan (Frova) 2.5 mg by mouth to treat recurrent migraine headaches. Which statement, if made by the patient, would indicate a need for further teaching?
    a. "I need to lie down in a dark room after taking the Frova because it takes several hours before it relieves the headache."
    b. "I may experience the same number of headaches for the first weeks that I take propranolol because it takes weeks to take effect."
    c. "I should take a double second dose of Frova an hour after the first dose if the first dose is ineffective."
    d. "Propranolol will decrease the number and intensity of my migraine attacks."

12. Match the drugs for prevention of migraines to the reasons to withhold the drug and contact the prescriber regarding the drug.

_____ a. amitriptyline (tricyclic antidepressant)
_____ b. candesartan (ARB)
_____ c. divalproex (antiseizure)
_____ d. estrogen (hormone)
_____ e. propranolol (beta blocker)
_____ f. topiramate (antiseizure)
_____ g. verapamil (CCB)

1. abdominal pain and amylase 500 international units/L
2. apical pulse 48 beats/min
3. pH 7.32; HCO_3 19 mEq/L; pCO_2 35 mm Hg
4. positive Homan's sign and swelling L calf
5. post-void bladder scan 600 mL
6. potassium 5.6 mEq/L
7. SBP drop 30 mm Hg when change from sit to stand

13. A patient is receiving lithium carbonate for prevention of cluster headaches. This drug has a narrow therapeutic index. Which of the following drug levels would fall into the safe and effective range?
    a. 0.1 mEq/L
    b. 0.2 mEq/L
    c. 0.5 mEq/L
    d. 0.8 mEq/L

CASE STUDIES AND PATIENT TEACHING

(Use a separate piece of paper for your responses.)

Case Study 1

A 49-year-old female nursing assistant is seen in the emergency department (ED) with a chief complaint of severe, frequent headaches that begin midmorning and grow progressively worse throughout the day. She admits to occasional nausea and vomiting. Advil has been minimally successful in treating the headaches. Her history includes the following: 2 months ago she noticed one black, tarry stool; she is on low-dose oral contraceptives for perimenopausal symptoms; and she is frequently asked to work double shifts. Her headaches are pulsatile and usually unilateral. All of the patient's laboratory findings are within normal limits. Sumatriptan (Imitrex) 6 mg subcutaneously is prescribed to be administered now along with a prescription for Imitrex STAT dose Pen 6 mg to be taken as directed.

1. Describe what the nurse should include in teaching this patient about administering the self-injecting pen.

2. The patient attempts to fill the prescription at the hospital outpatient pharmacy, but her insurance does not cover sumatriptan. Dihydroergotamine is prescribed in place of the sumatriptan. What teaching needs to be provided by the ED nurse regarding the administration of dihydroergotamine?

3. What teaching regarding preventing toxicity from dihydroergotamine should be provided to this patient?

4. The patient tells the nurse that a friend takes ergotamine. Her friend got hooked on ergotamine and had to go to the hospital to get off of it. What would the nurse include when comparing ergotamine and dihydroergotamine?

5. The patient is instructed to seek follow-up with her primary care provider (PCP). The PCP discusses the use of prophylactic drugs to prevent the migraine headaches. What drugs might be considered?

Case Study 2

A 20-year-old college student comes to the college health center with a complaint of frequent moderate headaches. The nurse is responsible for collecting data before the patient is seen by the nurse practitioner.

1. What subjective and objective data should the nurse obtain?

2. The patient complains of light sensitivity but no nausea or vomiting. The nurse practitioner prescribes Excedrin Migraine. What in the patient's history needs to be explored before the patient begins regular use of a product containing aspirin?

3. Developmentally, why were ergotamine or sumatriptan not prescribed for this patient?

4. What nonpharmacologic measures to prevent migraine headaches should be taught?

31

Antipsychotic Agents and Their Use in Schizophrenia

Answers can be reviewed online at http://evolve.elsevier.com/Lehne/.

OBJECTIVES

See page 28 for the Objectives.

CRITICAL THINKING AND STUDY QUESTIONS

1. Match the following categories to a corresponding class of symptoms.

_____ a. Cognitive
_____ b. Negative
_____ c. Positive

1. Diminished emotional response
2. False beliefs
3. Thinking is not logical
4. Disheveled appearance
5. Cannot remember
6. Suspiciousness
7. Cannot pay attention
8. Does not interact with others
9. False perceptions

2. Second-generation antipsychotic (SGA) drugs are commonly preferred over first-generation antipsychotics (FGA) primarily because they
   a. are perceived as being more effective.
   b. cost less.
   c. do not affect thinking.
   d. only cause minor adverse effects.

3. A highly potent antipsychotic differs from low potency drugs in that it
   a. is more likely to cure the disorder.
   b. produces desired effects at low doses.
   c. provides more symptom relief.
   d. treats positive and negative symptoms.

4. A patient who is receiving chemotherapy for breast cancer is prescribed chlorpromazine (Thorazine). There is no mention of other medical or psychiatric disorders in the patient's history. It is important for the nurse to assess for
   a. delusions.
   b. hallucinations.
   c. nausea.
   d. tics.

5. Which of the following extrapyramidal adverse effects of antipsychotic drugs would the nurse expect to only occur after an extended period of drug therapy?
   a. Repetitive, slow, twisting movements of the tongue and face
   b. Severe spasms of the mouth, face, neck, or back
   c. Slow movement, tremor, and rigidity
   d. Uncontrollable need to be in motion

* 6. The priority nursing focus for a patient experiencing acute dystonia is
   a. airway clearance.
   b. anxiety.
   c. pain.
   d. safety.

* ▶ 7. Which of these findings, if identified in a patient who has been receiving a neuroleptic antipsychotic, should the nurse report to the prescriber immediately?
   a. Agitation
   b. Difficulty speaking
   c. Involuntary movements of the tongue
   d. Sudden, whole-body muscle contractions

8. The best prescribing approach to prevent tardive dyskinesia is
   a. to always try SGA drugs first.
   b. prophylactic administration of anticholinergic drugs.
   c. to increase the dose of the FGA as soon as symptoms are noted.
   d. to use the lowest dose of FGA for the shortest time.

9. Which of the following interventions for neuroleptic malignant syndrome would most likely reduce body temperature by treating the cause of the hyperthermia?
   a. Acetaminophen (Tylenol)
   b. Acetylsalicylic acid (aspirin)
   c. Dantrolene (Dantrium)
   d. Increasing fluid intake

▶ 10. The nurse is assessing orthostatic blood pressure and pulse of a patient who is prescribed a neuroleptic antipsychotic drug. Which of the following assessment findings would be reason to withhold the drug and consult the prescriber?
   a. BP lying 110/66 mm Hg and pulse 76 beats/min; 2 minutes later BP standing 108/70 mm Hg and pulse 80 beats/min
   b. BP lying 116/70 mm Hg and pulse 72 beats/min; 2 minutes later BP standing 116/68 mm Hg and pulse 122 beats/min
   c. BP lying 120/84 mm Hg and pulse 70 beats/min; 2 minutes later BP standing 110/76 mm Hg; pulse 72 beats/min
   d. BP lying 146/90 mm Hg and pulse 73 beats/min; 2 minutes later BP standing 138/88 mm Hg; pulse 78 beats/min

* ▶ 11. Which of the following symptoms of an adverse effect, if identified in a patient who is receiving thioridazine (Mellaril) or haloperidol (Haldol), should the nurse report to the prescriber immediately?
   a. Fainting, not associated with sudden position changes
   b. Milk secretion from a male
   c. Red skin
   d. Sore throat

12. Second-generation antipsychotics (SGAs) were formerly called
   a. atypical antipsychotics.
   b. high-potency antipsychotics.
   c. low-potency antipsychotics.
   d. typical antipsychotics.

13. Because trifluoperazine can produce the adverse effect of agranulocytosis, it is important for the nurse to monitor which of the following laboratory test results?
   a. AST and ALT
   b. BUN and creatinine
   c. Hb and Hct
   d. WBC and neutrophils

14. It is important for the nurse to teach patients who are prescribed any neuroleptic antipsychotic drug to avoid taking which of the following over-the-counter medications?
    a. Acetaminophen (Tylenol)
    b. Acetylsalicylic acid (aspirin)
    c. Diphenhydramine (Benadryl)
    d. Pseudoephedrine (Sudafed)

15. A patient is prescribed haloperidol decanoate (Haldol) 50 mg IM every 4 weeks. When selecting a site for administration, the nurse knows the site that is no longer recommended for intramuscular (IM) injection is the
    a. deltoid.
    b. dorsogluteal.
    c. vastus lateralis.
    d. ventrogluteal.

▸ 16. Which of the following laboratory results should be reported promptly to the prescriber of haloperidol (Haldol)?
    a. BUN 18 mg/dL
    b. FBS 286 mg/dL
    c. Potassium 3.2 mg/dL
    d. Triglycerides 100 mg/dL

17. It is important for the nurse to assess for excessive hunger, thirst, and urination if a patient is prescribed
    a. chlorpromazine (Thorazine).
    b. haloperidol (Haldol).
    c. molindone (Moban).
    d. olanzapine (Zyprexa).

18. Morning fasting blood sugars via glucometer are ordered a patient who is receiving clozapine. Which of the following findings is most likely associated with clozapine?
    a. FBS 50 mg/dL
    b. FBS 75 mg/dL
    c. FBS 100 mg/dL
    d. FBS 125 mg/dL

▸ 19. Which of these findings would be of most immediate concern for the nurse who is caring for a patient who is admitted for an acute psychotic episode and who has been receiving clozapine (Clozaril)?
    a. Blood pressure drop of 10 mm Hg systolic when changing from lying to standing position
    b. Residual of 150 mL of urine after voiding
    c. Temperature 104°F (40°C)
    d. Weight gain of 2 lbs in 1 month

▸ 20. Which of the following laboratory test results would be of most immediate concern when a patient is prescribed clozapine and develops chest pain and shortness of breath?
    a. BNP 75 picograms/mL
    b. CRP 3 mg/mL
    c. HDL 80 mg/dL
    d. Postprandial blood glucose 175 mg/dL

21. The nurse has reason to believe that a paranoid schizophrenic patient is checking her risperadone (Risperdal) 2-mg tablets. It would be appropriate for the nurse to consult with the prescriber regarding discontinuing the tablets and changing the order to
    a. Haldol IM.
    b. Risperdal M-TAB.
    c. Risperdal IM.
    d. Risperdal tabs every 12 hours as needed.

22. A bipolar patient has revealed to the nurse that her appearance is very important to her. This patient would most likely be adherent to which of the following second-generation drugs?
    a. Aripiprazole (Abilify)
    b. Clozapine (Clozaril)
    c. Olanzapine (Zyprexa)
    d. Quetiapine (Seroquel)

23. A patient who has been stabilized on oral risperidone (Risperdal) receives an intramuscular injection of Risperdal Consta before discharge. How long does the patient need to continue oral therapy?
    a. 3 hours
    b. 3 days
    c. 3 weeks
    d. 3 months

24. A patient's daughter has read that clozapine (Clozaril) is the most effective second-generation antipsychotic. Which of the following should the nurse include in the explanation of why this drug is not used until other agents have failed?
    a. Clozaril can cause hypoglycemia.
    b. Clozaril can have an effect on white blood cell production.
    c. Use of Clozaril has a high incidence of tardive dyskinesias.
    d. Orthostatic hypotension is common with use of Clozaril.

▸ 25. What laboratory tests are important for the nurse to monitor when caring for a patient who is prescribed risperidone (Risperdal)? (Select all that apply.)
   a. ALT and/or AST
   b. Cholesterol
   c. Creatinine
   d. Hemoglobin A$_{1C}$
   e. INR
   f. Platelets
   g. Triglycerides
   h. WBC count

26. The nurse notes what appears to be a pill in the stool of a patient who is receiving paliperidone (Invega). The nurse should
   a. assess the patient for toxicity.
   b. continue nursing care.
   c. crush the tablet when administering and mix with applesauce.
   d. report the finding to the prescriber.

▸ 27. Why is it important for the nurse to know the half-life of antipsychotic drugs?

CASE STUDIES AND PATIENT TEACHING

(Use a separate piece of paper for your responses.)

Case Study 1

An 82-year-old woman who resides in a nursing facility is admitted to the hospital with pneumonia. She has a history of agitation and is ordered haloperidol 0.5 mg every 8 hours as needed when nonpharmacologic measures cannot control agitation. Two hours after administering the drug orally, the nurse notes the patient is moaning. Her eyes are rolled upward, and her back is arched.

✳ 1. What action should the nurse take first?

2. What assessment data are important for the nurse to collect and communicate to the prescriber?

Intravenous benztropine (Cogentin) 1 mg is prescribed STAT. The drug is available as 1 mg/mL and can be administered undiluted over at least 1 minute. The nurse decides to be cautious and administer the drug over 2 minutes.

3. How much drug should the nurse administer every 10 seconds?

4. What observations during infusion would be a reason to stop infusing the drug?

Case Study 2

The nurse is preparing for a group family session focusing on antipsychotic drugs.

1. What information should be presented regarding prevention, identification, and when to seek medical treatment for these common adverse effects?
   a. Blurred vision
   b. Constipation
   c. Dry mouth
   d. Orthostatic hypotension
   e. Photophobia
   f. Sedation
   g. Sexual dysfunction
   h. Tachycardia
   i. Urinary hesitancy

Case Study 3

A 52-year-old woman is admitted to the hospital for symptoms of schizophrenia. She has been hospitalized previously and was discharged on haloperidol (Haldol) 5 mg 3 times a day. Her husband reports that her symptoms had been controlled until she stopped taking her medication 3 days ago because of blurred vision, dry mouth, and chronic constipation. During the admission procedure she appeared to be responding to voices. The psychiatrist prescribes risperidone (Risperdal) orally disintegrating tablets 1 mg twice a day (day 1) with further orders to follow after laboratory test results are obtained.

1. What laboratory test results are important for the nurse to communicate to the psychiatrist when consulting for further medication orders?

2. The next day the psychiatrist increases the dose to 2 mg twice a day on day 2 and 3 mg twice a day on subsequent days. On the fourth day, the patient's husband discusses with the nurse his concern that his wife does not appear to be improving. How should the nurse respond?

3. After 10 days, the patient reports that the voices have decreased. The nurse is providing drug teaching to the patient and her husband. The patient is concerned about adverse effects and asks how risperidone (Risperdal) is different from haloperidol (Haldol). Because the patient's concentration can be limited, the nurse develops a teaching handout including common adverse effects for the patient and her husband. Complete this teaching handout.

risperidone (Risperdal)		
Administration directions:		
Possible adverse effects	**How to decrease chance that effect will occur**	**What to do if the effect occurs**

4. The patient's husband is concerned about his wife adhering to drug therapy. What information should the nurse offer to increase the likelihood that the patient will take the drug as prescribed?

Case Study 4

The nurse is leading a group session where antipsychotic pharmacotherapy is being discussed. A patient asks the nurse why everyone isn't prescribed the newer SGA if they can afford them. "Newer is better."

1. What information should the nurse include in this discussion?

32
Antidepressants

Answers can be reviewed online at http://evolve.elsevier.com/Lehne/.

OBJECTIVES

See page 28 for the Objectives.

CRITICAL THINKING AND STUDY QUESTIONS

*   1. When assessing a patient who is receiving an antidepressant, which of the following questions would be most important for the nurse to ask?
    a. "Are you concerned about weight gain when you take medications?"
    b. "Are you having any thoughts about doing anything that could harm yourself?"
    c. "Do you experience dizziness when you stand up?"
    d. "Have you had any difficulty voiding?"

2. Patient compliance with antidepressant drug therapy is most likely to be increased if the nurse explains
    a. drug interactions.
    b. expected timing of therapeutic response.
    c. the reason for limiting the number of units of the drug supplied with each prescription.
    d. the seriousness of adverse effects.

3. Which of the following characteristics of depression, if improved first by pharmacotherapy, would most likely increase the risk of suicide in a severely depressed patient?
    a. Feelings of helplessness
    b. Lack of appetite
    c. Lack of energy
    d. Loss of pleasure in normally fun activities

*   4. When a patient who is receiving an antidepressant verbalizes suicidal ideation, which action should the nurse take first?
    a. Administer the antidepressant.
    b. Ask the patient why he or she feels this way.
    c. Notify the prescriber.
    d. Provide a safe environment.

5. Tricyclic antidepressants are often the drug of first choice for depression because they are
    a. effective and inexpensive.
    b. have less adverse effects than other antidepressants.
    c. more effective than other antidepressants.
    d. not toxic if taken in excessive doses.

6. A patient who did not experience relief of depression after taking a tricyclic antidepressant was instructed to stop taking his prescription for amitriptyline hydrochloride (Elavil) 2 weeks ago. He has now been prescribed an MAO inhibitor. Because of possible interactions if the patient did not stop taking the amitriptyline when instructed, the nurse should assess for which of the following possible reactions?
    a. Fatigue
    b. Flushed skin
    c. Increase in blood pressure (BP)
    d. Excessive sweating

7. The nurse is doing discharge teaching for a patient who was prescribed amitriptyline hydrochloride (Elavil) for depression. Because of the possibility of causing hypertension, the nurse would caution the patient to consult the prescriber or pharmacist before taking any over-the-counter
    a. antacids.
    b. antidiarrheal drugs.
    c. cold medication.
    d. pain medications.

8. Tricyclic antidepressant (TCA) and selective serotonin reuptake inhibitor (SSRI) properties include (Select all that apply.)
    a. effect on neurotransmitters occurs rapidly.
    b. effect on neurotransmitters occurs slowly.
    c. serious adverse effects can occur if combined with MAO inhibitor antidepressants.
    d. therapeutic effects occur rapidly.
    e. therapeutic effects occur slowly.

▶ 9. The nursery nurse notes that a neonate, whose mother has been taking fluoxetine (Prozac) for major depression throughout pregnancy, is tremulous and very irritable. Which of the following assessment findings, noted when the neonate is crying, would be of most concern to the nurse?
   a. Difficulty calming
   b. Flexed extremities
   c. Respiratory distress
   d. Tachycardia

10. The nurse notes bruxism in the history of a patient who is prescribed an SSRI. The nurse assesses the patient for
   a. abnormal mouth movements.
   b. jaw pain.
   c. restlessness.
   d. tremors.

11. The nurse would be most concerned about the potential for hyponatremia if a patient exhibited nausea and anorexia and was prescribed fluoxetine (Prozac) and
   a. candesartan.
   b. enalapril.
   c. hydrochlorothiazide.
   d. spironolactone.

✳ 12. Which of these laboratory test results, if identified in a patient who is receiving fluoxetine and warfarin, should the nurse report to the prescriber immediately?
   a. AST 30 international units/L
   b. Creatinine 0.8 mg/dL
   c. INR 4.5
   d. Platelets 250,000/m³

13. The nurse should question which of the following orders?
   a. Fluoxetine (Prozac) 20 mg by mouth once a day at bedtime
   b. Fluoxetine 10 mg twice a day by mouth 8:00 AM and 12:00 PM
   c. Fluoxetine (Sarafem) 20 mg by mouth days 14 to 28 of menstrual cycle
   d. Discontinue fluoxetine today (Monday) and start enteric-coated fluoxetine (Prozac Weekly) 90 mg by mouth once a week next Monday

14. Paroxetine (Paxil CR) differs significantly from paroxetine hydrochloride (Paxil) in
   a. better absorption when administered with food.
   b. dose.

   c. length of action.
   d. less nausea.

15. The nurse would be especially vigilant to assess the patient for unexplained bleeding when a patient is prescribed fluoxetine and
   a. an antihistamine.
   b. lithium.
   c. low-dose aspirin therapy.
   d. a thiazide diuretic.

✳ 16. The nurse is reviewing laboratory test results for a patient whose drug regime includes desvenlafaxine (Pristiq). Which of the following results should be reported immediately to the prescriber?
   a. eGFR 90 mL/min
   b. hCG 900 milli-international units/mL
   c. Osteoarthritic changes in the spine
   d. Sodium 140 mEq/L

17. Which of these conditions, if identified in the history of a patient receiving duloxetine (Cymbalta), would be a concern to the nurse?
   a. Diabetic neuropathy
   b. Glaucoma
   c. Hypernatremia
   d. Musculoskeletal pain

18. Which of the following foods could be included in the diet of a patient who is prescribed the MAO inhibitor isocarboxazid (Marplan)?
   a. Cheddar cheese
   b. Chocolate
   c. Fava beans
   d. Roast beef

▶ 19. A patient complains to the nurse that he has been experiencing erectile dysfunction since he was prescribed paroxetine (Paxil). The best response by the nurse would be to
   a. encourage the patient to share this concern with the prescriber.
   b. instruct the patient to not take the antidepressant on weekends.
   c. suggest the patient ask the prescriber to change his prescription to bupropion (Wellbutrin).
   d. withhold the drug until the issue is resolved.

✳▸ 20. Which of the following laboratory results would be of greatest concern to the nurse when a patient is receiving nefazodone?
   a. AST 356 international units/L
   b. BUN 22 mg/dL
   c. Na 146 mEq/L
   d. WBC 11,000/mm³

✳ 21. The nurse has received reports on patients who have recently been prescribed the following antidepressant medication and are experiencing the noted adverse effects. Which patient is of highest priority for the nurse?
   a. Amitriptyline—sleepiness and constipation
   b. Fluoxetine—nausea and diarrhea
   c. Tranylcypromine (Parnate)—headache and vomiting
   d. Venlafaxine—anorexia and sweating

22. It is most important for the nurse to teach a patient who has been prescribed trazodone (Desyrel) to
   a. drink at least 2500 mL of fluid each day.
   b. increase fluid and fiber in diet to prevent constipation.
   c. report any symptoms of a urinary tract infection.
   d. seek medical care if an erection does not subside after ejaculation with sexual intercourse.

23. A patient has been taking St. John's Wort for minor depression. The nurse should teach the patient
   a. to protect the skin from sun exposure.
   b. to research has proven the product is as effective as antidepressant drugs for mild depression.
   c. that the substance has not been proven to be effective.
   d. that the substance is completely safe because it is natural and not a drug.

24. Match antidepressants to their associated adverse effects.

   _____ a. Bupropion   1. Anticholinergic effects
   _____ b. MAO inhibitors   2. Cardiotoxicity
   _____ c. Mirtazapine   3. CNS stimulation
   _____ d. SSRI   4. Headache
   _____ e. TCA   5. Hypertensive crisis from eating foods containing tyramine
          6. Hyponatremia
          7. Insomnia

   8. Nausea
   9. Orthostatic hypotension
   10. Sedation
   11. Seizures
   12. Sexual dysfunction

CASE STUDIES AND PATIENT TEACHING

(Use a separate piece of paper for your responses.)

Case Study 1

A 28-year-old mother of two, who is a high school science teacher, comes to the community mental health center at her family's urging because of lack of interest in usual activities, difficulty concentrating, excessive sleepiness, and feeling "down" every day for the past 3 months. Desipramine (Norpramin) 50 mg at bedtime is prescribed.

1. Developmentally, what are the advantages of this particular TCA for this patient?

2. The patient is hopeful that the medication will help. She asks "If the drugs work, why do I have to meet with the doctor every week?" What is the basis of the response to this question?

3. What symptoms should the patient, family members, and/or caregivers be told to report?

4. The patient asks why the drug is supposed to be taken at bedtime. How should the nurse respond?

5. What teaching should the nurse provide regarding these common adverse effects of tricyclic antidepressants?
   a. Sedation
   b. Orthostatic hypotension
   c. Anticholinergic effects

6. The patient is concerned about cost because the prescriber has prescribed only 1 week's supply at a time. What would be the rationale for such a small prescription amount?

7. The patient is admitted for an inguinal herniorrhaphy. When providing history information, the patient states that she has been taking desipiramine

(Norpramin) 200 mg at bedtime for 3 months. She tells the nurse that some nights she forgets to take the medication, but does not feel bad the next day. She states that she thinks she must not need the medication any more. How should the nurse respond?

Case Study 2

A patient who has been experiencing major depression has been admitted to a psychiatric unit and prescribed a TCA and cognitive behavioral therapy. She asks the nurse what is involved in this therapy.

1. What should the nurse include in a summary of this therapy?

The patient does not experience relief of symptoms despite compliance with cognitive-behavioral therapy and pharmacotherapy with a TCA for over 1 year. Later the patient was switched to an SSRI antidepressant. The patient has been admitted to the inpatient psychiatric unit and received electroconvulsant therapy 3 times a week for the past 2 weeks.

2. What should be included in the nurse's assessment and documentation?

3. The psychiatrist has explained that the discharge treatment plan includes prescribing phenelzine (Nardil), an MAO inhibitor antidepressant. The patient discontinued taking fluoxetine (Prozac) before admission and is anxious to start taking the new antidepressant. How should the nurse respond to the patient's concern?

4. What teaching would be important for the nurse to provide to the patient's significant others on discharge?

5. What teaching should the nurse provide about the prescribed phenelzine (Nardil)?

Case Study 3

An adolescent who had been irritable, refusing to go to school or eat meals for several months is admitted to an adolescent psychiatric unit. Cognitive behavioral therapy is started and the psychiatrist prescribes a SSRI antidepressant.

1. What precautions teaching would the nurse provide because of the risk of serotonin syndrome?

The patient's insurance only allows 10 days of inpatient hospitalization, and the patient is to be discharged to the care of his parents. All antidepressants have a black box warning for suicide risk, especially in children and adolescents.

2. The nurse would caution the parents that suicide risk is greatest at what point in antidepressant therapy?

3. What actions should be taken because of this risk?

4. What rationale would support the use of antidepressants in this case?

33

Drugs for Bipolar Disorder

Answers can be reviewed online at http://evolve.elsevier.com/Lehne/.

OBJECTIVES

See page 28 for the Objectives.

CRITICAL THINKING AND STUDY QUESTIONS

1. Which of the following statements about bipolar disorder (BPD) are true? (Select all that apply.)
   a. All patients alternate between mania and depression, but length of episodes vary.
   b. Cause is an unstable personality.
   c. It is a chronic condition.
   d. Involves atrophy of brain regions involved with emotion.
   e. Manic episodes are always distressing to the patient.
   f. Requires treatment for life.

* 2. A patient is admitted with an acute mixed episode of BPD. The patient is started on valproic acid and bupropion. A priority nursing concern is
   a. electrolyte imbalances.
   b. hydration.
   c. safety.
   d. toxicity.

▸ 3. A nurse is reviewing laboratory tests of a patient receiving lithium carbonate for an acute episode of BPD. Which of the following results should the nurse report to the prescriber immediately?
   a. ALT 30 international units/L
   b. Creatinine 2.7 mg/dL
   c. Sodium 132 mEq/L
   d. Potassium 4 mEq/L

▸ 4. The nurse is caring for a patient on a medical-surgical unit who is receiving lithium for BPD, which is currently not symptomatic. Which of the following treatments could increase lithium levels and cause toxicity? (Select all that apply.)
   a. Colonic cleansing preparation for colonoscopy
   b. Foley catheter insertion
   c. Frequent dressing change on a diabetic wound
   d. Hemodialysis
   e. Nasogastric suctioning
   f. Repeated hypoglycemic episodes with diaphoresis

5. The most common cause of lithium toxicity is
   a. overdose of medication.
   b. renal failure.
   c. sodium depletion.

▸ 6. When administering valproic acid (Depakote), which of the following observations would be a reason to hold the medication and contact the prescriber? (Select all that apply.)
   a. Constant midepigastric pain radiating to the back
   b. LMP 38 days ago
   c. Nausea, vomiting, and very dark colored urine
   d. Pale conjunctiva
   e. Petechiae
   f. Temperature 102.4°F
   g. Warm, hot skin and fruity breath

▸ 7. The CBC on a patient who is scheduled to receive the first dose of carbamazepine includes hemoglobin 14.5 gm/dL, platelets 170,000/mm^3, reticulocyte count 2%, and WBC 6600/mm^3. The nurse should
   a. administer the medication as ordered.
   b. hold the medication and assess the patient.
   c. hold the medication and consult the prescriber.
   d. hold the medication and page the prescriber STAT.

▶ 8. When administering lithium carbonate, which of the following assessments would indicate that therapy has achieved the desired effect?
    a. Displays flight of ideas
    b. Exhibits pressured speech
    c. Sits and watches TV for 8 hours per day
    d. Sleeps 8 hours per night

9. A patient has decided to try fish oil to treat her BPD. It is important for this patient to decrease intake of
    a. dairy products.
    b. processed grains.
    c. red meat.
    d. vegetable oils.

CASE STUDIES AND PATIENT TEACHING

(Use a separate piece of paper for your responses.)

Case Study 1

A 35-year-old female who has a history of BPD, hypertension, osteoarthritis, and environmental allergies has stopped taking her prescribed valproic acid (Depakote). She is brought to the hospital because she has become increasingly hyperexcitable over the past 5 days. She has talked on the phone almost continuously because she says she is trying to start a business. She has called friends and relatives all over the country at all hours of the night to tell them her news. She went on a spending spree to buy new clothes and equipment for her business venture and accumulated almost $10,000 worth of bills before she was caught for writing bad checks. Her husband was called when she tried to purchase a car, and the bank reported that she had insufficient funds to cover the check. She was brought to the hospital in an acute manic state. On admission she moves about restlessly, waving her arms in a threatening manner while loudly berating her husband and the hospital staff. She demands to be released from "this jail" and curses the nurse who interviewed her.

1. Why might this patient have stopped taking her medication?

2. Lithium carbonate 300 mg is prescribed 4 times a day. Why must lithium be taken in divided daily doses?

3. The patient complains that she cannot play cards or write a letter. What should the nurse do?

4. The nurse has explained the importance of monitoring plasma lithium levels every 2 to 3 days until therapeutic levels have been reached and maintained and every 1 to 3 months once maintenance level dose has been established to the patient and family. What should the nurse teach about other times that the patient should consult the prescriber about the need for additional monitoring?

5. What measures can the nurse teach the patient to prevent fluctuations in lithium levels?

6. What is the therapeutic range of plasma lithium for maintenance therapy, and at what point are lithium levels critical?

7. Adherence to drug therapy is often an obstacle to managing BPD. How can the nurse increase the likelihood of this patient taking her medication and participating in therapy as prescribed?

8. What teaching does the nurse need to provide to the patient and family relating to prescribed and over-the-counter drugs that relate to the patient's medical history?

9. What nonpharmacologic measures can the nurse teach the patient and family that may help modulate mood?

34
Sedative-Hypnotic Drugs

Answers can be reviewed online at http://evolve.elsevier.com/Lehne/.

OBJECTIVES

See page 28 for the Objectives.

CRITICAL THINKING AND STUDY QUESTIONS

1. Match the effect of benzodiazepines with the affected area of the brain.

_____ a. Anterograde amnesia	1. Cerebral cortex and hippocampus
_____ b. Confusion	2. Cortical areas
_____ c. Muscle relaxation	3. Limbic system
_____ d. Promote sleep	4. Supraspinal motor areas
_____ e. Reduce anxiety	

2. Lipid solubility of benzodiazepines (Select all that apply.)
   a. causes induction of hepatic metabolizing enzymes.
   b. decreases the risk that the drug will cause congenital defects.
   c. extends plasma half-life.
   d. increases absorption.
   e. improves distribution to CNS.

▶ 3. Although benzodiazepines are weak respiratory depressants, the nurse must be cautious with what situations that increase the risk that respiratory depression will cause significant problems?

4. Most benzodiazepines are
   a. absorbed from the GI tract very slowly.
   b. direct GABA agonists.
   c. prodrugs.
   d. short acting.

▶ 5. A patient asks for a sleeping pill at 2200. She states that she can fall asleep but awakens during the night and has difficulty getting back to sleep. The medication administration record (MAR) lists triazolam (Halcion) 0.125 mg hs PRN. The nurse should
   a. administer the triazolam.
   b. administer the triazolam and communicate the need to assess for effectiveness.
   c. contact the prescriber and discuss the need for a slower onset hypnotic.
   d. hold the triazolam because it is not effective in this situation.

6. Why are patients who are prescribed alprazolam (Xanax) for anxiety at greater risk for developing dependence on the drug than other benzodiazepines?

✳ 7. The nurse in the emergency department (ED) administers progressive doses of flumazenil (Romazicon) to a patient who has overdosed on a benzodiazepine and alcohol. A nursing priority in this situation is
   a. adequate fluids.
   b. monitoring breathing.
   c. reducing anxiety.
   d. renal function.

✳ 8. The immediate nursing priority when administering long-acting benzodiazepine as prescribed is
   a. gastric distress.
   b. potential for abuse.
   c. respiratory depression.
   d. safety.

89

9. When caring for a patient in the morning who has received zolpidem (Ambien) for sleep the night before, the nurse would monitor for symptoms of a common adverse effect?
   a. Dizziness
   b. Hypertension
   c. Sweating
   d. Tremors

10. Characteristics of benzodiazepine-like drug zolpidem (Ambien) include (Select all that apply.)
    a. can intensify the effects of alcohol.
    b. metabolized into an inactive compound.
    c. moderate muscle relaxation.
    d. prevents seizures.
    e. prolongs periods of uninterrupted sleep.
    f. promotes falling asleep.
    g. rapid onset.
    h. reduces REM sleep.
    i. reduced doses needed for people with liver impairment.
    j. significant rebound insomnia if suddenly discontinued.

11. A patient falls asleep without difficulty but frequently awakens during the night. The nurse would consult the prescriber if which of the following drugs was prescribed for sleep? (Select all that apply.)
    a. eszopiclone (Lunesta)
    b. ramelton (Rozerem)
    c. temazepam (Restoril)
    d. zaleplon (Sonata)
    e. zolpidem (Ambien CR)

12. Tolerance to barbiturates does not produce cross-tolerance to
    a. alcohol.
    b. benzodiazepines.
    c. general anesthetics.
    d. opiates.

13. A child who received a severe head injury is in a barbiturate-induced coma. The child's parents ask the nurse why he is being kept unconscious. They want the drug to be stopped so they can see if he will respond. The best explanation is that this therapy
    a. decreases the brain's need for oxygen and glucose.
    b. lowers the patient's blood pressure and pulse.
    c. produces amnesia so the child will not remember the accident.
    d. relaxes skeletal muscle so the patient is not uncomfortable.

14. Barbiturates are contraindicated for a patient with porphyria. Symptoms of porphyria include
    a. confusion, disorientation, and weakness.
    b. hypotension, bradycardia, and bradypnea.
    c. nausea, abdominal colic, behavioral and neuromuscular disturbances.
    d. restlessness, insomnia, and hyperthermia.

15. The nurse should assess for which symptoms in a patient with a suspected barbiturate overdose?
    a. Apnea and hyperthermia
    b. Bradypnea and constricted pupils
    c. Hypertension and hypothermia
    d. Hypotension and dilated pupils

✳ 16. A nursing priority for a patient during immediate care after overdose on a barbiturate is to monitor
    a. bowel sounds.
    b. deep tendon reflexes.
    c. peripheral pulses.
    d. urine output.

17. Patients with depression sometimes experience insomnia. The nurse recognizes that in addition to being a symptom of the disorder, insomnia is an adverse effect of some antidepressants. Which antidepressant is effective in treating depression-associated insomnia?
    a. Bupropion (Wellbutrin)
    b. Fluoxetine (Prozac)
    c. Fluvoxamine (Luvox)
    d. Trazodone (Desyrel)

18. An elderly patient occasionally uses diphenhydramine (Sominex) for insomnia. A nursing teaching to prevent a very common adverse effect is
    a. increase fiber in diet.
    b. limit fluids.
    c. low-fat diet.
    d. take medication with food.

19. A patient asks the nurse about use of melatonin for insomnia. Teaching should include (Select all that apply.)
    a. existing research suggests 2 mg of a controlled-release formula taken 2 hours before bedtime is most effective.
    b. it is a dietary supplement and is not closely regulated.
    c. it relieved insomnia in a study of blind insomniacs.

d. studies have shown that melatonin is effective in preventing jet lag.

e. there is no guarantee that product purchased contains the exact amount of melatonin as listed on the label.

CASE STUDIES AND PATIENT TEACHING

(Use a separate piece of paper for your responses.)

Case Study 1

An 18-year-old college student comes to the outpatient department of a local mental health center. She expresses worries about upcoming exams, states that she cannot sleep, cannot concentrate on her studies, has felt her heart pound, is dizzy, and has trouble catching her breath. These symptoms are unusual for her and began several weeks ago.

1. What additional data should the nurse collect about the patient's symptoms?

2. The patient is placed on alprazolam (Xanax) 0.25 mg 3 times a day with instructions to return to the mental health center in 2 weeks. Practically all responses to benzodiazepines, such as Xanax, result from actions in the CNS. Briefly describe the mechanism of action of benzodiazepines and barbiturates and explain why benzodiazepines are preferred over barbiturates and other general CNS depressants for anxiety and insomnia.
   a. Benzodiazepines
   b. Barbiturates

3. Why is it imperative that patients on benzodiazepines be cautioned against combining them with alcohol?

4. What information should be included in the nurse's health teaching plan for this patient?

Case Study 2

A 73-year-old man who lives alone is brought into the emergency department (ED) with multiple contusions and abrasions. He contacted the police and reported an intruder after awakening in the morning and finding his home in disarray, his clothing torn, and bruises over his body. The police report that there is no evidence of forced entry and all portals of entry were

locked. The patient has no memory of what occurred during the night. When taking the history, the nurse discovers that the patient took triazolam (Halcion) 0.25 mg at 0100.

1. What possible adverse effects of this drug could have caused this situation?

Case Study 3

The nurse is preparing to administer an intravenous (IV) benzodiazepine for status epilepticus.

1. Describe precautions that the nurse needs to take in this situation.

Case Study 4

A patient with a known history of alcohol abuse is brought into the ED unconscious. His wife states that he has been taking chlordiazepoxide (Librium) for alcohol withdrawal. His wife found him unresponsive, smelling of alcohol, with an empty pill bottle beside him. Assessment includes respirations 6 per minute. A decision to administer an antidote to the benzodiazepine is made before blood levels of the drug are available.

1. Why are blood levels of a benzodiazepine not extremely significant?

2. Flumazenil (Romazicon) 0.2 mg followed by a second dose of 0.3 mg 30 seconds later is prescribed by intravenous push. The drug is available in 0.1 mg/mL. How much drug should the nurse administer every 5 seconds?

3. After the second dose, the patient becomes responsive, and vital signs stabilize within normal limits. Why is it important for the nurse to continue to closely assess this patient?

Case Study 5

A patient who has been receiving benzodiazepine therapy for a long time has been notified that her insurance will no longer cover the medication.

1. What are possible effects of sudden discontinuation of the drug?

2. What can the nurse do to help this patient?

35
Management of Anxiety Disorders

Answers can be reviewed online at http://evolve.elsevier.com/Lehne/.

OBJECTIVES

See page 28 for the Objectives.

CRITICAL THINKING AND STUDY QUESTIONS

1. Which of the following statements about anxiety disorders and their treatment are true? (Select all that apply.)
   a. Acute anxiety, generalized anxiety, obsessive-compulsive, panic, phobia, and post-traumatic stress disorders are all primary anxiety disorders.
   b. Benzodiazepines are approved for use for three major anxiety disorders—generalized anxiety disorder, obsessive-compulsive disorder, and phobias.
   c. Cognitive behavioral therapy combined with drug therapy is effective for panic disorder.
   d. Depression often co-exists with anxiety disorders.
   e. Generalized anxiety disorder (GAD) is an acute condition.
   f. Onset of relief from anxiety with lorazepam (Ativan) and buspirone (BuSpar) is rapid.
   g. Principle adverse effects of buspirone (BuSpar) include sedation and psychomotor slowing.
   h. Selective serotonin reuptake inhibitors (SSRIs) are effective against anxiety even when depression is not present.

   i. Supportive, cognitive behavioral, and/or relaxation therapy is usually all that is needed in mild to moderate anxiety disorders.
   j. Symptoms of situational anxiety may be intense, but they are temporary.

✳ 2. A nurse is admitting a patient who is scheduled for outpatient cataract surgery. The patient had been instructed to take her levothyroxine (Synthroid) with a sip of water in the morning before coming to the hospital. The patient reveals that she was extremely anxious so she also took a lorazepam (Ativan), but only with the same sip of water "about 1 hour ago." Which of the following nursing actions would be of the greatest priority?
   a. Assessing for abuse of benzodiazepines
   b. Determining if the patient had signed all of the needed consents before coming to the hospital
   c. Ensuring that the patient understands the preoperative teaching
   d. Notifying anesthesia of the medications taken this morning

3. The nurse is preparing to administer buspirone (BuSpar) to a patient who has been taking the drug for 2 months for situational anxiety following a divorce. Important nursing considerations include
   a. assessing for suicidal ideation because of increased incidence of suicide in patients taking this drug.
   b. safety precautions because of sedation.

c. teaching to avoid drinking grapefruit juice.

d. teaching to not discontinue this drug suddenly.

4. Match the drug with the possible effects.

_____ a. Atypical antidepressant (venlafaxine) withdrawal

_____ b. Benzodiazepines (alprazolam and lorazepam)

_____ c. Buspirone (BuSpar)

_____ d. Monoamine oxidase (MAO) inhibitors

_____ e. SSRI (paroxetine and escitalopram)

_____ f. Trichloroacetic acid (TCA)

1. Abrupt discontinuance can produce
2. No abuse potential
3. CNS depressant
4. Can be used as needed (PRN)
5. Do not use with MAO inhibitor
6. Dysrhythmias can occur with overdose
7. Foods can cause hypertensive crisis
8. Hypertension
9. Can increase anxiety early in therapy
10. Nausea common adverse effect
11. Rapid onset
12. Sedates and slows movement
13. Slow onset
14. Spacey feeling

5. The nurse is caring for a patient who has been diagnosed with panic disorder. Teaching should include which of the following statements?

a. Avoid strenuous exercise because it increases anxiety.

b. Drug therapy helps the patient be more comfortable with situations and places they have been avoiding.

c. It is important to maintain adequate, regular sleep habits.

d. Symptoms usually only last 1 to 2 hours.

6. The nurse notes that a patient becomes very upset when the nurse rearranges any object in the room. The nurse would expect to find which diagnosis in the patient's history?

a. Obsessive-compulsive disorder (OCD)

b. Panic disorder

c. Social anxiety disorder (SAD)

d. Situational anxiety

▶ 7. When administering sertraline (Zoloft) for OCD, which of the following outcomes would indicate that therapy has achieved the desired effect?

a. Goes to market without experiencing palpitations, chest pain, dizziness, and fear of losing control

b. Rides in elevators without experiencing an anxiety attack

c. Sleeps 7 to 8 hours per night

d. Touches people without fear of contamination

8. Match the disorder with the symptom.

_____ a. Agoraphobia

_____ b. GAD

_____ c. OCD

_____ d. Panic disorder

_____ e. Post-traumatic stress disorder (PTSD)

_____ f. Social anxiety disorder

1. Anxiety when thinks cannot leave a room or situation
2. Chronic uncontrollable worrying
3. Intense irrational fear of embarrassment
4. Persistent uncontrollable thinking and repetitive actions
5. Re-experiencing, avoidance and/or emotional, numbing, and hyperarousal
6. Sudden anxiety attacks that may include fear of dying or going crazy

9. Experiencing which of the following is most likely to precipitate PTSD?

a. earthquake

b. flood

c. rape

d. war

10. Meta-analysis of studies of treatment for PTSD suggests

a. drug therapy helps.

b. drug therapy does not help.

c. repeated re-imagining the traumatic events makes symptoms worse.

d. there is no evidence that drug therapy helps.

CASE STUDIES AND PATIENT TEACHING

(Use a separate piece of paper for your responses.)

Case Study 1

A 58-year-old woman with a history of 70 pack-years of tobacco use is admitted with exacerbated chronic obstructive pulmonary disease. (COPD)The patient is very demanding. During care the patient states that she constantly worries about things that might go wrong. She has not been sleeping and has difficulty completing daily tasks because of weakness and fatigue.

1. What should the nurse do?

2. The nurse tries nonpharmacologic interventions to relieve the patient's anxiety without success. The prescriber orders alprazolam (Xanax) 0.5 mg 3 times a day. What should the nurse include in her teaching about this benzodiazepine drug?

3. A daughter comes to visit and expresses concern about her mother receiving a benzodiazepine drug. She states that her mother has a history of alcohol abuse, but has not had a drink for several years. How should the nurse respond to this information?

4. A consult is ordered, and the patient is diagnosed with GAD and history of alcohol abuse. Alprazolam (Xanax) is discontinued, and buspirone (BuSpar) 7.5 mg twice a day is ordered. Why is this drug a good choice for this patient?

5. The patient complains that the drug is not working. She asks if she can take an extra dose. How should the nurse respond?

36

Central Nervous System Stimulants and Attention-Deficit/Hyperactivity Disorder

Answers can be reviewed online at http://evolve.elsevier.com/Lehne/.

OBJECTIVES

See page 28 or the Objectives.

CRITICAL THINKING AND STUDY QUESTIONS

1. Indications for the use of central nervous system (CNS) stimulants include (Select all that apply.)
   a. attention-deficit/hyperactivity disorder (ADHD).
   b. as an antidote for CNS depressant poisoning.
   c. depression.
   d. narcolepsy.
   e. obesity.

2. An 8-year-old child being treated with methylphenidate (Ritalin) for ADHD is taken back to an examination room by the nurse in the pediatrician's office. What subjective and objective data should the nurse collect?

3. The elementary school nurse cares for a 5-year-old child who receives a CNS stimulant drug for ADHD. The child comes into the office complaining of not feeling well. Which of the following assessment findings would be a concern?
   a. BP 120/84 mm Hg
   b. Heart rate 100 beats/min
   c. Respirations 25 breaths per minute
   d. Weight gain of 2 lb since last year

4. A patient asks the nurse why her physician will not prescribe amphetamines to help her lose weight. Her mother took them and lost weight. The nurse's response should be based on the knowledge that amphetamines
   a. are ineffective for weight loss.
   b. can cause hypotension and bradycardia.
   c. can cause physical and psychologic dependence.
   d. can unmask latent bipolar disorder.

▶ 5. A patient with a history of narcolepsy, treated with Dexedrine Spansules, is first day postoperative after a right knee replacement. He has become agitated and is refusing all treatments including pain medications. He accuses the staff of trying to hurt him. The nurse should
   a. consult the prescriber of the dexedrine.
   b. consult the surgeon.
   c. continue nursing care, the symptoms will abate within hours.
   d. restrain the patient so that he does not injure the surgical site.

6. A child who has been prescribed Metadate CD for ADHD is having difficulty swallowing the medication. The nurse suggests
   a. crushing the medication and mixing it in a small amount of applesauce.
   b. notifying the prescriber; the medication must be taken whole.
   c. opening the capsule and sprinkling the beads in a small amount of soft food and telling the child to be careful not to chew the beads.
   d. opening the capsule and mixing the contents with 1 ounce of fluid.

7. A child who has been diagnosed with ADHD responded poorly to methylphenidate (Ritalin) 10 mg twice a day. If the prescriber stops the methylphenidate and prescribes dexmethylphenidate (Focalin), what dose of dexmethylphenidate would be equivalent to the Ritalin?
   a. Equal to the total methylphenidate dose but once a day
   b. One-half the methylphenidate dose
   c. The same as the methylphenidate dose
   d. Twice the methylphenidate dose

8. A 5th grade student with ADHD has been prescribed Daytrana transdermal methylphenidate patch. He normally awakens at 7:30 AM, attends school from 8:30 AM until 2:45 PM and does his homework as soon as he gets home from school. He goes to bed at 9:00 PM. The nurse will teach the parents that the best time to apply the patch is
   a. 5:30 AM.
   b. 8:00 AM.
   c. 4:00 PM.
   d. 9:00 PM.

9. A nurse's aide is experiencing a headache aura. Caffeine often helps prevent a full-blown migraine. She asks the nurse which of the following beverages has the most caffeine?
   a. Pepsi Cola 12 oz
   b. Snapple iced tea 12 oz
   c. Sprite 12 oz
   d. Sunkist orange soda 12 oz

10. Research suggests that moderately heavy caffeine consumption (500 mg/day) during human pregnancy is associated with
   a. birth defects.
   b. chromosomal damage.
   c. first trimester spontaneous abortion.
   d. sudden infant death syndrome (SIDS).

▶ 11. A loading dose of caffeine citrate (Cafcit) 60 mg has been prescribed for a neonate who weighs 6 lb 10 oz and is experiencing prolonged periods of apnea and bradycardia. The drug comes in a concentration of 20 mg/mL. How much caffeine citrate should the nurse administer?
   a. 0.66 mL
   b. 3 mL
   c. 20 mL
   d. None without consulting the pharmacy and/or prescriber. The dose is higher than the recommended dose.

✳ 12. Which of these assessment findings, if identified in a patient who is receiving pemoline (Cylert), should the nurse report to the prescriber immediately?
   a. Anorexia and insomnia
   b. Dark urine and nausea
   c. Headache and abdominal pain
   d. Lethargy and listlessness

13. Modafinil (Provigil) has been prescribed for a 22-year-old woman who works rotating shifts. When teaching about this drug, should the nurse include which of the following instructions? (Select all that apply.)
   a. Do not take with food because absorption of the drug will be decreased.
   b. Make the patient aware of orthostatic blood pressure precautions.
   c. Take as soon as you awaken because the drug can cause insomnia.
   d. Use a second form of birth control if using oral contraceptives.

✳ 14. A patient who is having a seizure is carried into the emergency department. Those accompanying him reveal that he is using drugs. Because there is a risk that the drugs were contaminated with strychnine, the nursing priority is
   a. airway clearance.
   b. breathing.
   c. cardiac output.
   d. tissue perfusion.

15. Atomoxetine (Strattera) is a newer drug for ADHD. Which of the following statements about this drug are true?
   a. It is approved for use in ADHD in adults.
   b. It has a moderate potential for abuse.
   c. It has a risk of liver injury.
   d. It takes 2 to 3 weeks before therapeutic effects develop.
   e. Patients doing well on stimulant drugs should be switched to Strattera because it is safer and more effective.
   f. Patients with an atypical form of the CYP2D6 metabolizing enzyme of cytochrome P450 need higher doses of the drug to be effective.
   g. Sexual dysfunction and urinary retention are possible adverse effects in adults.

CASE STUDIES AND PATEINT TEACHING

(Use a separate piece of paper for your responses.)

Case Study 1

The school nurse cares for a 7th-grade child who recently was diagnosed with ADHD, combined type. The mother had rejected the diagnosis previously because she does not like the idea of using medication. The child is prescribed methylphenidate (Ritalin) 10 mg 3 times a day. The mother speaks with the nurse when she delivers the medication and forms to the school. She verbalizes concern that she will be "drugging" her son and asks why behavioral therapy would not be sufficient.

1. Based on current research, how will the nurse explain the rationale for drug therapy?

2. The nurse has been administering the second dose at 11:00 AM. The nurse is planning for the individual education plan (IEP) meeting with teachers, a counselor, and parents. She notes that the child has not been gaining weight. The child admits that he is not very hungry. In the meeting, the nurse learned that the mother gives the child methylphenidate at 6:30 AM before she leaves for work. The child eats his breakfast at school. The last dose is administered at 5:00 PM with dinner. What changes can be made to help improve the appetite of this child?

3. Most teachers at the IEP meeting share that the child's behavior has improved since starting medication. However, his organization and study skills are still very weak. Based on the expected therapeutic response to methylphenidate, what information can the nurse provide?

4. The fourth-period (10:15 to 11:00 AM) teacher states that the child is very sleepy in his class. What could have been happening to cause this sleepiness?

5. Several weeks later the child's mother comes in to see the nurse stating that the pediatrician has recommended that her son be switched to Metadate CD 20 mg once a day. She is concerned because "this is a newer drug, and they don't know enough about it." How should the nurse respond?

6. The child does well at school on Metadate CD but has difficulty once home getting his homework done and socially at after-school activities. The prescriber puts the child on Concerta. How does the nurse explain the difference between Concerta and Metadate CD?

7. What teaching should be provided about administration of Concerta?

Case Study 2

A 25-year-old female is seeking medical help for amphetamine dependence. She was prescribed amphetamines for weight loss several years ago and lost 100 lb. She is now 5 feet 6 inches and weighs 130 lb. She continued taking amphetamines after she reached her goal weight and now wants to stop taking the drug, but says she cannot do it alone. When she stops taking the amphetamines, she experiences withdrawal symptoms and becomes frightened so she continues to use the drug.

1. What is the current medical opinion about taking amphetamines for weight loss?

2. What signs and symptoms would you expect the patient to exhibit when she is using amphetamines?

3. It is important to decrease the amphetamine slowly since the patient has previously experienced withdrawal symptoms. What withdrawal symptoms should the nurse be alert for when a patient is withdrawing from amphetamine use, and what nursing interventions can help the patient cope with these symptoms?

37
Drug Abuse I: Basic Considerations

Answers can be reviewed online at http://evolve.elsevier.com/Lehne/.

OBJECTIVES

See page 28 for the Objectives.

CRITICAL THINKING AND STUDY QUESTIONS

1. Why is it important for nurses to be knowledgeable of the developmental level of patients and the beliefs of different cultures and individuals relating to drugs?

2. Addictive behavior (Select all that apply.)
   a. involves physical, psychologic, or social harm.
   b. involves reinforcement of pleasure or reduction in intensity of an unpleasant experience.
   c. involves activation of the brain's endorphin reward circuit.
   d. is a chronic relapsing illness.
   e. is a treatable disease.
   f. is present if the patient is physically dependent on a psychoactive substance.
   g. requires a pre-existing psychopathology.

3. Match the following terms and definitions.

6	a. Cross-dependence	1. A particular dose elicits a less intense response
5	b. Cross-tolerance	2. Abstinence syndrome will develop if drug is stopped

2	c. Physical dependence	3. Intense subjective need for a drug
3	d. Psychologic dependence	4. Symptoms often opposite of the normal effects of the drug
4	e. Tolerance	5. When higher doses of a drug are needed because the person has abused another drug—usually in the same class
4	f. Withdrawal syndrome	6. When one drug can prevent withdrawal from another drug

4. Psychologic factors that have been associated with tendencies toward drug abuse would make it important for the nurse to provide drug abuse prevention for children who have been diagnosed with (Select all that apply.)
   a. ADHD.
   b. anxiety.
   c. depression.
   d. developmental delay.

5. An example of addiction is an individual who experiences abstinence if he stops taking
   a. amphetamines used to reduce symptoms of ADHD.
   b. OxyContin used for cancer pain.
   c. phenobarbital used to prevent seizures.
   d. tobacco used to reduce stress.

6. Drugs that the nurse can administer and that have the highest potential for abuse and dependence are classified by the Controlled Substances Act as
   a. schedule I.
   b. schedule II.
   c. schedule III.
   d. schedule IV.
   e. schedule V.

7. A patient has been prescribed hydrocodone 5 mg and acetaminophen 500 mg (Vicodin), a schedule IV drug. Federal regulations regarding refills of this drug are that it
   a. cannot be refilled.
   b. may be refilled two times within 3 months.
   c. may be refilled five times within 6 months.
   d. may be refilled as many times as the prescriber specifies within 12 months.

8. When there are different laws on the state and federal level regarding prescribing controlled substances the
   a. most restrictive law takes precedence.
   b. least restrictive law takes precedence.
   c. federal law takes precedence.
   d. state law takes precedence.

CASE STUDIES AND PATIENT TEACHING

(Use a separate piece of paper for your responses.)

Case Study 1

The nurse is working on a drug and alcohol detoxification unit. Describe how the nurse's expertise can be applied to address the following issues of drug abuse:

1. Diagnosis and treatment of toxicity.

2. Diagnosis and treatment of secondary medical complications.

3. Facilitating withdrawal.

4. Educating and counseling drug abusers in hopes of maintaining long-term abstinence.

38

Drug Abuse II: Alcohol

Answers can be reviewed online at http://evolve.elsevier.com/Lehne/.

OBJECTIVES

See page 28 for the Objectives.

CRITICAL THINKING AND STUDY QUESTIONS

1. The nurse is caring for a patient with a history of chronic alcohol abuse. The patient is prescribed thiamin to prevent Wernicke's encephalopathy. The nurse should assess for symptoms of this disorder. Select all that apply.
   a. abnormal ocular movements.
   b. confabulation.
   c. confusion.
   d. inability to convert short-term memory to long-term memory.
   e. nystagmus.
   f. polyneuropathy.

2. Research suggests consumption of one alcoholic drink per day has been associated with
   a. atrophy of the cerebrum.
   b. lower levels of HDL.
   c. improving the quality of sleep.
   d. preservation of cognitive functioning in the elderly.

▸ 3. A patient who has been a heavy drinker for 30 years is admitted with constant severe

midepigastric pain radiating to the flank. Which of the following laboratory test results should be reported immediately to the prescriber?
a. Amylase 500 international units /L
b. BNP 33 pg/mL
c. Bilirubin 1 mg/dL
d. Protein 6.5 gm/dL

4. For the average person with normal liver functioning, alcohol levels in the blood will begin to increase if a person consumes in 1 hour (Select all that apply.)
a. one (1.5 ounces) shot of whiskey.
b. 8-ounce glass of wine.
c. two (12 ounces) beers.

5. Match the substance with the effect when combined with alcohol.
_3_ a. Acetaminophen
_1_ b. Antihypertensives
_4_ c. Benzodiazepines
_5_ d. Disulfiram
_2_ e. Nonsteroidal anti-inflammatory drug (NSAID)

1. Counteracts effects when alcohol dose is high
2. Increases risk of injury to GI mucosa
3. Increases risk of liver damage
4. Intensifies CNS depression
5. Produces nausea and vomiting; can produce death

6. Chronic alcohol consumption does not produce tolerance to
a. activation of the reward circuit.
b. decreased alertness.
c. diminished reflexes.
d. respiratory depression.

7. Which of the following benzodiazepine regimens has been shown to protect against seizures and breakthrough symptoms of alcohol withdrawal while promoting speedier withdrawal?
a. Administered as needed in response to symptoms
b. Administered as needed in response to symptoms in combination with another drug to reduce withdrawal symptoms
c. Administered around-the-clock on a fixed schedule
d. Administered around-the-clock in declining doses on a fixed schedule

8. Disulfiram (Antabuse) reactions can occur if a patient is exposed to alcohol and takes which of the following antimicrobial medications?
a. azithromycin (Zithromax)
b. gentamicin (Garamycin)
c. metronidazole (Flagyl)
d. cefazolin (Ancef)

9. A patient is admitted with a fractured hip and scheduled for surgery. It is important to inform the surgeon of the patient's history of alcohol abuse and use of naltrexone (ReVia) to assist with abstinence because
a. there are specific analgesic drugs that the patient should not receive.
b. the patient is at risk for addiction to opioids used for postoperative pain.
c. the patient should not receive any opioid analgesics for postoperative pain.
d. usual doses of opioid analgesics for postoperative pain may be ineffective.

10. It is important for the nurse to teach a patient who has been prescribed acamprosate (Campral) to support abstinence from alcohol because
a. full effects do not occur for about a week.
b. he needs to increase fluid and fiber in the diet to prevent diarrhea.
c. severe hypotension can occur if alcohol is used while taking this drug.
d. the drug blocks craving for alcohol.

11. Which of the following information is most important to share with the prescriber if a patient has just been prescribed topiramate (Topamax) to reduce the craving for alcohol?
a. Patient has a history of migraine headaches.
b. Patient had his last alcoholic drink yesterday.
c. Patient started drinking as a teen.
d. Patient did not start drinking until after he lost his job at age 40.

12. Dietary counseling for a patient with alcohol abuse should include adequate servings of what type of food to prevent thiamin deficiency?
a. Fruit
b. Green leafy vegetables
c. Milk
d. Pork

CASE STUDIES AND PATIENT TEACHING

(Use a separate piece of paper for your responses.)

Case Study 1

The nurse is caring for 45-year-old man with a history of alcohol abuse and cirrhosis of the liver who is newly admitted with gastrointestinal bleeding from ulcers.

1. What would be appropriate nursing diagnoses and related assessments for this patient?

2. The patient's blood alcohol level is 0.320%. Chlordiazepoxide (Librium), a drug that is believed to enhance the action of gamma-aminobutyric acid (GABA) transmission in the central nervous system (CNS), was ordered at 100 mg IM STAT. The drug is then ordered by mouth at high doses with the dose decreasing every 3 days. What is the rationale for this treatment regimen?

3. What would be an appropriate nursing outcome for this patient relating to the reason for administrating chlordiazepoxide (Librium)?

4. The patient has been admitted once before for detoxification. He was discharged at that time on a maintenance dose of chlordiazepoxide (Librium). Based on the believed effects of alcohol on the CNS, why would this patient revert back to alcohol abuse?

5. After detoxification the patient states he is motivated to quit. He asks for disulfiram (Antabuse) to help him refrain from drinking. What teaching should the nurse provide to the patient and family about this drug?

6. Shortly after discharge, the patient stops taking the drug and resumes drinking. One morning, his wife is so disgusted about his return to drinking that she crushes 2 disulfiram tablets and puts them in his breakfast. The patient drinks alcohol and goes into shock and dies. What are possible consequences for the wife?

Case Study 2

Senior-level student nurses have just finished clinical hours in a local hospital emergency department (ED) and are having a postconference. They are discussing a 21-year-old male patient who was brought in during their shift and was resuscitated in the ED after acute overdose of alcohol. A fellow college student accompanying the patient reported that he had drunk four shots in 15 minutes while playing a drinking game. They had not eaten anything for over 3 hours before starting the game.

1. The nursing students identify which of the following as a priority nursing problem for this patient at this time?
   a. Airway clearance
   b. Anxiety
   c. Knowledge deficit
   d. Sensory perceptual alterations

2. The parents of the patient arrived at the ED. The patient's father asked how this could happen. He has had more than five drinks in an evening and has been fine. What factors contributed to the adolescent's extreme intoxication?

3. Why would discussion about alcohol's effects on the heart, liver, stomach and kidneys developmentally not be likely to motivate this patient to abstain from alcohol?

4. Developmentally, discussion of what adverse effects of alcohol might motivate this young man to drink responsibly?

5. If the patient were a female, what teaching should the nurse provide about the possible effects of alcohol use during pregnancy?

Answers can be reviewed online at http://evolve.elsevier.com/Lehne/.

OBJECTIVES

See page 28 for the Objectives.

CRITICAL THINKING AND STUDY QUESTIONS

✳ 1. A priority concern of the nurse when caring for an opioid addict who is experiencing abstinence syndrome is
   a. central nervous system (CNS) depression.
   b. preventing respiratory arrest.
   c. relapse to opioid use.
   d. timing of doses of nalmefene (Revex).

✳ 2. A patient who has a history of heroin abuse is brought into the emergency department (ED) unresponsive with pinpoint pupils. The nurse assesses that the patient has stopped breathing. In addition to supporting respirations, the patient is prescribed intravenous (IV) naloxone HCl (Narcan). The nurse notes an improvement in level of consciousness, respiratory rate, and effort within minutes of administration of naloxone. The priority action by the nurse 30 to 40 minutes after administration of the drug is
   a. assessing the patient for withdrawal symptoms.
   b. identifying the abused opioid.
   c. monitoring of pulse and blood pressure.
   d. reassessing for respiratory depression.

3. The nursing supervisor notes that an unusually high number of older, adult patients have become restless and irritable after receiving oral meperidine (Demerol) prescribed for postoperative pain. He suspects that a staff nurse may be replacing the meperidine tablets with another pill before administration and stealing the meperidine and that the patient's symptoms are due to uncontrolled pain. Appropriate actions would include
   a. assessing employees for opiate abuse symptoms including pupil constriction.
   b. meeting with the staff and sharing suspicions.

   c. researching effects of aging on metabolism of meperidine and possible adverse effects.
   d. reviewing nurse's applications for addresses suggesting low socioeconomic status.

▶ 4. Which of the following would be the most accurate indicator to the nurse that the dose of methadone prescribed to minimize abstinence syndrome is inadequate?
   a. The nurse notes that the patient has difficulty arising in the morning.
   b. The nurse notes that the patient is experiencing vomiting and diarrhea.
   c. The patient is exhibiting kicking motions.
   d. The patient states that the dose is inadequate.

5. Which of the following statements, if made by a patient who has been prescribed clonidine to assist with withdrawal from addiction to oxycodone (OxyContin), would indicate a need for further teaching?
   a. "I'm glad that I won't feel like I need the drug."
   b. "I need to be careful not to jump up out of bed too quickly."
   c. "I should have less muscle pain if I take this drug."
   d. "The medication should help prevent vomiting and diarrhea."

6. Which of the following outcomes best reflects the goal of administering methadone for suppressive therapy?
   a. The patient does not experience abstinence syndrome.
   b. The patient does not experience euphoria when taking opioids.
   c. The patient does not experience respiratory depression.
   d. The patient will not crave opioids.

7. A patient has been prescribed sublingual buprenorphine-naloxone (Suboxone) for long-term management of heroin addiction. It is important for the nurse to teach the patient that the drug should not be crushed, dissolved, and injected IV because this could cause
   a. an overdose.
   b. heroin-induced euphoria.
   c. respiratory depression.
   d. withdrawal symptoms.

8. Which of the following is associated with maintenance therapy with methadone?
   a. Early death
   b. Inability to form relationships with other people
   c. Lack of productivity at work
   d. Increased incidence of chronic disease

9. A known drug user is admitted to the ED. Assessment findings include bradypnea, pinpoint pupils, and unresponsive to painful stimuli. Overdose of which of the following drugs is known to cause these symptoms? (Select all that apply.)
   a. cannabis (marijuana)
   b. cocaine
   c. dexedrine (Adderall)
   d. heroin
   e. LSD
   f. methadone (Dolophine)
   g. methylphenidate (Ritalin)
   h. MDMA (Ecstasy)
   i. nalmefene (Revex)
   j. oxycodone (OxyContin)
   k. temazepam (Restoril)

* 10. A suspected barbiturate overdose patient is brought into the ED unresponsive with pinpoint pupils. A priority nursing intervention is
   a. administering an antidote.
   b. administering phenobarbital.
   c. maintaining respirations.
   d. preventing shock.

▶ 11. When responding to acute overdose of cocaine, which of the following outcomes would best indicate that therapy has been successful?
   a. Adequate cardiac output
   b. Sensory perceptions normal
   c. Effective breathing pattern
   d. Temperature 98°F to 99°F

▶ 12. The nurse is caring for a patient who has been admitted for amphetamine abuse. Assessment findings include T 99.4°F, BP 178/102 mm Hg, P 110 beats/min, respirations 25 breaths per minute, productive cough, rhinorrhea, and coryza. The nurse should consult the prescriber before administering which of the following medications for cold and allergy symptoms?
   a. chlorpheniramine (Chlor-Trimeton)
   b. dextromethorphan (Benylin)
   c. guaifenesin (Humibid)
   d. pseudoephedrine (Sudafed)

13. Intravenous dantrolene (Dantrium) is prescribed if needed for a patient who has been admitted with adverse effects of taking MDMA (Ecstasy). Which of the following assessment findings would warrant administration of the dantrolene?
   a. Extreme anxiety and confusion
   b. Hallucinations and delusions
   c. Spasmodic jerking and elevated temperature
   d. Suicidal thoughts and behavior

14. A patient who has taken phencyclidine (PCP) is brought to the ED exhibiting combative behavior and hallucinations. An appropriate nursing intervention is
   a. inserting an NG tube.
   b. reducing external stimuli.
   c. sodium bicarbonate administration.
   d. talking down.

▶ 15. A 9-month-old child is admitted to the ED after eating cigarettes. Which of the following assessment findings would be of most concern to the nurse?
   a. Apical pulse 145 beats/min
   b. Blood pressure 66/48 mm Hg
   c. Respirations 15 per minute
   d. Temperature 37°C

16. The nurse would withhold which of the following smoking cessation aid drugs and contact the prescriber if the patient exhibited seizure activity?
   a. bupropion (Zyban, Wellbutrin)
   b. nicotine patch (Nicotrol, Nicoderm CQ)
   c. nicotine lozenge (Commit)
   d. nortriptyline (Aventyl, Pamelor)

CASE STUDIES AND PATIENT TEACHING

(Use a separate piece of paper for your responses.)

Case Study 1

A student nurse is working with a clinical group in the drug abuse section of the healthcare facility. A 43-year-old woman shares her story of drug abuse. She began drinking in high school and by tenth grade was getting drunk several times a week. She married an alcoholic and drank with him for many years. She then began taking diazepam (Valium) with her alcohol. She says she had hangovers in the mornings so she would have a beer or two and some amphetamines to "get myself together." She would also take a few aspirins for the headache and go to work feeling sick. As a rule, she would leave work at 5:00 PM, stop by the liquor store, then go home to watch TV, drink, and take a few diazepam to calm down. After a few years of this, she began to get crack cocaine from the streets. She was unable to do her job because she was either high or was in need of a fix, so she was fired. She stayed home and drank and found she was having difficulty buying the drugs. She would get into violent arguments with her husband. He physically abused her, and she finally left him and sought help at a women's shelter. She tried to stop using drugs many times over the years, but could only stop for a few days before she began to feel ill. She started stealing to support her habit. After being arrested for stealing, she was required to enter a treatment program.

1. How has tolerance and physical dependence contributed to this person's drug abuse?

2. What assessments should the nurse perform to assess for drug withdrawal?

3. What interventions might the nurse employ to decrease the adverse effects of withdrawal?

Case Study 2

A school nurse is developing a program relating to preventing use of marijuana for 12- to 14-year old students. Complete the following teaching plan.

Prevention of Marijuana Abuse	
Teaching approaches based on thinking of 12- to 14-year-old according to Piaget	
Teaching approaches based on psychosocial developmental stage according to Erikson	
Desired environment for teaching	
Desired outcomes	
Developmentally appropriate content	
Method of teaching	

Case Study 3

1. Debate the pros and cons of legalizing marijuana.

Case Study 4

The nurse is creating a plan to prevent and/or address tobacco abuse using the Nola Pender revised Health Promotion Model (see below).

1. Complete the following charts relating to the developmental stage as it influences promoting abstinence. Consider the personal sociocultural factors of the age group to identify behavior-specific cognitions and affect influencing tobacco use.

INDIVIDUAL CHARACTERISTICS AND EXPERIENCES

- Personal sociocultural factors
  - Characteristics of the workers including race, ethnicity, education, and sociocultural factors that influence beliefs, affect, and performance of a health-promoting behavior

1.

Developmental Stage	Personal sociocultural factors that influence tobacco use	How these characteristics influence ability and willingness to attempt health-promoting behavioral change
Young Adult		
Adult		
Older Adult		

BEHAVIOR-SPECIFIC COGNITIONS AND AFFECT

- Perceived benefits of action
  - Positive effects the person thinks they will experience from not smoking
- Perceived barriers to action
  - Negative effects the person thinks they will experience if they smoke
- Perceived self-efficacy
  - Belief that the person can be successful
- Activity related affect
  - Positive and negative effects experienced when smoking or when being encouraged to smoke
- Interpersonal influences
  - Behaviors, beliefs, or attitudes of others that can influence the person's decision to smoke or not smoke
- Situational influences
  - Environmental factors that can influence the person's decision to smoke or not smoke

Reference

Pender, N, et al: *Health promotion in nursing practice,* 4th ed., Upper Saddle River, NJ, Prentice Hall, 2002.

2.

Behavior-specific cognitions and affect relating to substance abuse	Young Adult	Nursing Interventions
Perceived benefits of action		
Perceived barriers to action		
Perceived self-efficacy		
Activity related affect		
Interpersonal influences		
Situational influences		

3.

Behavior-specific cognitions and affect relating to tobacco use	Young Adult	Nursing Interventions
Perceived benefits of action		
Perceived barriers to action		
Perceived self-efficacy		
Activity-related affect		
Interpersonal influences		
Situational influences		

4.

Behavior-specific cognitions and affect relating to substance abuse	Older Adult	Nursing Interventions
Perceived benefits of action		
Perceived barriers to action		
Perceived self-efficacy		
Activity-related affect		
Interpersonal influences		
Situational influences		

40

Diuretics

Answers can be reviewed online at http://evolve.elsevier.com/Lehne/.

OBJECTIVES

See page 28 for the Objectives.

CRITICAL THINKING AND STUDY QUESTIONS

1. Match the following terms and descriptors.

   _____ a. Filtration
   _____ b. Reabsorption
   _____ c. Active tubular secretion
   _____ d. Solutes
   _____ e. Water

   1. Most significant regulator of urine composition
   2. Moves passively following osmotic gradient
   3. Filtered then reabsorbed by active transport
   4. Nonselective
   5. Uses pumps selective for organic acids and organic bases for active transport

2. The kidney produces approximately 180 L (180,000 mL) of filtrate each day. How much is normally excreted as urine in a day?
   a. 0.9 L
   b. 1.8 L
   c. 3.6 L
   d. 4.5 L

3. Most diuretics work by
   a. blocking synthesis of pumps responsible for sodium and potassium transport in the distal nephron.
   b. acting on the collecting duct to increase permeability to water.
   c. blocking sodium and chloride reabsorption.
   d. blocking reabsorption of sodium in the distal nephron and increasing potassium reabsorption.

4. Diuretics that produce the most significant diuresis affect reabsorption in the
   a. thick segment of the ascending Loop of Henle.
   b. early distal convoluted tubule.
   c. late distal convoluted tubule.
   d. collecting ducts.

5. Diuretics can affect blood levels of (Select all that apply.)
   a. acids and bases.
   b. calcium.
   c. chloride.
   d. glucose.
   e. lipids.
   f. magnesium.
   g. potassium.
   h. sodium.
   i. uric acid.
   j. water.

6. A patient with heart failure (HF) who weighs 176 lb has been prescribed a high-ceiling diuretic with the goal of loss of 1000 mL of additional urine output in the next 24 hours. If this goal is met, the nurse would expect the patient's weight to be
   a. 168 lb.
   b. 170 lb.
   c. 172 lb.
   d. 174 lb.

7. A patient in chronic renal failure has been retaining fluid despite dialysis. Which diuretic would the nurse expect to administer?
   a. bumetanide (Bumex)
   b. hydrochlorothiazide (Oretic, HydroDIURIL)
   c. metolazone (Zaroxolyn)
   d. spironolactone (Aldactone)

8. Research the mechanism of action of the diuretics furosemide (Lasix) and spironolactone (Aldactone). Explain why a prescriber may prescribe a lower dose of each of these medications instead of a higher dose of one of the drugs.

▶ 9. A patient with left-sided HF has been prescribed a high-ceiling diuretic. The assessment that most accurately reflects a therapeutic effect of this drug is
   a. drop in systolic blood pressure of 10 mm Hg.
   b. normal heart sounds.
   c. clear lung sounds.
   d. pulse 80 and regular.

▶ 10. A patient who has been diagnosed with HF and type 2 diabetes mellitus (DM) has been prescribed furosemide (Lasix) 20 mg by mouth once a day. Based on the effect of furosemide on the patient's DM, it is important for the nurse to assess this patient for
   a. irritability, paresthesias, and muscle weakness.
   b. diaphoresis, shakiness, and tachycardia.
   c. increased thirst; confusion; and dry, hot skin.
   d. nausea, vomiting, and diarrhea.

▶ 11. A patient is receiving a diuretic. The nurse takes orthostatic BP readings before administering the diuretic. Which change in orthostatic BP should be reported to the prescriber?
   a. 150/90 mm Hg lying; 125/70 mm Hg sitting
   b. 140/82 mm Hg lying; 125/72 mm Hg sitting
   c. 130/90 mm Hg lying; 118/78 mm Hg sitting
   d. 116/70 mm Hg lying; 110/68 mm Hg sitting

12. A patient has been prescribed a high-ceiling diuretic. Which of the following foods are important to include in the diet to prevent hypokalemia? (Select all that apply.)
   a. Bananas
   b. Beans
   c. Cheese
   d. Red meat
   e. Oranges
   f. Pork
   g. Raisins
   h. Spinach
   i. Yogurt

13. A patient has been prescribed a high-ceiling diuretic. The nurse should monitor lab tests for (Select all that apply.)
   a. hypocalcemia.
   b. hypochloremia.
   c. hypoglycemia.
   d. hypokalemia.
   e. hypomagnesemia.
   f. hyponatremia.
   g. increased HDL.

   h. decreased triglycerides.
   i. elevated LDL.
   j. elevated uric acid.

14. An over-the-counter medication that can counteract the effects of diuretics is
   a. acetaminophen.
   b. ibuprofen.
   c. iron.
   d. multiple vitamins.

15. The recommended diuretic for initial therapy of essential hypertension is a(n)
   a. high-ceiling (loop) diuretic.
   b. osmotic.
   c. potassium-sparing diuretic.
   d. thiazide.

16. It is important for the nurse to assess for ototoxicity when a patient has been prescribed a high-ceiling diuretic and a(n)
   a. aminoglycoside antibiotic.
   b. cephalosporin antibiotic.
   c. macrolide antibiotic.
   d. penicillin antibiotic.

▶ 17. The nurse is reviewing the lab values for a patient who has been prescribed lithium carbonate for bipolar disorder and furosemide for HF. Which of the following electrolyte results would be a reason for concern?
   a. Chloride 100 mEq/L
   b. Magnesium 1.8 mEq/L
   c. Potassium 4.1 mEq/L
   d. Sodium 128 mEq/L

18. Patients with hypertension often need more than one antihypertensive drug. The nurse is doing an admission history and assessment. The patient states that she is taking several drugs for "high blood pressure." The nurse would assess for what symptoms that suggest hyperkalemia if the patient has been prescribed spironolactone (Aldactone) and Enalapril (Vasotec) or Triamterene (Dyrenium)?
   a. Disorientation and seizures
   b. Muscle weakness and hypotension
   c. Confusion and heavy legs, and tall T waves on ECG
   d. Skeletal muscle weakness and absent bowel sounds

19. A female patient did not mention that she is taking Yasmin, an oral contraceptive that contains the potassium-saving ingredient drosperinone when being seen to adjust drug therapy for hypertension. She was prescribed valsartan (Diovan). She is admitted to the ED with chest pain. Which ECG finding suggests that the combination of drugs is causing hyperkalemia?
    a. Prolonged ST interval
    b. Tall tented T waves
    c. Depressed ST segments
    d. Extra P waves

▸ 20. Which of the following laboratory results should be reported to the prescriber if a patient is prescribed hydrochlorothizide 50 mg once a day and metformin/glyburide (Glucovance) 500 mg/2.5 mg twice a day?
    a. FBS 90 mg/dL
    b. HbA$_{1c}$ 8.2%
    c. Potassium 4 mEq/L
    d. Sodium 136 mg/dL

✳ 21. A 20-year-old female has been prescribed spironolactone (Aldactone) for primary polycystic ovary syndrome (POS). Developmentally, what would be a priority nursing diagnosis?

22. The nurse is preparing to administer mannitol (Osmitrol) to a patient. The nurse notes crystals in a clear solution. The nurse should
    a. administer the solution.
    b. discard the solution.
    c. use an in-line filter.
    d. warm the solution to dissolve the crystals, cool to body temperature, and use an in-line filter.

23. Because of the risk of hyperkalemia, the nurse consults the prescriber and monitors potassium levels if a patient was prescribed spironolactone and a drug with which of the following suffixes? (Select all that apply.)
    a. –cycline
    b. –floxacin
    c. –olol
    d. –pril
    e. –sartan
    f. –statin

CASE STUDIES AND PATIENT TEACHING

(Use a separate piece of paper for your responses.)

Case Study 1

An 80-year-old nonsmoking woman has been taking spironolactone (Aldactone) 100 mg/day for about 6 years to control her moderate hypertension and mild HF. She comes to the emergency department with bilateral crackles (rales) in the lower and middle lobes and a blood pressure of 190/120 mm Hg. She is short of breath, very anxious, tachycardic (HR 134 beats/min), and diaphoretic. Her family assures you that she has been taking her medication. The family tells you she has been getting worse over the past 2 weeks since having friends bring her lunches of hot dogs and potato chips every day. Pulmonary edema is diagnosed. Orders include STAT intravenous push furosemide (Lasix) 40 mg and morphine sulfate 2 mg, 3 L of oxygen via nasal cannula, electrolytes, and complete blood count, and an indwelling Foley catheter.

1. How will furosemide (Lasix) help relieve this patient's symptoms?

2. What information must the nurse know about furosemide (Lasix) administration before administering the drug intravenous push?

3. The drug handbook states that 40 mg of furosemide (Lasix) can be administered undiluted over 1 to 2 minutes; do not exceed 4 mg/min in patients with renal impairment. The nurse is unsure of the patient's renal status and plans to administer the drug over 10 minutes (4 mg/min). The furosemide (Lasix) vial states 40 mg/4 mL. The 5-mL syringe is marked with a line every 0.2 mL. The nurse will administer 0.2 mL (one line) of furosemide (Lasix) over what time period?

4. Why was the Foley catheter ordered?

5. It has been 45 minutes since the patient received her furosemide (Lasix). Her Foley catheter is in place. She says that she is very thirsty. What assessments should be made at this point?

6. Lab results, drawn before she received any medication, have returned. Her sodium is 140 (135 to 145 mEq/L), chloride is 110 (98 to 106 mEq/L), and potassium is 3.5 (3.5 to 5 mEq/L). Knowing that she received her furosemide (Lasix) after these lab values were drawn, what should be included in the nurse's plan of action?

7. The patient improves significantly within the first 6 hours. Her blood pressure is 138/90 mm Hg, pulse 102, respirations 20, and rales are heard only in her bases bilaterally. She asks you how this could have happened since she had been taking her medicine as prescribed. What should the nurse discuss with the patient as possible reasons for her condition?

8. What nursing assessments would be made on at least a daily basis while she is in the hospital?

9. The patient continues to improve and is being discharged home on furosemide (Lasix) 20 mg twice a day and spironolactone (Aldactone) 50 mg daily. What teaching should be provided regarding dietary patterns, activity, and signs and symptoms of further problems?

10. What information should the nurse provide to prevent problems with drug interactions?

11. The patient will need to be started on digoxin. What must the nurse remember now that the patient is on digoxin and furosemide (Lasix)? What laboratory values need to be monitored?

Case Study 2

A 42-year-old female patient who has recently been diagnosed with essential hypertension has described to the nurse a recent concern of overactive bladder. The prescriber has just prescribed hydrochlorothiazide (HydroDIURIL) to treat the hypertension.

1. List some nursing concerns and teachings.

Answers can be reviewed online at http://evolve.elsevier.com/Lehne/.

OBJECTIVES

See page 28 for the Objectives.

CRITICAL THINKING AND STUDY QUESTIONS

1. Match the effect of the situation on fluid volume and ion concentration.

_____ a. Hypertonic contraction
_____ b. Hypotonic contraction
_____ c. Isotonic contraction
_____ d. Volume expansion

1. Vomiting, diarrhea
2. Heart failure (HF), cirrhosis
3. Extensive burns, older adult
4. Diuretics, chronic renal failure

2. Total osmolality of plasma is equal to approximately
   a. the osmolality of sodium.
   b. twice the osmolality of sodium.
   c. the osmolality of potassium.
   d. twice the osmolality of potassium.

3. When infusing an intravenous (IV) solution in cases of isotonic contraction, it is most important for the nurse to
   a. assess for crackles (rales) in the lung fields.
   b. calculate the infusion rate in drops per minute and hang by gravity.
   c. infuse the fluid quickly.
   d. infuse 0.45% sodium chloride.

4. Intravenous solutions of 5% dextrose in water are technically isotonic in the bag but are hypotonic in the body because
   a. the body uses the dextrose for energy.
   b. the kidneys rapidly excrete the dextrose.
   c. $C_6H_{12}O_6$ is metabolized in the blood to H_2O and CO_2.
   d. dextrose in a nonabsorbable sugar.

5. Match the following conditions with the appropriate descriptor. (Answers may be used more than once.)

_____ a. Metabolic acidosis
_____ b. Respiratory acidosis
_____ c. Metabolic alkalosis
_____ d. Respiratory alkalosis

1. Can occur if ventilator set too high (respirations too rapid)
2. Lung changes from smoking are a risk for this condition
3. May be associated with prolonged gastric suctioning
4. Seen in uncontrolled diabetes mellitus
5. Treat with rebreathing CO_2
6. Treat with O_2, deep exhalations, and sodium bicarbonate
7. Treat NaCl plus KCl to increase excretion of bicarbonate

6. A 15-year-old girl with bulimia abuses laxatives. She is admitted to the hospital after experiencing extreme leg weakness. Potassium chloride 40 mEq by mouth twice a day has been prescribed. The nurse reviews the most recent laboratory tests before administering the patient's medications. Results include Na 137 mEq/L, K 3.7 mEq/L, and Cl 100 mEq/L. The nurse should
   a. page the prescriber STAT.
   b. administer the medication.
   c. hold the medication and contact the prescriber.
   d. administer the medication and contact the prescriber.

7. The nurse is administering furosemide (Lasix) and sustained-release potassium chloride (K-Dur) to a patient with HF. The nurse notes that the patient is chewing the potassium

chloride. The patient states she cannot swallow the large pill. The nurse should
   a. crush the pill and mix it with applesauce or pudding.
   b. instruct the patient to drink at least 8 ounces of water with the potassium pill.
   c. contact the prescriber.
   d. page the prescriber STAT.

▶ 8. A patient is admitted with a serum glucose level of 750 mg/dL. Intravenous regular insulin is prescribed to lower the patient's blood sugar. When administering the IV insulin, the nurse needs to assess the patient for which symptoms of a possible electrolyte disorder that can be caused by this treatment?
   a. Skeletal muscle weakness and absent bowel sounds (hypokalemia)
   b. Disorientation, psychosis, and seizures (hypomagnesemia)
   c. Muscle weakness, hypotension, and sedation (hypermagnesemia)
   d. Confusion, anxiety, heavy legs, and tall T waves on ECG (hyperkalemia)

9. Which of the following medications used to treat hypertension can increase the risk of hyperkalemia if prescribed with potassium or with each other?
   a. amlodipine (Norvasc)
   b. atenolol (Tenormin)
   c. carvedilol (Coreg)
   d. diltiazem (Cardizem)
   e. enalapril (Vasotec)
   f. hydrochlorothiazide (Oretic)
   g. ramipril (Altace)
   h. spironolactone (Aldactone)
   i. triamterene (Dyrenium)

10. Oral magnesium supplementation may not be effective if the patient
   a. has impaired renal functioning.
   b. is a diabetic.
   c. has hypertension.
   d. experiences diarrhea.

11. The nurse reviews laboratory test results that include a magnesium level of 1 mEq/L on a newly admitted patient. It is most important for the nurse to promptly inform the prescriber if the patient has a history of
   a. asthma.
   b. AV heart block.
   c. gastroesophageal reflux disease (GERD).
   d. rheumatoid arthritis.

12. Because of the risk of neuromuscular blockade when administering magnesium, the nurse must have access to what IV medication?
   a. Calcium gluconate
   b. Potassium chloride
   c. Sodium chloride
   d. Sodium polystyrene sulfonate

CASE STUDIES AND PATIENT TEACHING

(Use a separate piece of paper for your responses.)

Case Study 1

A patient is admitted with prolonged diarrhea. An IV solution of 0.45% sodium chloride with 40 mEq of potassium chloride is prescribed at 80 mL/hr.

1. What laboratory tests does the nurse need to monitor when administering potassium supplements?

2. What assessments does the nurse need to perform to ensure safe infusion of the potassium solution?

3. What measures should the nurse take to ensure accurate infusion of the prescribed dose of fluid and electrolytes?

4. Which of the following findings would be a reason for the nurse to stop the IV infusion and notify the prescriber? (Select all that apply.)
   a. Blood pressure 100/65 mm Hg
   b. Blood urea nitrogen (BUN) 28 mg/dL
   c. Creatinine 4.2 mg/dL
   d. Potassium 3.5 mEq/L
   e. Pulse 58 beats/min
   f. Serum glucose 220 mg/dL
   g. Sodium 140 mEq/L
   h. One-hour urine output of 10 mL

5. The nurse receives the electrolyte report for the sample drawn this morning. Results include pH 7.31, sodium 142 mEq/L, potassium 5.7 mEq/L, chloride 102 mEq/L, and magnesium 1.8 mEq/L. What treatments might be prescribed?

Case Study 2

A postoperative patient has been NPO for 4 days with a nasogastric tube set to low intermittent suction. The patient develops muscle cramping and disorientation. Serum Mg is 1.0 mEq/L. The prescriber orders an IV solution of 10% magnesium sulfate to infuse at 100 mL/hr.

1. What should the nurse do before initiating this IV therapy?

2. The prescriber changes the infusion rate to 90 mL/hr. What critical assessment should the nurse perform while administering magnesium?

3. What assessment findings would warrant the nurse stopping the infusion?

Case Study 3

A 165-pound patient is admitted to the burn unit with burns over 36% of her total body surface area (TBSA). Because of evaporative and intracellular fluid loss, burns over 15% of TBSA require more rapid fluid replacement than other cases of hypertonic

contraction. This facility uses the modified Parkland (Baxter) formula for fluid replacement. Crystalloid replacement is Lactated Ringer's solution 4 mL/kg × %TBSA/24 hours.

1. What is the total amount of lactated Ringers solution that needs to be infused in the first 24 hours?

2. Half of the fluid is to be administered during the first 8 hours. What rate in mL/hour should the nurse program into the IV pump?

3. What assessments should the nurse perform to identify fluid overload?

4. One fourth of the fluid is to be administered during the next 8 hours. What rate in mL/hour should the nurse program into the IV pump?

42

Review of Hemodynamics

Answers can be reviewed online at http://evolve.elsevier.com/Lehne/.

OBJECTIVES

See page 28 for the Objectives.

CRITICAL THINKING AND STUDY QUESTIONS

1. Which of the following statements about the circulatory system are true? (Select all that apply.)
   a. Arteries readily stretch in response to pressure changes.
   b. Arterioles determine blood flow to tissue.
   c. Conditions that decrease chest expansion with breathing decrease blood return to the heart.
   d. Conditions that cause an inability of skeletal muscle to contract (or severe weakness) can cause peripheral edema.
   e. Normal adult blood volume is 8 L.
   f. The heart of a normal adult pumps the entire blood volume in approximately 1 minute.
   g. The majority of the blood in the body is in the arteries and the heart.
   h. Vasodilation increases resistance to blood flow.

2. Individuals who have plaque occluding their arteries experience an increase in vessel resistance. The nurse should assess for which of the following that is/are the body's attempt to compensate?
   a. Peripheral edema
   b. Rise in blood pressure (BP)
   c. Shifting of point of maximal impulse (PMI)
   d. Slowing of heart rate

3. Drugs that can be used to lower her BP decrease venous resistance by
   a. dilating veins.
   b. reducing blood volume.
   c. reducing right atrial pressure.
   d. stimulating auxiliary muscle pumps.

4. A patient with early heart failure (HF) has an average heart rate of 90 beats/min and a stroke volume of 55 mL. This patient's per minute cardiac output is
   a. extremely low.
   b. low.
   c. normal.
   d. high.

5. A patient who experiences orthostatic (postural) hypotension gets up to go to the bathroom during the night to void. In addition to instructing him to change positions slowly, the nurse teaches him to try to void sitting down. What is the rationale for this teaching?
   a. Voiding can cause dehydration and hypotension.
   b. Voiding can cause tachycardia and hypertension.
   c. Voiding involves stimulation of beta-adrenergic receptors in the heart, and a rebound tachycardia can occur.
   d. Voiding involves stimulation of the vagus nerve, which can cause bradycardia and further hypotension.

▸ 6. The nurse is researching a drug. The handbook states that it decreases afterload. Before the nurse administers this medication to a patient, which of these assessments would be most critical to assess?
   a. BP for hypotension
   b. Pulse for tachycardia
   c. Respirations for tachypnea
   d. Temperature for fever

✳ 7. The nurse is assessing a patient who is receiving medication for acute HF. Which of the following assessments would be the most critical?
   a. BP 165/90 mm Hg
   b. Expiratory wheezes of bronchi and bronchioles
   c. Loud inspiratory and expiratory gurgling sounds throughout lung fields
   d. Pulse 100 beats/min

8. Drugs can cause vasodilation by
   a. blocking parasympathetic receptors.
   b. blocking sympathetic receptors.
   c. stimulating parasympathetic receptors.
   d. stimulating sympathetic receptors.

▸ 9. The nurse is reassessing a patient 1 hour after administering a vasodilator to treat hypertension. Assessment findings include BP 110/70 mm Hg (down from 136/88 mm Hg), pulse 88 (up from 80 beats/min), and respirations 22 (down from 20). The nurse should (Select all that apply.)
   a. continue collecting additional assessment data.
   b. document the findings.
   c. explain orthostatic BP precautions.
   d. page the prescriber STAT.
   e. prepare for a cardiac arrest.
   f. raise all four bed side rails for safety.
   g. reassess the vital signs within 1 hour.

▸ 10. A patient is receiving a vasodilator that has a high incidence of orthostatic hypotension. Before administering the medication and after the patient has rested supine for 10 minutes, the nurse assesses the BP and pulse. Results are BP 145/80 mm Hg, P 68 beats/min. The nurse assists the patient to stand, providing safety and after 1 minute reassesses the BP and pulse. Which of the following readings would be of most concern to the nurse?
   a. BP 110/70 mm Hg, pulse 92 beats/min
   b. BP 120/70 mm Hg, pulse 78 beats/min
   c. BP 130/70 mm Hg, pulse 88 beats/min
   d. BP 140/82 mm Hg, pulse 70 beats/min

CASE STUDIES AND PATIENT TEACHING

(Use a separate piece of paper for your responses.)

Case Study 1

A patient newly diagnosed with coronary artery disease (CAD) has been prescribed a nitroglycerin patch 12 hours on and 12 hours off. The nurse is explaining the medication to the patient and her daughter. Nitroglycerin is a drug that causes extensive venous vasodilation. The drug handbook states that the therapeutic effect is to decrease the workload of the heart. The patient wants to know how this helps her heart.

1. How should the nurse explain this effect?

2. The patient verbalizes understanding of nitroglycerin, but states she is afraid to take off the patch because she might have a heart attack. The rationale for not using nitroglycerin patches continuously is
   a. absorption is decreased if left on too long.
   b. skin irritation occurs.
   c. tolerance to the drug's effect develops.
   d. toxicity develops.

Case Study 2

The student nurse is caring for a patient in HF. The heart is enlarged, weak, and its muscle fibers are stretch beyond the point of effective recoil. The student nurse must do a teaching project.

1. Describe how the student nurse could use a balloon to demonstrate the pathophysiology of HF to the patient.

43

Drugs Acting on the Renin-Angiotensin-Aldosterone System

Answers can be reviewed online at http://evolve.elsevier.com/Lehne/.

OBJECTIVES

See page 28 for the Objectives.

CRITICAL THINKING AND STUDY QUESTIONS

1. The nurse recognizes that the generic names of angiotensin II receptor blocker (ARB) drugs end in
   a. -mycin.
   b. -olol.
   c. -pril.
   d. -sartan.

2. The nurse recognizes that the generic names of angiotensin-converting enzyme (ACE) inhibitor drugs end in
   a. -mycin.
   b. -olol.
   c. -pril.
   d. -sartan.

3. A nurse is teaching how drugs that block the effects of angiotensin II can be beneficial for heart failure patients. What information would not be incorporated into the teaching?
   a. The drug helps the heart function primarily by slowing the heart rate.
   b. The drug can help heart function by decreasing sodium and water resorption by the kidneys, which would raise blood pressure.
   c. The drug can decrease the formation of extra heart muscle mass.
   d. The drug can help heart function by preventing thickening of the arterial wall and resultant hypertension.

4. Which of the following would not stimulate renin release by the kidneys?
   a. Dehydration
   b. Hemorrhage
   c. Hypernatremia
   d. Stimulation of beta$_1$-adrenergic receptors

5. Angiotensin-converting enzyme (ACE) is chemically the same as the enzyme kinase II, which stimulates the breakdown of bradykinin. A patient may experience which adverse effect from taking an ACE inhibitor reflecting accumulation of bradykinin?
   a. Dehydration
   b. Dry cough
   c. Hyperkalemia
   d. Hyponatremia

6. Drugs that block the renin-angiotensin-aldosterone system lower blood pressure by
   a. constricting arteries.
   b. constricting veins.
   c. increasing excretion of potassium.
   d. increasing excretion of water.

▶ 7. When the nurse is scheduled to administer lisinopril to a patient, which of these lab values should be reviewed? (Select all that apply.)
   a. ALT
   b. BUN
   c. Calcium
   d. Creatinine
   e. CRP
   f. Fasting blood sugar
   g. Sodium
   h. Potassium
   i. Uric acid
   j. Urine protein

8. The nurse receives laboratory test results including AST 22 international units/L, ALT 33 international units/L, BUN 20 mg/dL, and creatinine 3.2 mg/dL on a patient who is scheduled to receive an ACE inhibitor drug. Which of the following ACE inhibitors could be administered without concern of toxicity?
   a. captopril
   b. enalapril
   c. fosinopril
   d. lisinopril

9. The nurse teaches the patient who is prescribed an ACE inhibitor that orthostatic blood pressure precautions are especially important when the
   a. drug prescribed is lisinopril (Prinivil, Zestril).
   b. first dose or an increase in dosage is taken.
   c. patient is taking a dose of an ACE inhibitor in the morning.
   d. potassium level is greater than 4 mEq/L.

▶ 10. Which of these ECG findings would suggest hyperkalemia in a patient who is prescribed an ACE inhibitor and who was using a salt substitute?
   a. Flat T waves
   b. Prolonged QT interval
   c. Shortened QT interval
   d. Tall, peaked T waves

11. A patient who has been taking an ACE inhibitor for hypertension is concerned because she has just discovered that she is 7 weeks pregnant. The nurse knows that research suggests that if the patient stops taking the ACE inhibitor now, the risk for adverse effects on the fetus are
   a. low.
   b. medium.
   c. high.
   d. unknown.

✳ 12. When a patient is prescribed enalapril (Vasotec), which of these assessment findings would warrant an immediate response by the nurse?
   a. Cough
   b. Neutrophil count 60%
   c. Swelling around the mouth
   d. Unilateral renal artery bruit

▶ 13. A patient is prescribed lithium for bipolar disorder and losartan (Cozaar) for hypertension. The nurse should assess for which electrolyte laboratory result that could increase the risk for lithium toxicity?
   a. Sodium greater than 145 mEq/L
   b. Sodium less than 135 mEq/L
   c. Potassium greater than 5 mEq/L
   d. Potassium less than 3.5 mEq/L

14. A patient who was previously prescribed an ACE inhibitor has now been prescribed an ARB. The nurse knows that research suggests this medication change will decrease the patient's risk of developing
   a. angioedema.
   b. death from heart failure.
   c. death from kidney failure.
   d. hyperkalemia.

15. Advantages of the direct renin inhibitor aliskiren (Tekturna) over ARBs is
   a. less incidence of cough.
   b. fewer gastrointestinal (GI) adverse effects.
   c. unclear (ie, There are no clear advantages.).
   d. no drug interactions.

16. Spironolactone (Aldactone) is less selective than eplerenone (Inspra). The nurse knows that this means that spironolactone
    a. causes more adverse effects.
    b. has less drug interactions.
    c. is less effective.
    d. produces therapeutic effects more rapidly.

17. The nurse assesses a hypertensive, diabetic patient who is prescribed eplerenone (Inspra) for early symptoms of the most likely electrolyte imbalance, which includes
    a. flushed, dry skin.
    b. hyperactive bowel sounds.
    c. irritability.
    d. weak hand grasps.

∗ 18. When taking a history from a patient who is prescribed an ACE inhibitor, ARB, or eplerenone (Inspra), which of the following questions would be most important for the nurse to ask?
    a. "Are you bothered by a frequent nonproductive cough?"
    b. "Do you eat 4 to 5 servings of fruits and vegetables each day?"
    c. "Have you ever been diagnosed with iron deficiency anemia?"
    d. "What spices do you use to season your food?"

19. A patient who has been prescribed quinapril (Accupril) for hypertension has not had the expected reduction in blood pressure. Regular use of which of the following over-the-counter medications may be contributing to lack of therapeutic effect of the ACE inhibitor?
    a. Acetaminophen
    b. Calcium carbonate
    c. Ibuprofen
    d. Milk of magnesia

CASE STUDIES AND PATIENT TEACHING

(Use a separate piece of paper for your responses.)

Case Study 1

A 68-year-old male was admitted to the medical unit with complaints of a 10-lb weight gain over the past week, swollen ankles, and increasing shortness of breath. Although furosemide (Lasix) was partially effective, the prescriber chooses to add an ACE inhibitor. The patient is prescribed captopril (Capoten) 12.5 mg by mouth, three times a day. His blood pressure is currently 140/74 mm Hg. Significant history includes an anterior myocardial infarction 12 months ago and renal artery stenosis involving the right kidney.

1. What question should the nurse ask when consulting the prescriber about this new medication order?

2. What teaching should the nurse provide about timing of the doses of captopril (Capoten)?

3. What assessments and actions should the nurse perform when administering the first dose of captopril (Capoten)?

4. What teaching should the nurse provide to the patient and family about reasons to contact the prescriber?

5. The patient's wife states that her sister used to take captopril (Capoten), but her sister's prescriber discontinued the ACE inhibitor and prescribed the newer drug valsartan (Diovan). She would like her husband to be prescribed valsartan because it is newer and better. How should the nurse respond?

Answers can be reviewed online at http://evolve.elsevier.com/Lehne/.

OBJECTIVES

See page 28 for the Objectives.

CRITICAL THINKING AND STUDY QUESTIONS

1. The suffix of the generic name of dihydropyridine calcium channel blockers (CCB) is
   a. (-azosin).
   b. (-lol).
   c. (-pine).
   d. (-sartan).

2. The drop in blood pressure (BP) produced by the CCB activates baroreceptors and stimulates the sympathetic nervous system. Which of these CCB is most likely to have the adverse effect of reflex tachycardia?
   a. diltiazem (Cardizem)
   b. nifedipine (Procardia)
   c. verapamil (Calan)

3. The nurse is caring for a patient who is scheduled to receive verapamil (Calan) and atenolol (Tenormin), a beta$_1$-adrenergic blocker at 0900. It is important for the nurse to assess for what critical adverse effects based on the combination of these two drugs before administration? (Select all that apply.)
   a. Bradycardia
   b. Crackles of pulmonary edema
   c. Muscle pain
   d. Shortness of breath
   e. Thrombocytopenia
   f. Urinary output of at least 45 mL/hr
   g. Weight gain of 3 pounds in 24 hours

▶ 4. The nurse is caring for a patient who is scheduled to receive verapamil (Calan SR) 180 mg and atenolol (Tenormin) 50 mg, a beta$_1$-adrenergic blocker at 0900. The patient has had a gastric tube (G-tube) inserted and drugs are to be administered via the tube. Which of the

following actions should the nurse take before administering these two drugs?
   a. Change the time of the drug administration so that they are administered via the G-tube at least 2 hours apart.
   b. Consult the prescriber.
   c. Crush both tablets separately.
   d. Flush the G-tube with 5 to 15 mL of water between administering the drugs.

▶ 5. A patient is prescribed diltiazem (Cardizem). Which of the following assessment findings would be a reason to hold the medication and contact the prescriber?
   a. BP 150/85 mm Hg
   b. Constipation
   c. Dizziness with position changes
   d. Pulse 50 beats/min

▶ 6. Which of the following dermatologic findings on an older adult would warrant consultation with the prescriber regarding administration of diltiazem (Cardizem)?
   a. Burrows and erythematous papules between the fingers
   b. Erythematous oozing vesicles on the chin and inside of elbows
   c. Silvery scaling plaques on the elbows
   d. White cheesy plaque on the tongue

7. The nurse is administering the Verelan PM form of verapamil. The patient states she takes all of her medications in the morning when she awakens. The nurse's response should be based on the knowledge that Verelan PM
   a. produces maximal effects in the morning when most cardiac events occur.
   b. is given at night so it peaks during sleep to prevent orthostatic hypotension.
   c. should not be administered with any other medication.
   d. should be taken at night because it causes sedation.

8. A patient on a surgical unit has been prescribed intravenous (IV) diltiazem (Cardizem) for atrial fibrillation. The nurse should
   a. move the resuscitation cart into the patient's room.
   b. arrange for the patient to be transferred to a unit where constant monitoring of BP and electrocardiogram is possible.
   c. continuously monitor the patient's oxygen saturation and pulse during infusion.
   d. have another nurse check the calculated drip rate before hanging the medication by gravity feed.

9. A patient taking both verapamil (Calan) and digoxin (Lanoxin) is at greater risk for digitalis toxicity. The nurse should assess and monitor the patient for early symptoms of digitalis toxicity, which include
   a. anorexia and nausea.
   b. confusion and slurred speech.
   c. hypertension and tachycardia.
   d. photophobia and halos around bright objects.

▸ 10. The nurse is administering medications on a medical-surgical unit in a hospital. The medication administration record states that the patient should receive Cardizem LA 120 mg once a day. The patient's drug supply includes Cardizem SR. The nurse should
   a. administer the medication.
   b. administer the medication and notify the prescriber of the change.
   c. contact the pharmacy.
   d. hold the medication and contact the prescriber.

▸ 11. Diltiazem is prescribed for IV infusion for a patient in atrial fibrillation. A dose of 5 mg/hr has been prescribed. The pharmacy has supplied the drug in a concentration of 0.45 mg/mL. How many mL/hr will the nurse program into the IV infusion pump?

12. Which of the following drugs might be prescribed to counteract the reflex tachycardia associated with administration of dihydropyridine calcium channel blockers (CCB)?
   a. digoxin (Lanoxin)
   b. enalapril (Vasotec)
   c. furosemide (Lasix)
   d. metoprolol (Lopressor)

13. A patient who has experienced palpitations (reflex tachycardia) while taking nifedipine (Procardia) 20 mg three times a day has had his prescription changed to nifedipine (Procardia XL) 60 mg once a day. The patient asks the nurse how taking the same medication once a day instead of three times a day will help prevent palpitations. The nurse's response should include that
   a. rapid-acting formulas of nifedipine are more potent than sustained-release formulas.
   b. blood levels of rapid-acting formulas of nifedipine rise more rapidly than with sustained-release formulas.
   c. sustained-release formulas of nifedipine cause a more gradual drop in BP.
   d. sustained-release formulas of nifedipine suppress the automaticity of the heart like verapamil.

14. Because of its selectivity for blockade of calcium channels in cerebral blood vessels, which CCB is used for prevention of cerebral artery spasm following subarachnoid hemorrhage?
   a. nicardipine (Cardene)
   b. nimodipine (Nimotop)
   c. felodipine (Plendil)
   d. isradipine (DynaCirc)

15. A patient has been prescribed extended-release nifedipine (Procardia). Teaching regarding administration should include which of the following?
   a. Administer 1 hour before or 2 hours after meals.
   b. Do not crush or chew tablet.
   c. Take with grapefruit juice to improve absorption.
   d. Must be taken on an empty stomach.

▸ 16. The recommended initial dose of diltiazem (Cardizem) IV push is 0.25 mg/kg for adult patients. What is the recommended safe dose for a patient that weighs 178 lb?

CASE STUDIES AND PATIENT TEACHING

(Use a separate piece of paper for your responses.)

Case Studies 1

A 75-year-old female, nonsmoker, with a history of hypertension, esophageal cancer, and diabetes type 2 comes to the emergency department with fatigue and extreme shortness of breath. She is diagnosed with atrial fibrillation. The prescriber orders verapamil (Calan) 5 mg IV push.

1. Verapamil is available as 5 mg/2 mL to be administered no faster than 2 minutes. The nurse administers 0.1 mL every 5 seconds. Is this a safe rate of administration?

2. The nurse is administering the verapamil (Calan) IV push. While administering the medication, the nurse notes a sudden reduction in heart rate and prolongation of the PR interval on the cardiac monitor. What should the nurse do?

3. Thirty minutes after injecting the IV verapamil, the patient requests assistance with getting up and using the toilet to void. The nurse should
   a. assist the patient to the bathroom.
   b. secure a bedside commode.
   c. provide assistance with using a bedpan.
   d. get an order for a Foley catheter.

4. The patient is stabilized and the prescriber has prescribed verapamil (Calan) 120 mg three times a day. The nurse is reviewing the patient's laboratory tests. Which of the following laboratory values would require consultation with the prescriber regarding administration of verapamil? (Select all that apply and explain why.)
   a. Alanine aminotransferase (ALT) 250 units/L
   b. Blood urea nitrogen (BUN) 28 mg/dL
   c. Creatinine 3.2 mg/dL
   d. Fasting glucose (FBS) 250 mg/dL
   e. Hemoglobin (Hb) 10 mg/dL
   f. International ratio (INR) 1.8
   g. Potassium (K+) 3.3 mEq/L
   h. Sodium (Na+) 146 mg/dL

5. The nurse is reviewing the patient's prescribed medications. In addition to verapamil 80 mg three times a day, the patient is taking nateglinide (Starlix) 120 mg, a medication that increases production of insulin by the pancreas and lowers the blood sugar to treat the patient's diabetes mellitus. Both verapamil and nateglinide are metabolized by the CYP3A4 hepatic enzyme. Verapamil inhibits the action of this enzyme. Because of this interaction, the nurse knows the patient is at increased risk for
   a. hyperglycemia.
   b. hypoglycemia.

6. What teaching should the nurse provide that can prevent problems with common adverse effects of verapamil?

45

Vasodilators

Answers can be reviewed online at http://evolve.elsevier.com/Lehne/.

OBJECTIVES

See page 28 for the Objectives.

CRITICAL THINKING AND STUDY QUESTIONS

1. Hydralazine, minoxidil, diltiazem, nifedipine, verapamil, and diazoxide (Select all that apply.)
   a. decrease cardiac afterload.
   b. decrease tissue perfusion.
   c. have a high risk of postural hypotension.
   d. increase cardiac output.
   e. increase the force of cardiac contraction.
   f. reduce the force at which blood is returned to the heart.
   g. vasodilate arteries.
   h. vasodilate veins.

* 2. A priority nursing problem when the nurse is caring for a patient who is receiving an arterial vasodilator is
   a. activity intolerance.
   b. altered tissue perfusion
   c. decreased cardiac output.
   d. fluid volume excess.

3. Which of the following drugs is commonly prescribed for patients with heart failure along with hydralazine (Apresoline)?
   a. Atenolol
   b. Hydrochlorothizide
   c. Isosorbide dinitrate
   d. Minoxidil

* 4. When caring for a patient who is prescribed minoxidil, it is most important for the nurse to assess for
   a. abnormal hair growth.
   b. bradycardia.
   c. fluid volume deficit.
   d. shortness of breath.

▶ 5. A patient with severe hypertension is prescribed minoxidil (Loniten). The nurse should contact the prescriber STAT if assessment findings include
   a. distended neck veins, muffled heart sounds, and narrow pulse pressure.
   b. exertional dyspnea, 1+ ankle edema, and anxiety.
   c. headache, dizziness, and blurred vision.
   d. shift of point of maximal impulse (PMI) to left, bruits over carotid arteries, and wheezing.

6. The nurse is caring for a nonambulatory patient who is receiving hydralazine (Apresoline). When monitoring for adverse effects, the nurse would expect that edema would first appear
   a. around the medial malleolus of the ankle.
   b. in the fingers.
   c. in the sacral area.
   d. on the dorsal aspect of the feet.

▶ 7. Laboratory test results on a patient receiving hydralazine (Apresoline) include elevated antinuclear antibodies (ANA). When notifying the prescriber of these lab results, which of the following assessment findings is most significant to also include in the report?
   a. Blood pressure 150/90 mm Hg
   b. Pulse 90 beats/min
   c. Respirations 22/min
   d. Temperature 101°F (38.3°C)

8. Which of the following elevated laboratory results is most likely to be related to administration of diazoxide (Hyperstat)? (Select all that apply.)
   a. Amylase
   b. ANA
   c. Calcium
   d. Capillary blood sugar
   e. High-density lipoproteins
   f. Low-density lipoproteins
   g. Uric acid

9. What lab tests should be monitored in a patient who is receiving diazoxide (Hyperstat)? (Select all that apply.)
   a. Amylase and lipase
   b. Creatinine and eGFR
   c. Fasting and postprandial glucose
   d. Uric acid and ESR

▶ 10. The nurse is administering nitroprusside (Nitropress) in a cardiac care unit. The prescriber also orders administration of oral antihypertensives. The patient's blood pressure is still elevated, but dropping slowly. The nurse should
   a. administer both medications.
   b. hold both the nitroprusside and oral antihypertensives until the prescriber can be consulted.
   c. hold the nitroprusside and administer the oral antihypertensives until the prescriber can be consulted.
   d. hold the oral antihypertensives and administer the nitroprusside until the prescriber can be consulted.

11. A patient who weighs 110 lb is receiving intravenous (IV) nitroprusside sodium (Nipride) 300 mcg/min. An important nursing assessment at this dose is for
   a. adequate fluid intake and urinary output.
   b. anorexia, nausea, and vomiting.
   c. fever, flushing, and chills.
   d. palpitations, disorientation, and respiratory depression.

12. The nurse is preparing to administer nitroprusside sodium (Nipride). The solution has just been prepared in the pharmacy, but has a faint brown discoloration. The nurse should
   a. administer the medication.
   b. consult the prescriber before administering the solution.
   c. discard the solution and get a new bag from the pharmacy.
   d. warm the IV bag and reassess to see if the brown color clears.

13. A patient who is receiving nitroprusside is receiving a concurrent dose of IV thiosulfate. The nurse knows that thiocyanate levels must be monitored and should not exceed what level?
   a. 0.01 mg/mL
   b. 0.1 mg/mL
   c. 1 mg/mL
   d. 10 mg/mL

14. Match the mechanism of action of drugs that act on the renin-angiotensin-aldosterone system.
   _____ a. ACE inhibitor
   _____ b. ARB
   _____ c. DRI

   1. (-kiren) inhibit enzyme that forms angiotensin I
   2. (-pril) block conversion of angiotensin I to angiotensin II
   3. (-sartan) block receptors for angiotensin II

CASE STUDIES AND PATIENT TEACHING

(Use a separate piece of paper for your responses.)

Case Study 1

A 55-year-old patient has just been admitted to the intensive care unit in a hypertensive crisis. He is confused, lethargic, and his blood pressure is 240/160 mm Hg. The healthcare providers are concerned that he may have a massive cerebrovascular accident (stroke or CVA) if his blood pressure is not brought down immediately. An IV push of diazoxide (Hyperstat) 2 mg/kg is prescribed. Recommended dose is 1 to 3 mg/kg up to a maximum of 150 mg per dose. The patient weighs 220 lb.

1. What dose of diazoxide is safe and therapeutic?

2. The drug comes in a concentration of 15 mg/mL and should be administered by rapid IV push over 3 minutes. How many milliliters should the nurse administer per 5 seconds if 100 mg is ordered?

3. What assessments does the nurse need to perform and how frequently should these assessments occur?

4. The patient's wife informs the nurse that her husband is a "brittle" diabetic. Why is it important to share this information with the prescriber?

5. Why must a patient on diazoxide (Hyperstat) stay recumbent for at least 30 minutes after discontinuing diazoxide injection, but only normal postural hypotension precautions are needed with nitroprusside?

Case Study 2

A 78-year-old woman is being seen in the emergency department in hypertensive crisis. She is 5 feet 2 inches and weighs 125 lb. Her BP is 230/130 mm Hg, and she is very edematous. She has a history of alcohol abuse. IV nitroprusside sodium (Nipride) at 0.3 mcg/kg/min is prescribed.

1. What assessments of the solution and precautions should the nurse take when administering this medication?

2. Knowing that nitroprusside sodium (Nipride) creates a rapid response (within 1 to 2 minutes), what and how often should the nurse assess to follow the results of the drugs and the patient's response?

3. The patient suddenly becomes diaphoretic and complains of nausea, palpitations, and headache. What should the nurse do?

4. The patient has improved significantly. The prescriber orders hydralazine, metoprolol, and hydrochlorothiazide on a long-term basis to control her blood pressure. Explain the rationale for this combination of medications.

5. The nurse checks the drug handbook, and the dose recommendation for adults for hydralazine is listed as 10 to 50 mg 4 times a day or 100 mg 3 times a day. What are possible reasons for the low dose being extended to every 8 hours?

46

Drugs for Hypertension

Answers can be reviewed online at http://evolve.elsevier.com/Lehne/.

OBJECTIVES

See page 28 for the Objectives.

CRITICAL THINKING AND STUDY QUESTIONS

1. The nurse knows it is important to teach lifestyle modifications to patients at risk for hypertension. Which of the following mean of two blood pressure (BP) readings taken 5 minutes apart, if identified on three or more separate occasions, would be classified by JNC 7 as prehypertension? (Select all that apply.)
   a. 110/70 mm Hg
   b. 118/86 mm Hg
   c. 120/80 mm Hg
   d. 128/92 mm Hg
   e. 130/85 mm Hg
   f. 137/74 mm Hg
   g. 138/92 mm Hg
   h. 146/76 mm Hg

2. When possible, the nurse should assess the patient's BP with the patient
   a. lying flat in bed.
   b. lying in bed with the head elevated at least 45 degrees.
   c. sitting, with feet dangling.
   d. sitting, with feet on the floor.

3. The nurse is reviewing a patient's history and notes "essential hypertension." This older term is synonymous with
   a. isolated systolic hypertension.
   b. prehypertension.
   c. primary hypertension.
   d. secondary hypertension.

4. Pheochromocytoma causes hypertension because a tumor of the adrenal gland secretes excessive amounts of
   a. dopamine.
   b. epinephrine.
   c. gamma-aminobutyric acid (GABA).
   d. serotonin.

5. It is important for the nurse to discuss adverse effects of the antihypertensive drugs that are prescribed because adverse effects often
   a. affect compliance.
   b. are life threatening.
   c. are necessary if the antihypertensive is at a dose that is effective.
   d. indicate the cause of hypertension.

6. The teaching plan for a patient taking antihypertensive drugs should include
   a. cigarette smoking will cause antihypertensive drugs to be ineffective.
   b. following dietary and exercise recommendations will prevent the need for antihypertensive drugs.
   c. symptoms of hypertension usually do not occur until organ damage has occurred.
   d. treatment with antihypertensive drugs can cure hypertension.

7. When administering an antihypertensive drug to a patient who has a history of hypertension and type 2 diabetes mellitus, what would be an appropriate outcome for therapy?
   a. BP 100/60 to 110/70 mm Hg
   b. BP 110/70 to 130/80 mm Hg
   c. BP 120/80 to 130/85 mm Hg
   d. BP 128/80 to 138/90 mm Hg

8. The nurse is teaching a prehypertensive patient about healthy eating. Which of the following snacks would be most beneficial for BP control?
   a. Broccoli
   b. Celery
   c. Cheddar cheese
   d. Red pepper

9. Match the action of the following antihypertensives with the logical adverse effects for which the nurse should assess.
   _____ a. Arterial dilators
   _____ b. Beta blockers
   _____ c. Diuretics
   _____ d. Venodilators
   1. Dizziness and fainting
   2. Peripheral edema
   3. Slow heart rate
   4. Urinary output, electrolyte levels, and dehydration

10. A patient is hypertensive and receiving drug therapy. When would the nurse expect reflex tachycardia to be most likely to occur?

11. Match the drugs affecting the renin-angiotensin-aldosterone system (RAAS) with the actions.
    _____ a. Angiotensin-converting enzyme (ACE) inhibitors
    _____ b. Aldosterone
    _____ c. ARBs
    _____ d. Beta blockers
    1. Suppress renin release by the kidneys
    2. Prevent conversion of angiotensin I to angiotensin II
    3. Prevent activation of angiotensin receptors
    4. Block angiotensin II receptors

12. Which of the following laboratory results should be reported to the prescriber if a patient is receiving a thiazide or loop diuretic?
    a. Blood urea nitrogen (BUN) 20 mg/dL
    b. Hemoglobin A$_{1C}$ 5.5%
    c. Potassium (K$^+$) 3.2 mEq/L
    d. Uric acid 20 mg/dL

13. The nurse would teach a patient who is on which of the following diuretics to avoid use of potassium-containing salt substitutes and excessive consumption of bananas and orange juice?
    a. ethacrynic acid (Edecrin)
    b. furosemide (Lasix)
    c. hydrochlorothiazide (HydroDiuril)
    d. triamterene (Dyrenium)

14. Acebutolol (Sectral), carteolol (Cartrol), penbutolol (Levatol), and pindolol (Visken) are beta blockers that have intrinsic sympathomimetic activity. This results in less
    a. bradycardia at rest.
    b. bronchoconstriction.
    c. heart block.
    d. hypoglycemia.

15. When a patient has been prescribed an alpha$_1$ blocker, including doxazosin (Cardura), it is most important for the nurse to teach the patient to
    a. change positions slowly.
    b. include adequate potassium in the diet.
    c. monitor urinary output.
    d. seek medical care if chest pain occurs.

16. A patient would most likely experience reflex tachycardia if receiving which of the following antihypertensive drugs?
    a. ACE inhibitors
    b. Beta blockers
    c. Direct-acting vasodilators
    d. Nondihydropine calcium channel blockers

▸ 17. Nurses can make a significant contribution toward assisting a patient with controlling BP by
    a. identifying obstacles to adherence to therapy.
    b. suggesting drugs that can be effective.
    c. teaching the patient to assess their BP sitting and standing.
    d. telling the patient to exercise at least 30 minutes a day.

✳ 18. The nurse has administered an ACE inhibitor. Response to which of the following adverse effects, if it occurred, would be a priority?
    a. Cough that is non-productive
    b. High-pitched breathing
    c. Inspiratory crackles (rales)
    d. Expiratory gurgles (rhonchi) overlarge airways

19. The intervention that is most likely to decrease adverse effects of hypertension in African American adults is
    a. explaining measures to respond to adverse effects of antihypertensive drugs.
    b. identifying adverse effects of antihypertensive drugs.
    c. prescribing of the appropriate drug for hypertension.
    d. promoting regular screening of BP.

20. The nurse would expect pharmacotherapy for an African American patient with hypertension to include a(n)
    a. ACE inhibitor.
    b. calcium channel blocker.
    c. diuretic.
    d. vasodilator.

21. A positive hCG would be of most concern if the patient is prescribed
    a. captopril (Capoten).
    b. hydrochlorothiazide (HydroDiuril).
    c. prazosin (Minipress).
    d. propranolol (Inderal).

22. The best treatment for severe preeclampsia is
    a. delivery of the fetus.
    b. labetalol (Normodyne).
    c. lisinopril (Zestril).
    d. methyldopa (Aldomet).

▸ 23. A nurse has been administering magnesium sulfate to a patient with eclampsia. The nurse would notify the obstetrician if the magnesium level is
    a. 4 mEq/L.
    b. 5.5 mEq/L.
    c. 7 mEq/L.
    d. 8.5 mEq/L.

CASE STUDIES AND PATIENT TEACHING

(Use a separate piece of paper for your responses.)

Case Study 1

A 48-year-old African American male who is 5 ft 9 in tall and weighs 220 lb with a history of type 2 diabetes mellitus comes to the emergency department (ED) with a frontal headache and generalized complaints of "not feeling well." Upon examination, his BP is 210/120 mm Hg, pulse is 98, and respirations are 24 and labored.

1. What risk factors does this patient have for a cardiovascular event?

2. When is it important to lower this patient's BP within 1 hour rather than slowly as for most hypertensive patients?

3. The ED resident writes an order for intravenous nitroprusside 80 mg/min. Is this dose within the recommended dosage?

4. The resident changes the order to 80 mcg/min. What precautions should the nurse take while administering this medication?

5. The patient is stabilized and discharged on hydrochlorothiazide (HydroDiuril) and diltiazem (Cardizem). On the follow-up visit, the patient's BP is 160/90 mm Hg. The patient asks why the prescriber does not just give him a high enough dose to bring his BP down to normal. How should the nurse respond?

Case Study 2

The industrial nurse is creating a health promotion plan for factory workers relating to lifestyle changes that can prevent or minimize hypertension. Most workers are 25 to 55 years old. Based on developmental knowledge of the target population, use the Nola Pender revised Health Promotion Model (see below) to complete the following charts.

Consider the personal sociocultural factors of the age group to identify behavior-specific cognitions and affect influencing tobacco use.

INDIVIDUAL CHARACTERISTICS AND EXPERIENCES

- Personal sociocultural factors
  - Characteristics of the workers, including race, ethnicity, education, and sociocultural factors that influence beliefs, affect, and performance of a health-promoting behavior

Characteristics of 25- to 55-year-old factory workers who are regularly employed, but are struggling to pay all home expenses	How these characteristics influence ability and willingness to attempt health-promoting behavioral changes

BEHAVIOR-SPECIFIC COGNITIONS AND AFFECT

- Perceived benefits of action
  - Positive effects the person thinks they will experience from the lifestyle changes
- Perceived barriers to action
  - Negative effects the person thinks they will experience if they do not implement positive lifestyle changes
- Perceived self-efficacy
  - Belief that the person can be successful with lifestyle changes
- Activity-related affect
  - Positive and negative effects experienced when trying to change a behavior
- Interpersonal influences
  - Behaviors, beliefs, or attitudes of others that can influence the person's decision to change a behavior
- Situational influences
  - Environmental factors that can influence the person's decision to change a behavior

Reference

Pender, N, et al: *Health promotion in nursing practice,* 4th ed., Upper Saddle River, NJ, Prentice Hall, 2002.

Behavior-specific cognitions and affect	Recommended dietary changes	Developmentally appropriate plans to institute change
Perceived benefits of action		
Perceived barriers to action		
Perceived self-efficacy		
Activity-related affect		
Interpersonal influences		
Situational influences		

Behavior-specific cognitions and affect	Regular aerobic exercise	Nursing Interventions
Perceived benefits of action		
Perceived barriers to action		
Perceived self-efficacy		
Activity-related affect		
Interpersonal influences		
Situational influences		

Repeat this exercise with a patient during your clinical experience.

47

Drugs for Heart Failure

Answers can be reviewed online at http://evolve.elsevier.com/Lehne/.

OBJECTIVES

See page 28 for the Objectives.

CRITICAL THINKING AND STUDY QUESTIONS

1. Which of the following statements, if made by a patient with heart failure (HF), would indicate a need for further teaching?
   a. "If blood cannot get through my heart the backup of fluid will make it hard for me to breathe."
   b. "My heart is stretching so much it is loosing the ability to squeeze out the blood."
   c. "The changes in my heart started when I began to feel tired and short of breath."
   d. "When my heart beats too fast, it cannot fill properly."

2. Elevation of B-natriuretic peptide (BNP) suggests HF because BNP is released when the heart
   a. beats faster.
   b. chambers stretch.
   c. does not get enough oxygen.
   d. muscle thickens.

* 3. The nurse would be most concerned if a patient with HF exhibits which of the following symptoms?
   a. Swollen ankles
   b. Urine output of 825 mL in 24 hours
   c. Visible distention of the jugular veins when the patient is supine
   d. Weight gain of 2 lb in 24 hours

4. The nurse cannot hear the apical pulse of a patient with the diagnosis of HF when assessing at the 5th ICS at the midclavicular line. Which direction should the nurse move the stethoscope diaphragm/bell to be more likely to hear the pulse?
   a. Toward the clavicle
   b. Toward the left side
   c. Toward the sternum
   d. Toward the waist

5. Loop diuretics are the type of diuretic most commonly administered to hospitalized patients in HF because they
   a. are effective when kidney function declines.
   b. block receptors for aldosterone.
   c. do not increase the risk of digitalis toxicity.
   d. seldom cause hypotension.

6. Benefits of ACE inhibitors in HF include (Select all that apply.)
   a. improving renal blood flow.
   b. increasing renal excretion of sodium, potassium, and water.
   c. promoting proper functioning of baroreceptors.
   d. reducing peripheral vascular resistance.
   e. reducing venous congestion and edema.
   f. stimulating the release of aldosterone.

▶ 7. A patient with HF is prescribed eplerenone (Inspra) and enalapril (Vasotec). Which of the following symptoms, if exhibited by the patient, would warrant consultation with the prescriber regarding evaluation of the patient's potassium levels?
   a. Abdominal and muscle cramps
   b. Abdominal distention
   c. Diminished deep tendon reflexes
   d. Weakness and fatigue

8. Beta blockers differ from cardiac glycosides in that beta blockers
   a. decrease the rate of cardiac contraction.
   b. decrease the force of cardiac contraction.
   c. decrease the conduction of impulses through the heart.
   d. do not prolong life.

▶ 9. A maintenance intravenous (IV) infusion of inamrinone is prescribed for a patient who has a current infusion of 5% dextrose and 0.45% NaCl running at 45 mL/hr. The nurse should administer the inamrinone
   a. after flushing the primary line.
   b. as a secondary infusion through the primary line.
   c. over 2 to 3 minutes.
   d. via a second IV site.

10. Nitrates, including nitroglycerin and isosorbide, reduce the workload of the myocardium by
   a. decreasing the amount of blood returning to the heart.
   b. decreasing conduction of impulses through the heart.
   c. decreasing the volume of blood in the vascular system.
   d. increasing myocardial remodeling.

✳ 11. The nurse is preparing to administer hydralazine (Apresoline) for HF. Because this drug has been associated with drug-induced lupus-like syndrome, it would be a priority to report what symptom to the prescriber?
   a. Facial rash
   b. Heartburn
   c. Joint pain
   d. Smoky-colored urine

12. Before administering nitroglycerin to a new admission, it would be most important for the nurse to identify if the patient has recently self-medicated with a drug for
   a. erectile dysfunction.
   b. fever.
   c. itching.
   d. pain.

13. The nurse has diluted a single use vial of nesiritide (Natrecor) to 6 mcg/mL. How many mL should be administered to the patient who weighs 62 kg if 2 mcg/kg is prescribed?
   a. 5 mL
   b. 10 mL
   c. 20 mL
   d. 25 mL

14. A possible explanation for why digoxin has not demonstrated an improvement in mortality is that the drug does not
   a. decrease heart rate.
   b. improve heart remodeling.
   c. increase cardiac output.
   d. increase urine production.

▶ 15. When a patient with HF is prescribed digoxin and furosemide, the nurse should carefully assess the patient for early symptoms of the most likely electrolyte disturbance including
   a. anorexia and nausea.
   b. anxiety and abdominal cramps.
   c. bone pain and constipation.
   d. muscle spasms and convulsions.

▶ 16. What findings would warrant that the nurse not administer digoxin and notify the prescriber?
   a. Blood pressure 100/76 mm Hg
   b. Digoxin 2.4 ng/mL
   c. Heart rate 100 beats/min
   d. Potassium 5.3 mEq/L

17. The nurse would consult with the prescriber if a patient with HF who is experiencing pain is prescribed
    a. acetaminophen.
    b. imipramine.
    c. ibuprofen.
    d. morphine.

18. A fixed dose of hydralazine and isosorbide (BiDil) has been approved to treat HF in people of which descent?
    a. Hispanic
    b. Asian
    c. Mediterranean
    d. African

CASE STUDIES AND PATIENT TEACHING

(Use a separate piece of paper for your responses.)

Case Study 1

A 78-year-old female has been admitted to the nursing unit from the emergency department (ED) on a Sunday evening with a diagnosis of right intratrochanteric femur fracture. Open reduction and internal fixation of the fracture is planned for Monday morning pending medical clearance for surgery. The patient is placed in Buck's traction to relieve muscle spasm and maintain reduction of the fracture and has a Foley catheter inserted. The patient has a history of chronic HF, hypertension, type 2 diabetes mellitus, and chronic obstructive pulmonary disease. Current medication orders include aspirin 81 mg once a day, hydrochlorothiazide 25 mg once a day, atenolol (Tenormin) 50 mg once a day, ramipril (Altace) 5 mg once a day, glipizide/metformin (Metaglip) 2.5 mg 500 mg once a day, tiotropium (Spiriva) one inhalation per day, IV methylprednisolone 40 mg every 6 hours, and IV morphine 1 mg every 4 to 6 hours as needed. An IV solution of 5% dextrose in water is infusing at a rate of 83 mL per hour. Oxygen is being provided via nasal cannula at 2 L. The patient's daughter is very upset and tells the nurse that she thinks her mother fell because the doctor is drugging her with so many medications.

1. How should the nurse respond?

2. The 3 PM to 11 PM (1500 to 2300) nurse is making initial patient rounds. What assessments are a priority for the nurse to obtain at this time relating to the patient's cardiovascular status?

3. What problem may the nurse encounter in maintaining traction relating to the patient's history of HF?

Case Study 2

An 81-year-old male with chronic HF, who resides in a long-term care facility, has been treated with digoxin (Lanoxin) 0.25 mg, furosemide 80 mg, and potassium chloride (K-Dur) 20 mEq once a day by mouth for a long time. Recently, the prescriber added eplerenone (Inspra) 50 mg orally once a day to the medication regimen.

1. When consulting the prescriber about this patient, what questions might the nurse ask?

2. Why is it important for the nurse to monitor electrolyte and digoxin levels on this patient?

3. The long-term care nurse notes during report from the night shift that the patient has become increasingly restless, "coughs all night," and seems very fatigued when the staff is providing care. His appetite has been poor, even for things he normally enjoys. Assessment findings include BP 90/70 mm Hg; alternating weak and strong pulse at a rate of 118 beats/min, S3 ventricular gallop, rales throughout lung fields, and a 5-lb weight gain in the last week. What action should the nurse take at this time?

4. The patient is admitted to an acute care facility. Based on the knowledge of digoxin and its relationship to potassium, how could these blood levels have contributed to the patient's decompensation?

Case Study 3

A 64-year-old male patient is a direct admission to the nursing unit with the complaint of abdominal pain, nausea, and extreme weakness. The patient has a history of diabetes, chronic renal failure, and sleep apnea. Admission nursing assessment findings include temperature 99.3°F, BP 174/110 mm Hg, pulse 96 and irregular, PMI shifted to the left, JVD 4.5 cm above the angle of Louis, 3+ pitting edema in the lower extremities, and tenderness in the RUQ with abdominal palpation.

1. What nursing diagnosis is most appropriate for this patient?

2. The nurse obtains laboratory results from tests drawn on admission including BNP 1275 pg/mL; K⁺ 5.4 mEq/L, creatinine 2.7 mg/dL, BUN 42 mg/dL. The nurse contacts the prescriber who orders a stat electrocardiogram, which shows S-T changes. What action should the nurse take at this point?

3. The patient is transferred to the coronary care unit. Oxygen is administered along with furosemide (Lasix), morphine, nitroglycerin, and enalapril (Vasotec). What is the rationale for administration of these drugs?

4. The patient is stabilized and is transferred to the nursing unit. Prescribed drugs include carvedilol, enalapril, and furosemide. What laboratory values does the nurse need to monitor when a patient is receiving these drugs?

5. What teaching should the nurse provide to prepare this patient for discharge?

6. The patient lives in an apartment building with 12 stairs to climb to his apartment. After climbing the stairs, he needs to rest because he is short of breath. He can, however, perform most activities of daily living. According to the New York Heart Association (NYHA), what is this patient's HF classification?

48

Antidysrhythmic Drugs

Answers can be reviewed online at http://evolve.elsevier.com/Lehne/.

OBJECTIVES

See page 28 for the Objectives.

CRITICAL THINKING AND STUDY QUESTIONS

▶ 1. The priority nursing concern for a patient with a dysrhythmia is
   a. alteration in cardiac output.
   b. imbalance of fluid and electrolytes.
   c. inadequate peripheral tissue perfusion.
   d. ineffective breathing pattern.

2. Match the following electrolyte with its fast potential.

_____ a. Calcium   1. Blocking this ion from
_____ b. Potassium   entering slows depolari-
_____ c. Sodium   zation.
                      2. Blocking this ion from exit-
                         ing can reduce the force of
                         contraction.
                      3. Blocking this ion from exit-
                         ing increases the amount of
                         time when the cell cannot
                         be stimulated to contract.

▶ 3. Multiple P waves before the QRS complex on an ECG indicate
   a. atria are depolarizing faster than the ventricles.
   b. atrial impulses to the ventricles are being slowed.
   c. ventricles are depolarizing faster than the atria.
   d. ventricular impulses to the atria are being slowed.

4. Cells (ectopic) other than the sinoatrial node can dominate the pace of the heart if the discharges of the ectopic stimuli are
   a. atrial in origin.
   b. faster than the SA node.
   c. from the ventricles.
   d. slower than the SA node.

▶ 5. A patient has been prescribed an antidysrhythmic drug that prolongs the QT interval on ECG. The nurse should teach the patient the importance of reporting which of the following symptoms that suggests that the dangerous adverse effect, torsades de pointes, may be occuring?
   a. Ankle edema
   b. Feeling faint
   c. Headache
   d. Shortness of breath

6. A patient asks the nurse why she is receiving a different treatment for her dysrhythmia than her husband. The nurse's response should be based on the fact that selection of antidysrhythmic drug therapy selection is based on the patient's
   a. age.
   b. family history of dysrhythmia.
   c. response to drug therapy.
   d. sex.

▶ 7. An action that can slow an acute supraventricular dysrhythmia is instructing the patient to
   a. bear down as if having a bowel movement.
   b. breathe through pursed lips.
   c. pant like a dog.
   d. perform Kegel exercises.

▶ 8. A focused nursing assessment of a patient with atrial fibrillation should always include assessment of changes in
   a. appetite.
   b. deep tendon reflexes.
   c. kidney functioning.
   d. mental status.

▶ 9. Which of the following laboratory results for international normalized ratio (INR), if identified in a patient with atrial fibrillation who is receiving warfarin (Coumadin), would indicate that therapy has achieved the desired effect?
   a. INR 1
   b. INR 3
   c. INR 5
   d. INR 7

10. The nurse responds quickly when a ventricular tachydysrhythmia is identified because this type of dysrhythmia impairs the ability of the heart
   a. to contract rapidly enough to meet body needs.
   b. to eject an adequate amount of blood.
   c. valves to close properly.
   d. valves to open properly.

▶ 11. It would be most important for the nurse to promptly consult the physician if ventricular premature beats (VPBs) were noted during cardiac monitoring of a patient who has been admitted with the diagnosis of
   a. acute renal failure.
   b. chronic obstructive pulmonary disease.
   c. myocardial infarction.
   d. systemic lupus erythematosus.

12. Match the following antidysrhythmic drugs with their actions.

_____ a. Class I
_____ b. Class II
_____ c. Class III
_____ d. Class IV

1. Delay repolarization of fast potentials by blocking potassium (K$^+$) channels
2. Reduce calcium (Ca^{++}) entry during fast and slow depolarization and depress phase 4 repolarization of slow potentials
3. Slow impulse conduction in atria and ventricles by blocking sodium (Na$^+$) channels

▶ 13. A patient with a dysrhythmia, type 2 diabetes mellitus (DM), and heart failure (HF) is prescribed quinidine, metformin, furosemide, and digoxin. The nurse should be vigilant in monitoring for early adverse effects of digitalis toxicity, which may occur with this combination of drugs, including
   a. anorexia and nausea.
   b. cool, clammy skin.
   c. excessive urination and thirst.
   d. yellow tinted blurred vision.

14. A patient has received instructions regarding administration of quinidine. Which of these statements made by the patient would indicate the patient understood the directions?
   a. "I should take this medication 1 hour before or 2 hours after I eat food."
   b. "I should take this medication at bedtime."
   c. "I should take this medication first thing in the morning, 30 minutes before I eat or drink anything, and I should not lie down for at least 30 minutes after taking the drug."
   d. "I should take this medication with food."

▶ 15. Which of these assessment findings, if identified in a patient who is receiving quinidine, should the nurse report to the prescriber immediately?
   a. BP 150/88 mm Hg
   b. Difficulty hearing
   c. Three soft stools in 8 hours
   d. Wheezing at the end of expiration

16. A patient asks the nurse why he was instructed to take quinidine with food. An appropriate response by the nurse is that taking the drug with food
   a. decreases the incidence of diarrhea.
   b. increases absorption.
   c. prevents cinchonism.
   d. prevents ventricular tachycardia.

▶ 17. The nurse is monitoring the ECG of a patient who received the first dose of quinidine 45 minutes ago. The nurse notes that the QRS complex was widened 8% from pre-drug therapy findings. The nurse should
   a. administer a beta blocker.
   b. continue nursing care.
   c. discontinue monitoring the ECG.
   d. notify the prescriber immediately.

18. The nurse should assess patients receiving long-term therapy with procainamide for which of the following adverse effects? (Select all that apply.)
   a. Chest pain and dyspnea
   b. Elevated ANA and painful joint swelling
   c. Elevated platelet levels and increased thrombi formation
   d. Enlarged liver and elevated liver enzymes
   e. Sore throat, fever, and chills
   f. Ventricular tachycardia

▸ 19. The prescriber wrote an order to switch a patient from intravenous (IV) to oral procainamide. The IV drug was discontinued at 11:30 AM. When should the nurse administer the first dose of oral procainamide?
   a. Immediately
   b. 1:00 PM
   c. 2:30 PM
   d. 4:00 PM

20. When administering disopyramide (Norpace), the nurse should assess for which of the following anticholinergic adverse effects of the drug?
   a. Chest pain and palpitations
   b. Nausea, vomiting, and diarrhea
   c. Isolated systolic hypertension
   d. Postvoid residual greater than 100 mL of urine

21. Because of extensive first-pass effect, the nurse expects to administer lidocaine
   a. in a sustained-release formula.
   b. intravenously.
   c. orally, on an empty stomach.
   d. with a full glass of water.

▸ 22. The nurse is preparing to administer the cardioselective beta blocker acebutolol (Sectral). Which of the following assessments would indicate the need for immediate consultation with the prescriber?
   a. Apical pulse 155 beats/min
   b. Bronchial wheezes
   c. Capillary blood glucose 220 mg/dL
   d. One plus pitting edema of the dorsal aspect of the foot

23. In addition to monitoring the heart rate and rhythm, what must the nurse continuously monitor when administering the potassium channel blockers, bretylium, or amiodarone?
   a. Blood pressure
   b. Level of consciousness
   c. Intravenous site
   d. Respiratory effort

24. The patient must be informed of possible damage to the lungs when prescribed oral therapy with which of the following drugs?
   a. amiodarone (Cordarone)
   b. dofetilide (Tikosyn)
   c. propafenone (Rhythmol)
   d. propranolol (Inderal)

▸ 25. Because verapamil (Calan) can cause blockade of calcium channels in vascular smooth muscle, the nurse should teach a patient who is prescribed this drug to
   a. drink 2500 mL of fluid each day, especially water.
   b. increase fiber in diet.
   c. take orthostatic BP precautions.
   d. report bruising.

▸ 26. A patient who weighs 165 lb is prescribed IV diltiazem. The recommended initial bolus dose is 0.25 mg/kg. What is the recommended dose for this patient?

▸ 27. When a patient who is receiving adenosine exhibits facial flushing and chest pain, which action should the nurse take first?
   a. Administer oxygen.
   b. Assess vital signs.
   c. Discontinue the infusion.
   d. Initiate CPR.

28. In most cases the need for antidysrhythmic drugs exceeds the risks of adverse effects when
   a. the dysrhythmia is prolonged.
   b. the QT interval is excessively long.
   c. ventricular pumping is ineffective.
   d. the sinoatrial node discharges at a rate exceeding 160 beats/min.

▸ 29. A patient with a dysrhythmia, type 2 diabetes mellitus (DM), and heart failure (HF) is prescribed quinidine, metformin, furosemide, and digoxin. The patient complains of nausea, and the nurse notes that the patient has only consumed 10% to 25% of his meals over the past 48 hours. The nurse should review the most recent laboratory results for
   a. digoxin levels less than 0.8 ng/mL.
   b. fasting blood glucose less than 60 mg/dL.
   c. potassium levels less than 3.5 mEq/L.
   d. sodium levels less than 140 mEq/L.

CASE STUDIES AND PATIENT TEACHING

(Use a separate piece of paper for your responses.)

Case Study 1

An overweight 75-year-old retiree underwent open-heart surgery 5 days ago and postoperatively developed a cerebrovascular accident (CVA). His history includes hypertension, renal insufficiency, alcohol abuse, and a 2-pack-per-day smoking habit. He was progressing well postoperatively without any further complications. A physical therapist and nurse assisted the patient to transfer to a chair. Following transfer to a recliner, the patient complained to the physical therapist that his "heart felt like it was racing."

1. What assessments should the nurse perform at this time?

The monitor nurse walks in to check on the patient because the monitor revealed a heart rate of 185 beats/min. The nurse asks the patient to bear down to stimulate the vagus nerve and slow the heart rate. After obtaining a full set of vital signs, the nurse places a call to the attending physician. The physician orders a STAT 12-lead ECG. The attending physician arrives on the unit, examines the 12-lead ECG, and diagnoses ventricular tachycardia (v-tach). A bolus dose of lidocaine 100 mg is ordered.

2. What elements of the patient's history are important when the prescriber is determining the dose of lidocaine to be infused?

3. What precautions must the nurse take when administering this bolus dose?

4. The bolus dose is followed by an infusion of a solution of lidocaine. What patient data can the nurse provide to assist the prescriber with determining the amount of fluid in which to dilute the lidocaine?

5. One gram of lidocaine in 250 mL of 5% dextrose in water at a rate of 2 mg/min is prescribed. The IV pump is calibrated in mL per hour. What rate should be programmed into the pump?

6. Before infusing the drug, the nurse should examine the IV solution and not administer the drug if the solution contains what additives?

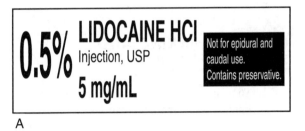

A

B

C

7. What should be included when the nurse reports to the prescriber the patient's response to lidocaine?

Answers can be reviewed online at http://evolve.elsevier.com/Lehne/.

OBJECTIVES

See page 28 for the Objectives.

CRITICAL THINKING AND STUDY QUESTIONS

1. The nurse is teaching a patient with hyperlipidemia dietary interventions to reduce her serum cholesterol. The patient's dietary history includes the following foods. Which food is likely to cause the greatest increase in the patient's circulating cholesterol?
   a. Avocado
   b. Honey
   c. Milk
   d. Olive oil

2. A 45-year-old female smoker with a family history of coronary heart disease (CHD) has been prescribed a lipid-lowering medication. Which of these outcomes would be most important for this patient?
   a. Cholesterol, total 170 mg/dL
   b. HDL 50 mg/dL
   c. LDL 90 mg/dL
   d. Triglycerides 120 mg/dL

3. A patient has received instructions regarding cholesterol and the body. Which of these statements made by the client would indicate the patient needs further teaching?
   a. "Drugs that decrease the liver's ability to produce cholesterol should be taken so that they peak during the night."
   b. "Drugs that prevent the absorption of cholesterol from food are more effective than drugs that limit the making of cholesterol by the liver."
   c. "It is more important to limit the amount of saturated fat in my diet than the total amount of cholesterol."
   d. "My cholesterol can be high even if I eat a low-fat diet and exercise regularly."

4. Recent laboratory results for a patient include HDL 85 mg/dL, LDL 145 mg/dL, and triglycerides 630 mg/dL. The nurse should assess the patient for
   a. abdominal pain and nausea.
   b. chest pain and shortness of breath.
   c. rash and pruritus.
   d. tachycardia and diaphoresis.

5. The nurse is preparing a seminar for a community health fair. Which of the following risk factors for CHD should be stressed because they correlate to the greatest risk of a major coronary event within 10 years? (Select all that apply.)
   a. Abdominal aortic aneurysm
   b. Diabetes insipidus
   c. Diabetes mellitus
   d. HDL cholesterol less than 50 mg/dL
   e. Older than 44 years of age
   f. Peripheral artery disease
   g. Smoker
   h. Systolic blood pressure greater than 120 mm Hg

6. The nurse is caring for a 68-year-old man who has been admitted for a left below-the-knee amputation because of peripheral vascular disease associated with type 2 diabetes mellitus. He is receiving a lipid-lowering drug. Which of these levels of LDL would be an appropriate outcome for pharmacotherapy?
   a. LDL 35 mg/dL
   b. LDL 50 mg/dL
   c. LDL 85 mg/dL
   d. LDL 115 mg/dL

7. A 42-year-old female is 5'4" tall, 202 lb, waist circumference is 42", resting BP is 155/72 mm Hg, P 72 BPM, R 24/min. Current screening laboratory results include FBS 95 mg/dL, triglycerides 328 mg/dL, HDL 49 mg/dL. This patient is at risk for CHD because she exhibits the symptoms of
   a. Addison's disease.
   b. atherosclerosis.
   c. diabetes mellitus.
   d. metabolic syndrome.

8. Clinical trials suggest that HMG-CoA reductase inhibitors (statins) benefit patients with atherosclerosis by
   a. increasing serum LDL.
   b. promoting the production of thrombin.
   c. reducing serum HDL.
   d. stabilizing endothelial plaque.

▶ 9. The nurse has reviewed the laboratory results for a patient who is scheduled to receive lovastatin (Mevacor) 40 mg. Results include AST 78 international units/L, CK 100 units/L, HDL 45 mg/dL, and LDL 245 mg/dL. The nurse should
   a. administer the drug and continue nursing care.
   b. hold the drug and assess for chest pain.
   c. hold the drug and assess for abdominal pain.
   d. hold the drug and notify the prescriber of the laboratory results.

▶ 10. A 38-year-old female has been diagnosed with hypercholesterolemia. The prescriber has ordered simvastatin (Zocor) 20 mg, once a day at hour of sleep, to be started after laboratory results are obtained. Which of the following laboratory results would be a reason to withhold the drug?
   a. ALT 7 international units/L
   b. Creatinine 1 mg/international units/dL
   c. CRP 3 mg/dL
   d. hCG 287 international units/L

✳ 11. A patient who is receiving lovastatin experiences chest pain. CK level is 580 units/mL (CK-MM 99%) and troponin T 0.02 g/mL. It is a priority for the nurse to monitor the functioning of which organ?
   a. Brain
   b. Heart
   c. Kidneys
   d. Lungs

▶ 12. A patient who is receiving nicotinic acid to elevate HDL and reduce triglycerides exhibits dry, hot, and flushed skin; thirst; hunger; and confusion. The nurse should
   a. assess for chest pain.
   b. assess for abdominal pain.
   c. continue nursing care.
   d. notify the prescriber.

13. The nurse has been caring for a patient admitted with dehydration. The patient has been taking cholestyramine (Questran) and complains of nausea. Which of the following assessment findings would be of most concern to the nurse?
   a. Bloating after medication administration
   b. Flatulence
   c. Increase in bowel sounds and "hush" sounds
   d. Indigestion

14. A patient has been prescribed cholestyramine in addition to other drugs for diabetes mellitus and hypertension. The cholestyramine should be administered
   a. 1 hour before other drugs.
   b. 2 hours before other drugs.
   c. 3 hours before other drugs.
   d. 4 hours before other drugs.

15. The nurse should teach a patient who has been prescribed colestipol (Colestid) to prevent the most common adverse effect by
   a. avoiding gas-producing vegetables.
   b. consuming 2500 mL of fluid each day.
   c. decreasing fat in the diet.
   d. taking the medication with milk.

16. The nurse would be most concerned about which of the following patients?
   a. A patient receiving lovastatin and experiencing a rash
   b. A patient receiving nicotinic acid and experiencing hot flashes with facial flushing
   c. A patient receiving colesevelam and experiencing nausea
   d. A patient receiving gemfibrozil and experiencing right upper quadrant pain

CASE STUDIES AND PATIENT TEACHING

(Use a separate piece of paper for your responses.)

Case Study 1

A 52-year-old white female underwent a thorough physical examination. She smokes one pack of cigarettes each day and leads a sedentary lifestyle because of knee pain from osteoarthritis. She takes acetaminophen every day for joint pain, but does not take any prescription medications. Her examination was unremarkable except for being overweight. Her vital signs included BP 140/80 mm Hg, pulse 78 beats/min, and respirations 22 and regular. Her family history is negative for coronary artery disease (CAD), myocardial infarction (MI), and cerebrovascular accident (CVA). Her diet is high in fat because of her intake of fast foods. Her laboratory results include cholesterol 285 mg/dL, HDL 33 mg/dL, and LDL 129 mg/dL.

1. What is her 10-year risk for CHD according to the Framingham Risk Prediction Score?

2. Because of the elevated cholesterol in addition to a low HDL, the patient is considered to be at an increased risk for CAD. The physician has placed her on a restricted diet in an attempt to lower serum cholesterol and has mentioned that if this does not correct the problem, he may need to place her on medication. She asks the nurse about nondrug therapies that she can implement in an attempt to lower her cholesterol. What should be included in the nurse's response?

3. The patient returns 3 months later and has shown no improvement in lipid levels despite therapeutic lifestyle changes. Atorvastatin 10 mg at bedtime is prescribed. When the patient gets to the pharmacy, the pharmacist informs her that her prescription plan does not cover atorvastatin, but he has called the prescriber and received an order to dispense lovastatin 20 mg once a day, to be taken with the evening meal. After going home, the patient calls the prescriber's office and asks to speak with the nurse. She is upset about the change in medication and asks why she has been given a different drug with a higher dose, to be taken at a different time of the day. How should the nurse respond?

Case Study 2

The middle school nurse is concerned about the incidence of obesity in the fifth and sixth grade population of the inner city school. The physical education faculty have collaborated with the nurse and identified that many of the children do not get outside for active play because of danger in the neighborhood. They are planning an activity to help the children make healthier choices.

1. What are possible developmentally appropriate health promotion strategies that could be included?

50

Drugs for Angina Pectoris

Answers can be reviewed online at http://evolve.elsevier.com/Lehne/.

OBJECTIVES

See page 28 for the Objectives.

CRITICAL THINKING AND STUDY QUESTIONS

▶ 1. The priority nursing concern for a patient with angina pectoris is
   a. alteration in cardiac output.
   b. impaired gas exchange.
   c. inadequate myocardial tissue perfusion.
   d. ineffective breathing pattern.

2. The goal of drug therapy for chronic stable angina is to
   a. constrict coronary arteries to increase blood pressure during stress.
   b. decrease myocardial need for oxygen during stress.
   c. increase myocardial blood flow during systole.
   d. prevent coronary artery spasms.

3. Match drugs for unstable angina pectoris with their therapeutic effect.

_____ a. ACE inhibitor
_____ b. Anticoagulant
_____ c. Antiplatelet
_____ d. Beta blocker
_____ e. Morphine
_____ f. Nitroglycerin-(NTG)

1. Decrease venous thrombus formation.
2. Prevent thrombocytes from sticking to plaque in arteries.
3. Reduce blood returning to heart by venous dilation, decreasing workload of heart.
4. Relieve pain, which decreases sympathetic stimulation and myocardial workload.
5. Slow heart rate, decreasing myocardial need for oxygen.
6. Vasodilate and increase fluid excretion, decreasing blood pressure.

4. A patient asks the nurse why nitroglycerin can be administered in so many ways. The basis of the nurse's response is that nitroglycerin
   a. does not undergo first-pass effect in the liver.
   b. has few adverse effects, so varying doses can be administered via different routes.
   c. is an inactive compound, so it does not matter which route it is administered.
   d. is lipid soluble, so it is readily absorbed via different routes.

5. Nitroglycerin has myocardial vasodilation effects in variant (Prinzmetal's) angina but not in chronic stable angina because in chronic stable angina myocardial arterioles are
   a. already maximally dilated.
   b. experiencing spastic vasoconstriction.
   c. occluded with thrombi.
   d. unable to diffuse oxygen into the cell.

6. A patient who has been using a nitroglycerin patch for angina has recently been prescribed diltiazem (Cardizem). Which statement, if made by this patient, would suggest that the patient understood teaching about the new drug?
   a. "I need to take this drug because nitroglycerin causes my blood pressure to go up."
   b. "If I take both of these drugs, I can use sildenafil (Viagra) if I experience erectile dysfunction."
   c. "This drug prevents my heart from racing, which can happen when people take nitroglycerin."
   d. "This drug will make the nitroglycerin work better."

7. A patient is prescribed a nitroglycerin patch that is to be applied at 0900 (9:00 AM) and removed at 2100 (9:00 PM). When preparing to administer the 0900 patch, the nurse notes that a nitroglycerin patch is still in place. The nurse should
   a. apply the new patch to a different site, but leave the old patch on until the nursing supervisor is contacted.
   b. consult with the prescriber.
   c. remove the old patch and apply the new patch to a different site.
   d. remove the old patch and change the timing of the medication so that the patch is removed at 0900 and applied at 2100.

8. During data collection from a patient who is not obtaining relief from nitroglycerin tablets, the nurse should ask the patient if she allows the tablet to completely dissolve while in her mouth because swallowing sublingual nitroglycerin tablets
   a. inactivates the drug.
   b. increases tolerance.
   c. prevents absorption.
   d. speeds excretion.

9. It is important for the nurse to teach a patient who has been prescribed nitroglycerin (NitroQuick) on an as needed basis to
   a. discard unused tablets after 12 months.
   b. store the tablets in a locked medicine cabinet in the bathroom.
   c. take a few tablets from the bottle and keep them in a plastic bottle in your purse or pocket for emergency use.
   d. write the date that the tablets are opened on the outside of the bottle.

10. When assessing a patient who is scheduled to receive the second dose of newly prescribed sustained-release nitroglycerin, the patient complains of a headache. The nurse should
    a. administer an ordered mild analgesic such as acetaminophen.
    b. crush the medication to speed absorption through the oral mucosa.
    c. notify the prescriber of the headache STAT.
    d. withhold the drug and consult the prescriber.

11. The nurse is aware that which of the following nitroglycerin preparations has a rapid onset and sustained effect?
    a. Sublingual tablets
    b. Sustained-release capsule
    c. Topical ointment
    d. Transdermal patch
    e. Translingual spray
    f. Transmucosal tablet

12. Intravenous (IV) nitroglycerin is prescribed at a rate of 5 mcg/min for a patient in the emergency department (ED). The drug is available in a premixed glass bottle with 5 mg/250 mL of 5% dextrose in water (D_5W). The IV pump is calibrated in mL/hr. At what rate should the nurse program the pump?

13. Cigarette smoking causes coronary artery disease by
    a. damaging the heart valves.
    b. increasing the heart rate.
    c. narrowing arteries.
    d. stretching the ventricles.

14. It would be most important for the nurse to report to the prescriber that a family member smokes cigarettes in the home if a patient is prescribed which of the following medications for angina?
    a. Amyl nitrate
    b. Beta blocker
    c. Diltiazem or verapamil
    d. Isosorbide
    e. Nitroglycerin

15. The nurse recognizes that a drug is a beta blocker if the generic name of the drug ends in
    a. -cillin.
    b. -lol.
    c. -pril.
    d. -sartan.

16. Beta blockers are useful to improve myocardial oxygen supply in angina because they slow the heart rate and force and
    a. dilate coronary arteries.
    b. dilate veins.
    c. lengthen the time that blood enters coronary arteries.
    d. reduce blood return to the heart.

17. The nurse would withhold a beta blocker and immediately contact the prescriber if it was discovered that the patient has a history of
    a. asthma.
    b. first-degree heart block.
    c. hyperglycemia.
    d. sick sinus syndrome.

18. The nurse would assess for bradycardia when an anginal patient is receiving which of the following drugs for angina?
    a. Diltiazem
    b. Isosorbide
    c. Metoprolol
    d. Nifedipine
    e. Nitroglycerin
    f. Verapamil

19. Which of the following would warrant notification of a prescriber when the nurse is caring for a patient who is receiving ranolazine (Ranexa)? (Select all that apply.)
    a. eGFR 95 mL/min
    b. Patient just diagnosed as HIV+
    c. Penicillin prescribed for upper respiratory infection
    d. Patient occasionally has grapefruit juice for breakfast
    e. Systolic BP decreases 8 mm Hg with position changes
    f. Unexplained fainting

CASE STUDIES AND PATIENT TEACHING

(Use a separate piece of paper for your responses.)

Case Study 1

A 75-year-old male with a history of stable angina, asthma, and hypertension is admitted to the hospital with substernal chest pain that was not relieved by 3 sublingual nitroglycerin (NTG) tablets. In the ED, the patient is prescribed diltiazem and an IV nitroglycerin drip.

1. What actions must the nurse take when administering IV nitroglycerin?

2. The patient's pain is relieved after receiving a dosage of 330 mcg/hr. He is admitted to the coronary care unit. His vital signs are stable, and he is currently without pain. Cardiac enzyme levels do not suggest myocardial cell death. The ECG shows normal sinus rhythm. The physicians believe that the patient is having classic angina and not a myocardial infarction (MI). The attending physician orders that the patient be weaned from the nitroglycerin drip and that nitroglycerin transdermal patches 10 mg/24 hr be started. He is also prescribed aspirin 81 mg, diltiazem-CD (30 mg) and ramipril (Altace) 2.5 mg, which he is to receive once a day. If the prescriber wants a continuous administration of nitroglycerin when changing the patient from the nitroglycerin drip to the patch, when, in relation to discontinuing the IV nitroglycerin, should the nurse apply the nitroglycerin patch?

3. What teaching should the nurse provide about administration of the nitroglycerin patch?

4. The patient has the nitroglycerin drip turned off, the nitroglycerin patch is applied, and the diltiazem-CD is administered. He asks the nurse what may have been the reason that his nitroglycerin sublingual tablets did not work. Based on knowledge of nitroglycerin sublingual tablets, what factors may have contributed to why the nitroglycerin tablets may not have relieved his anginal pain?

5. The nurse asks the patient's wife to bring his supply of sublingual nitroglycerin tablets in to the hospital. The wife pulls out a small plastic pill container from her purse. "Heart pills" is handwritten on a masking tape label. What teaching does the nurse need to provide?

6. The patient states that he guesses he will not need to get any more nitroglycerin sublingual tablets now that he is using the nitroglycerin patches. How should the nurse respond?

7. The nurse is reviewing medications during discharge instructions. The patient admits to adherence issues with taking his antihypertensive drug therapy because of experiencing erectile dysfunction. He asks what the nurse thinks about sildenafil (Viagra). What information should the nurse provide?

Case Study 2

A farmer who lives in a remote area was admitted with chest pain. He has been diagnosed with angina and is being discharged with a prescription for sublingual nitroglycerin tablets.

1. What teaching should the nurse provide about administration and storage of this drug?

2. The prescriber has written instructions that this patient should take the nitroglycerin before participating in stressful activity. What teaching should the nurse provide, considering farm work includes operation of potentially dangerous equipment?

3. The prescriber has instructed this patient to continue to take nitroglycerin up to 3 tablets 5 minutes apart, take an aspirin, and to seek emergency medical care if relief is not obtained after administration of the first sublingual nitroglycerin tablet. The patient's wife states that her mother took nitroglycerin and had been instructed to seek medical care if not obtaining relief after taking 3 tablets. Why are the prescriber's instructions logical for this patient?

4. The patient has been instructed to take 1 baby aspirin tablet per day. The patient verbalizes that this seems silly as 1 baby aspirin tablet will not do much to relieve his chest pain. How should the nurse respond?

Case Study 3

The occupational nurse is preparing for a health promotion fair at the manufacturing plant. Coronary artery disease (CAD) has been identified at a level higher than the national and state level in the community where the plant is located. The nurse wants to develop a teaching plan, including realistic interventions to help employees and their families prevent the incidence and adverse effects of CAD.

1. Complete this chart that could be used by the nurse as the basis for developing a presentation appropriate for this setting.

Coronary Artery Disease		
Risk Factors for CAD	**How this factor increases risk of CAD**	**Interventions to prevent, reverse, or minimize negative effects on heart**
Smoking		
High cholesterol		
Hypertension		
Diabetes		
Obesity		
Physical inactivity		

51

Anticoagulant, Antiplatelet, and Thrombolytic Drugs

Answers can be reviewed online at http://evolve.elsevier.com/Lehne/.

OBJECTIVES

See page 28 for the Objectives.

CRITICAL THINKING AND STUDY QUESTIONS

1. A patient asks why heparin cannot be administered orally. The basis of the nurse's response is heparin
   a. has a prolonged half-life when administered orally.
   b. can only be prepared as an oral solution and is bitter tasting.
   c. is destroyed by proteases in the gastrointestinal tract.
   d. is large and negatively charged, limiting absorption.

✳ 2. Which of these laboratory test results (which are flagged on the laboratory sheet as abnormal) would be a priority to report to the prescriber if a patient is prescribed heparin?
   a. aPTT 75 seconds
   b. BUN 22 mg/dL
   c. Platelet count 40,000/mm³
   d. WBC 11,000/mm³

▸ 3. A patient who has been receiving heparin tells the nurse that she thinks she could be pregnant. The nurse should
   a. administer the heparin as ordered and notify the prescriber of the possible pregnancy status.
   b. withhold the heparin.
   c. withhold the heparin until pregnancy status can be confirmed.
   d. withhold the heparin and consult the prescriber regarding administration of the antidote protamine sulfate.

▸ 4. A patient has been receiving long-term high-dose heparin therapy. What nursing teaching would be best to prevent a common adverse effect of this type of therapy?
   a. Avoid crowds
   b. Develop a plan for weight-bearing exercise as approved by healthcare provider
   c. Increase fluid and fiber in diet
   d. Regular use of any over-the-counter antacid

5. Protamine sulfate acts as an antidote to heparin by
   a. activating clotting factor Xa.
   b. activating thrombin.
   c. binding with the negatively charged groups on the heparin molecule.
   d. suppressing antithrombin activity.

▸ 6. A patient is scheduled for a below-knee amputation at 1000 (10:00 AM) the next day. Heparin 5000 units are scheduled to be administered subcutaneously (subQ) at 2100 (9:00 PM) today. The nurse should
   a. administer the medication.
   b. withhold the medication and contact the prescriber.

▸ 7. A patient who received 5000 units of heparin subQ at 0900 develops hematemesis at 1030. The prescriber orders 50 mg of protamine sulfate via slow intravenous (IV) push injection. Protamine sulfate is available as 10 mg/mL. If the nurse administers this dose over 10 minutes, how much should be administered every 15 seconds?

8. Heparin therapy is considered therapeutic when the results of the aPTT are
   a. 30 to 40 seconds.
   b. 40 to 50 seconds.
   c. 60 to 80 seconds.
   d. 90 to 120 seconds.

9. One unit of heparin will prevent 1 mL of sheep plasma from coagulating for what period of time?
   a. 1 hour
   b. 2 hours
   c. 4 hours
   d. 12 hours

10. It is important for the nurse to distinguish between concentrations of heparin used for IV flushing from concentrations used for subQ injection because the concentration for subQ use is how much greater than that for IV flushing?
    a. 1 to 25 times greater
    b. 10 to 100 times greater
    c. 25 to 400 times greater
    d. 100 to 2500 times greater

11. The nurse would consult the prescriber if which of the following drugs was prescribed, but there was no order for monitoring of aPTT?
    a. Fragmin
    b. Heparin
    c. Innohep
    d. Lovenox

12. The nurse is teaching a patient about rivaroxaban (Xarelto) prescribed for after right knee replacement. Which of the following statements, if made by the patient, suggests that he understands the teaching?
    a. "I should use a soft tooth brush and electric razor."
    b. "I should not touch the needle when injecting this drug."
    c. "I only need to have a blood test once a month when taking this drug."
    d. "If I have sudden shortness of breath, I should sit down and rest."

▶ 13. A patient who weighs 176 lb has been prescribed IV lepirudin (Refludan) 12 mg/hr after experiencing heparin-induced thrombocytopenia. Before the first dose, the nurse

reviews the patient's laboratory results, which include patient aPTT 47 seconds, reference aPTT 40 seconds, creatinine clearance 42 mL/min/1.73 m², AST 35 units/L, and ALT 22 international units/L. Which of the following is a possible concern to the nurse that should be communicated to the prescriber?
    a. Abnormal aPTT
    b. Dose too high for weight
    c. Liver dysfunction
    d. Renal insufficiency

▶ 14. The nurse should teach patients who are prescribed warfarin (Coumadin) to eat consistent amounts of which of the following foods? (Select all that apply.)
    a. Cabbage
    b. Citrus fruits
    c. Dairy products
    d. Green leafy vegetables
    e. Liver
    f. Mayonnaise
    g. Red meat

15. Which of the following should the nurse teach a patient about precautions before dental surgery when the patient is prescribed long-term warfarin therapy?
    a. No action is needed.
    b. Inform the dentist of the most recent international normalized ration (INR) results.
    c. Stop warfarin 3 days before dental surgery.
    d. Take half of the normal dose of warfarin for 3 days before dental surgery.

▶ 16. A patient is diagnosed with gastrointestinal (GI) bleeding during warfarin therapy. The nurse is preparing to administer IV phytonadione (Vitamin K₁). Assessment findings include INR 5.8, blood pressure 98/54 mm Hg, oxygen saturation 96%, respirations 25 breaths per minute, and temperature 102.8°F. The nurse should
    a. administer acetaminophen to reduce fever.
    b. administer aspirin to reduce fever.
    c. administer the IV phytonadione (vitamin K₁) very slowly.
    d. withhold the IV phytonadione (vitamin K₁) and contact the prescriber.

17. For what period of time should the nurse take precautions to prevent bleeding, including applying pressure to puncture sites for 5 min-

utes, after warfarin (Coumadin) therapy has been discontinued?
a. 6 hours
b. 8 to 12 hours
c. 2.5 days
d. 5 days

18. Which of the following statements, if made by a patient who has been prescribed low-dose aspirin therapy, would indicate a need for further teaching?
a. "I need to inform my pharmacist that I am taking aspirin therapy."
b. "I should quit smoking."
c. "I should not use a drug that reduces stomach acid while on aspirin therapy."
d. "If I use an enteric-coated aspirin, I don't need to worry about my stomach."

▶ 19. Which of the following adverse effects, if noted in a patient who has recently been prescribed ticlopidine (Ticlid), would be a reason for the nurse to contact the prescriber immediately?
a. Change in level of consciousness
b. Diarrhea
c. Dyspepsia
d. Itchy rash

▶ 20. The nurse is reviewing the laboratory tests of a patient who has been prescribed ticlopidine (Ticlid) for the past week. The WBC count is 3000/mm^3, and the neutrophil count is 30%. A nursing priority for this patient is
a. adequate cardiac output.
b. effective airway clearance.
c. maintaining skin integrity.
d. preventing infection.

▶ 21. Which of the following laboratory tests, if not ordered for a patient who has been recently prescribed clopidogrel (Plavix), would be a reason for the nurse to consult with the prescriber?
a. aPTT
b. INR
c. Platelets
d. PT

▶ 22. The nurse calculates the safe dose of tirofiban (Aggrastat) for a 220-lb patient undergoing balloon angioplasty per table 51-7. The drug comes in a solution of 12.5 mg/250 mL. The IV pump is calibrated in milliliters per hour. What rate will the nurse enter into the IV pump per hour?
a. 24 mL/hr
b. 48 mL/hr

c. 72 mL/hr
d. 96 mL/hr

▶ 23. The nurse teaches a patient who has been prescribed cilostazol (Pletal) that risk of the adverse effect of bleeding is increased if the patient includes in the diet which of the following foods?
a. Cabbage
b. Dairy products
c. Grapefruit juice
d. Green vegetables

24. Which of the following drugs should be available when streptokinase is being administered?
a. Aminocaproic acid (Amicar)
b. Phytonadione (Vitamin K$_1$)
c. Protamine sulfate

25. The critical care nurse monitors for the adverse effects of hypotension and fever in a patient who is receiving which of the following thrombolytic drugs?
a. Alteplase
b. Reteplase
c. Streptokinase
d. Tenecteplase

CASE STUDIES AND PATIENT TEACHING

(Use a separate piece of paper for your responses.)

Case Study 1

A 185-lb patient with a history of osteoarthritis, type 2 diabetes mellitus, hypertension, hyperlipidemia, and benign prostatic hyperplasia experiences pulmonary emboli after right total hip replacement surgery.

The prescriber orders include:
- *STAT baseline CBC, INR, aPTT, and platelets*
- *If baseline laboratory results are within normal limits:*
  - *One dose of heparin 100 units/kg IV push (round to nearest 100 units)*
  - *Heparin 25,000 units/250 mL 5% dextrose in water to infuse at 12 units/kg/hr*
  - *STAT aPTT 6 hours after start of heparin infusion*

1. Baseline laboratory results are within normal limits. How much heparin will the nurse administer as the initial IV push dose in units?

2. Heparin is available in concentrations of 100 units/mL and 5000 units/mL. Which concentration of heparin should the nurse use, and how many milliliters should the nurse administer IV push for the initial dose?

3. What is the initial dose and infusion rate of heparin based on the above orders?

Further heparin orders are by the following protocol (round to nearest 100 units):

aPTT (sec)	IV Bolus (units)	Hold Heparin (min)	IV Heparin Rate Change	Repeat aPTT and INR
Less than 50 sec	5000	0	+ 3 units/hr	4 hr
50–59 sec	0	0	+ 2 units/hr	6 hr
60–80 sec	0	0	none	Next AM
80–95 sec	0	0	−2 units/hr	6 hr
96–120 sec	0	30	−3 units/hr	4 hr
Greater than 120 sec	0	60	Contact prescriber	4 hr

4. The patient's aPTT results after 6 hours of heparin therapy is 30 seconds. Based on the protocol, the nurse should set the infusion pump to what rate?

5. After 12 hours, the patient's aPTT results are 75 seconds. What actions should the nurse take?

6. What precautions should the nurse take to prevent accidentally infusing too much IV heparin?

7. The hospital has a policy that heparin must be infused using a separate IV site and separate pump. Piggyback medication can never be added to the heparin line. The patient asks why she must have two IV sites. What would the nurse include in her explanation?

8. After 4 days, the IV heparin is discontinued, and the patient is ordered subQ heparin. How soon after discontinuation of the IV heparin do anticoagulant effects diminish and end?

9. Describe the technique for nursing administration of subQ heparin, including the rationale for each step.

10. What antidote should be available to the nurse when a patient is receiving heparin? How long does this antidote effect last?

Case Study 2

A 36-year-old, 132-lb female whose job requires frequent long airplane trips is admitted for treatment of a deep venous thrombosis (DVT) in the right thigh. The patient's husband asks why her primary care provider did not prescribe low-dose aspirin to prevent DVTs.

1. How should the nurse respond?

2. The patient is initially ordered a heparin drip by the emergency department physician. What is the most common adverse effect of heparin, and what symptoms of this adverse effect should be monitored by the nurse?

3. Heparin is pregnancy category C, which means that research studies suggest that risk to the developing fetus cannot be ruled out. If heparin does not cross the placenta, why is it not categorized as pregnancy class B?

4. The patient's primary care practitioner discontinues the IV heparin and orders enoxaparin 60 mg every 12 hours. How much time should elapse between the nurse discontinuing the heparin drip and starting the subQ enoxaparin (Lovenox)? Why?

Case Study 3

A patient is admitted with atrial fibrillation and is initially prescribed subQ heparin and warfarin.

1. Why are both anticoagulant drugs ordered for this patient?

2. Daily INR is ordered. What information does the nurse have to provide to the phlebotomist who will be collecting the blood sample for this test?

3. The patient asks what the INR measures. How should the nurse explain the results of this test?

4. After 4 days of both drugs, the patient is to be discharged with a prescription for warfarin (Coumadin). What is the antidote and dosing for an overdose of warfarin?

5. What patient information does the nurse need to provide the patient before he is discharged home on warfarin?

52

Management of ST-Elevation Myocardial Infarction

Answers can be reviewed online at http://evolve.elsevier.com/Lehne/.

OBJECTIVES

See page 28 for the Objectives.

CRITICAL THINKING AND STUDY QUESTIONS

1. A protocol in the emergency department (ED) is to administer 4 chewable 81-mg aspirin tablets (total 324 mg) to patients with suspected myocardial infarction. A student nurse asks the nurse why 4 chewable aspirin tablets are administered instead of 2 regular aspirin tablets (650 mg). Which of the following is the most accurate explanation for this protocol for the first dose of aspirin?
   a. Aspirin is an acid, and acids are more readily absorbed in the acid environment of the stomach.
   b. Chewable forms of aspirin are absorbed through the buccal mucosa bypassing hepatic first pass.
   c. Chewing breaks the tablet into smaller particles, which are more readily absorbed in the intestines.
   d. Exceeding 325-mg doses can offset the vasodilation and antiplatelet effects of lower doses.

2. A patient who is undergoing an acute ST-elevation myocardial infarction (STEMI) is prescribed metoprolol 50 mg by mouth every 6 hours. Which of the following assessment findings would be a reason to withhold the medication and immediately contact the prescriber?
   a. Altered taste
   b. Insomnia
   c. Rhinorrhea
   d. Wheezing

3. The ED triage nurse answers the call of a patient who has a history of angina pectoris and chronic obstructive pulmonary disease (COPD) who reports chest pain that has not been relieved

by three doses of nitroglycerin. The patient had been told by his physician that he should take chewable aspirin should this occur but he does not have any aspirin. The nurse should instruct this individual to
a. call 911.
b. call his physican for directions.
c. take ibuprofen and seek medical care.
d. turn on his home oxygen and rest.

4. Which of the following drugs prescribed for acute STEMI should be withheld and the prescriber consulted immediately if the patient's pulse is 118 beats/min?
a. Aspirin
b. Atenolol
c. Morphine
d. Nitroglycerin

5. The nurse knows that nitroglycerin decreases the workload of the heart by
a. dissolving existing clots.
b. preventing clot formation.
c. slowing the heart rate.
d. slowing venous return to the heart

6. When caring for a patient during a STEMI who is prescribed alteplase, the nurse would question the prescriber if which of the following drugs was also prescribed?
a. abciximab (ReoPro)
b. clopidogrel (Plavix)
c. lisinopril (Zestril)
d. low molecular weight (LMW) heparin (Lovenox)

7. Which of the following in the history of a patient who is experiencing STEMI would be most important to report to the prescriber who has just ordered captopril (Capoten)?
a. AST 120 international units/L
b. BUN 15 mg/dL
c. eGFR 42 mL/min
d. troponin T 0.8 ng/mL

CASE STUDIES AND PATIENT TEACHING

(Use a separate piece of paper for your responses.)

Case Study 1

A 57-year-old male who is vacationing locally is admitted to the ED with severe, crushing chest pain. The pain radiates into his left arm, and he is experiencing diaphoresis, weakness, and nausea. The ECG shows elevated ST segments in the inferior leads. Troponin T (TnT) is elevated three times above lower limits, and the total creatine kinase (CK) and the CK-MB isoenzyme are slightly elevated. The physician diagnoses STEMI. The physician decides to start thrombolytic therapy with alteplase (tPA).

1. What assessments should the nurse monitor relating to the risk of intracranial bleeding?

2. The nurse is directed to interview the patient's wife. What information does the nurse need to obtain to assist the physician with deciding if thrombolytic therapy is appropriate?

3. The following medications are ordered. What is the purpose of these drugs, and what assessment should the nurse perform relating to administration of these drugs?
a. Aspirin (ASA) 81-mg chewable tablets, 4 tablets STAT
b. Intravenous (IV) morphine 4 mg followed by 2 mg every 10 minutes as needed to control pain
c. Metoprolol 5 mg IV every 2 minutes for 3 doses then 50 mg orally every 6 hours × 48 hours
d. Nitroglycerin IV drip 10 mcg per minute

4. Why is it important for the nurse to assess if this patient has taken sildenafil in the past 24 hours?

5. The patient is being discharged with prescriptions for metoprolol (Lopressor) 100 mg once a day, captopril (Capoten) 25 mg every 8 hours, aspirin 81 mg once a day, and warfarin (Coumadin) 5 mg once a day. The patient's wife asks why he must have blood work (INR) done every week. How should the nurse respond?

6. When explaining warfarin therapy, the nurse shares the patient's INR results, which most recently were 1.8. The laboratory result form lists the normal INR as 0.85 to 1.2. How can the nurse explain that the target INR is 3, which appears to be abnormal?

Case Study 2

A nurse is leading an educational program for patients in a cardiac rehabilitation program.

1. What teaching regarding drugs and nonpharmacologic interventions can the nurse provide to decrease these risk factors for reinfarction?
   a. Diabetes
   b. Hyperlipidemia
   c. Hypertension
   d. Obesity and sedentary lifestyle
   e. Smoking cessation

2. What are reasons why the nurse should teach patients to seek medical care immediately if experiencing chest pain?

53
Drugs for Hemophilia

Answers can be reviewed online at http://evolve.elsevier.com/Lehne/.

OBJECTIVES

See page 28 for the Objectives.

CRITICAL THINKING AND STUDY QUESTIONS

1. Hemophilia (Select all that apply.)
   a. always produces a severe bleeding disorder.
   b. can result from a spontaneous gene mutation.
   c. interferes with the formation of a platelet plug.
   d. is inherited on the Y chromosome.
   e. has a risk factor of 50% for every boy born to a mother who is a carrier for the defective gene, no matter how many brothers have the disease.
   f. never occurs in females.
   g. affects 100% of daughters of hemophiliacs because they are carriers of the disease.
   h. treatment with clotting factor replacement is highly effective.

✳ 2. The nurse is caring for a 3-year-old boy who was admitted after a car accident. His laboratory tests indicate that he has 0.4% of the normal amount of clotting factor VIII. Which of the following symptoms would be of most concern to the nurse?
   a. Blood pressure 72/58 mm Hg
   b. Difficult to arouse
   c. Pulse 100 beats/min
   d. Swollen ankle

▶ 3. The nurse is teaching a patient with severe hemophilia and his family the importance of protecting joints from injury. The nurse teaches that because this body part is most commonly injured, it is most critical to prevent injury to the
   a. ankle.
   b. elbow.
   c. knee.
   d. skull.

▶ 4. The nurse needs to give an intramuscular immunization to a patient with a history of mild hemophilia B. The nurse should
   a. administer the immunization as usual.
   b. administer the immunization subcutaneously.
   c. apply pressure to the site for 5 to 10 minutes after the injection.
   d. only administer with an oral or nasal route.

5. The mother of a child with hemophilia calls the pediatrician's office. She has forgotten which medication she can give her son for mild pain and fever. The telephone triage nurse follows protocol and explains that the safest choice for hemophiliacs is
   a. acetaminophen (Tylenol).
   b. acetylsalicylic acid (aspirin).
   c. celecoxib (Celebrex).
   d. ibuprofen (Motrin).

✳ ▶ 6. A priority nursing diagnosis for a 9-year-old boy with hemophilia is
   a. anxiety.
   b. impaired parenting.
   c. ineffective coping.
   d. risk for injury.

7. The parents of a boy newly diagnosed with hemophilia express concern that their son will contract HIV, other infections, or have an allergic reaction from factor concentrates. The basis of the nurse's response is
   a. no case of virus transmission has been reported with any of the products now used in the United States.
   b. recombinant factor concentrate products carry a risk of contracting Creutzfeldt-Jakob disease (CJD).
   c. there is a risk of contracting HIV from plasma-derived factor concentrate, but the risk of bleeding is more serious.
   d. viruses for hepatitis A and parvovirus are lipid-coated viruses that are found in plasma-derived factor concentrate.

▶ 8. A nurse in the perioperative area is caring for a 12-year-old boy with hemophilia A who weighs 99 pounds. Intravenous push of 1000 units of recombinant factor concentrate is prescribed. The nurse should
   a. administer the factor concentrate as prescribed.
   b. administer the factor concentrate by continuous infusion.
   c. consult the prescriber because the dose is less than the recommended dose.
   d. consult the prescriber because the dose exceeds the recommended dose.

9. Calculations are available to predict patient response to infusion of factor concentrates. For each unit/kg of recombinant factor IX (BeneFix) administered, the patient's normal factor IX should increase
   a. 0.1%.
   b. 0.2%.
   c. 0.5%.
   d. 1%.

10. When the prescriber is determining the proper dose of factor concentrate, the most important patient factor to consider is
   a. age.
   b. clinical response.
   c. target percentage of normal factor levels.
   d. weight.

▶ 11. Desmopressin nasal spray 150 mcg is prescribed preoperatively for a 4-year-old boy with mild hemophilia A. The pharmacy only carries the spray that delivers 10 mcg/spray and is unable to obtain any other concentration. The nurse should
   a. administer 15 sprays of the medication.
   b. administer 150 mcg intravenously.
   c. consult with the prescriber regarding an intravenous dose order.
   d. consult with the prescriber regarding an oral dose order.

▶ 12. The nurse should teach the parents to assess for allergy symptoms when administering factor concentrate. What should the parents do first if the child experiences swelling around the face?
   a. Administer aminocaproic acid (Amicar).
   b. Administer diphenhydramine (Benadryl).
   c. Seek immediate emergency medical care.
   d. Slow the infusion.

13. Aminocaproic acid (Amicar) syrup may be prescribed to prevent bleeding from dental care for patients with
   a. hemophilia A and B.
   b. hemophilia A only.
   c. hemophilia B only.
   d. severe hemophilia A and B only.

14. The nurse knows that inhibitor antibodies to factor concentrate is most likely to occur in hemophiliacs of which of the following descent? (Select all that apply.)
   a. African American
   b. Asian
   c. Latino
   d. Middle Eastern
   e. Native American
   f. Northern European
   g. Scandinavian

15. When a patient is receiving factor VIIa (NovoSeven), he should be carefully assessed for
    a. allergy to pork.
    b. anorexia and nausea.
    c. chest pain and shortness of breath.
    d. muscle weakness and fatigue.

CASE STUDIES AND PATIENT TEACHING

(Use a separate piece of paper for your responses.)

Case Study 1

A 17-month-old boy has been newly diagnosed with hemophilia A. Review of his chart indicates he has not been immunized for hepatitis A.

1. What teaching needs to be provided relating to hepatitis immunization, and what information relating to immunizations does the nurse need to obtain regarding caregivers?

2. The mother asks why aspirin should not be given to her son. Describe what the nurse should explain.

3. The nurse provides a comprehensive list of over-the-counter drugs that contain salicylate. Which of these drugs would the nurse include on this list? (Select all that apply.)
    a. Alka Seltzer
    b. Anacin
    c. Aspergum
    d. Arthropan
    e. Ascriptin
    f. Disalcid
    g. Doan's original
    h. Dolobid
    i. Empirin
    j. Keygesic
    k. Momentum
    l. Pepto-Bismol
    m. St Joseph's baby aspirin
    n. Trilisate

4. The home health nurse goes to the boy's home to teach the mother how to administer recombinant factor VIII concentrate via a central venous catheter. What are nursing diagnoses that the nurse should consider when developing the plan of care for this family?

5. Administering factor concentrate carries a risk of complications. What should the nurse teach the caregiver to prepare for possible complications?

54

Drugs for Deficiency Anemias

Answers can be reviewed online at http://evolve.elsevier.com/Lehne/.

OBJECTIVES

See page 28 for the Objectives.

CRITICAL THINKING AND STUDY QUESTIONS

1. Match the following terms and definitions.

_____ a. Erythroblast
_____ b. Ferritinbone
_____ c. Hematocrit
_____ d. Hemoglobin
_____ e. Hemosiderin
_____ f. Iron-binding capacity (IBC) [total IBC (TIBC)]
_____ g. Mean corpuscular hemoglobin concentration (MCHC)
_____ h. Mean corpuscular volume (MCV)
_____ i. Myoglobin
_____ j. Proerythroblast
_____ k. Red blood cell distribution width (RDW)
_____ l. Reticulocyte
_____ m. Transferrin

1. Developing red blood cells (RBC) in marrow after incorporates hemoglobin
2. Developing RBC in bone marrow before incorporates hemoglobin
3. Immature nonnucleated RBCs
4. Iron-containing protein in muscle cells that stores oxygen
5. Measures color of RBCs
6. Measures size of RBCs
7. Oxygen-carrying protein of RBCs
8. Percentage of RBCs in a volume of blood
9. Saturation capacity of transferrin with iron
10. Storage form of iron
11. Storage form of iron in bone marrow
12. Transports absorbed iron to bone marrow
13. Variation in size of RBC

▶ 2. The nurse is caring for an anemic cancer patient who is receiving chemotherapy that prevents the reproduction of rapidly dividing cells, including the cancer cells, hair, RBC, and epithelium of the gastrointestinal (GI) tract. Which of the following laboratory results suggests that the anemia is getting worse?
   a. Hemoglobin 9 mg/dL
   b. Hematocrit 26%
   c. RBC 3.8×10^{12}/L
   d. Reticulocyte count 0.002%

3. It is important for the nurse to assess for symptoms of anemia in a patient who has a history of
   a. chronic obstructive pulmonary disease.
   b. chronic renal failure.
   c. diabetes insipidus.
   d. hypertension.

4. Normally the body prevents excessive buildup of iron in the body by
   a. decreasing intestinal absorption of iron.
   b. increasing metabolism of RBCs.
   c. increasing excretion of RBCs in bile.
   d. increasing excretion of RBCs in urine.

5. Which of the following foods should the nurse include in her dietary teaching for pregnant women regarding prevention of iron deficiency anemia? (Select all that apply.)
   a. Carrots
   b. Cheese
   c. Chicken
   d. Citrus fruit
   e. Egg white
   f. Egg yolk
   g. Fish
   h. Legumes
   i. Milk
   j. Red meat
   k. Squash
   l. Yogurt

6. Match the following terms and definitions.

_____ a. Hyperchromic
_____ b. Hypochromic
_____ c. Macrocyte
_____ d. Megaloblast
_____ e. Microcytic

1. Excessive color
2. Large erythroblast
3. Large erythrocyte
4. Pale
5. Small size cell

150

7. In iron deficiency anemia, the nurse would expect which of the following tests to be elevated from normal levels?
   a. Hematocrit (Hct)
   b. Hemoglobin (Hgb or Hb)
   c. (Total) Iron-binding capacity (IBC or TIBC)
   d. Mean corpuscular volume (MCV)

8. A common nursing diagnosis for patients with iron-deficiency anemia is
   a. body image disturbance.
   b. breathing pattern, ineffective.
   c. cardiac output, decreased.
   d. fatigue.

▶ 9. The school nurse has been consulted by a 5th grade teacher regarding a student who tires excessively as the day progresses, is pale, and whose academic performance has been declining. What action would be appropriate at this time?
   a. Contact the parents and inform them that their child is anemic.
   b. Contact the child's parents and tell them their child needs to be seen by their pediatrician.
   c. Make an appointment along with the teacher to speak with the parents about noted concerns.
   d. Tell the child that you think he is anemic and that he should tell his parents.

10. The most common adverse effect of administration of ferrous sulfate is
   a. discoloration of teeth.
   b. dyspepsia.
   c. hypotension.
   d. weak, rapid pulse.

11. A patient complains of intolerable nausea and heartburn from taking an oral iron preparation. The nurse should instruct the patient to
   a. consult with the prescriber.
   b. take a calcium carbonate antacid with the iron.
   c. take the iron with milk.
   d. take the iron with orange juice.

▶ 12. The nurse is providing care to a patient who is receiving an oral iron preparation. The patient's stool is greenish black. Initially the nurse should
   a. administer a dose of the iron preparation.
   b. consult the prescriber.
   c. determine if this stool is usual or a change for this patient.
   d. hold the iron preparation.

✳ 13. A patient with peptic ulcer disease has developed severe anemia. Iron dextran (DexFerrum) has just been prescribed. The nurse has administered a test dose. It is most critical to observe the patient for
   a. angioedema.
   b. hives.
   c. phlebitis at the site of injection.
   d. tissue damage from extravasation.

14. When iron must be administered by injection, how should it be administered?
   a. Intradermal
   b. Intrathecal
   c. Subcutaneous
   d. Z-track intramuscular

✳ 15. The dialysis nurse has administered iron sucrose (Venofer) and erythropoietin. A priority nursing concern relating to adverse effects is
   a. gastrointestinal cramping.
   b. infusion site discomfort.
   c. maintaining adequate tissue perfusion.
   d. taste alterations.

16. The nurse should teach the patient with pernicious anemia to report
   a. fatigue.
   b. joint pain.
   c. paresthesias.
   d. temperature >100.4°F (38°C).

▶ 17. A patient with pernicious anemia complains of numbness and tingling of the hands and feet. What data relating to possible neurologic damage should the nurse collect before notifying the prescriber of the patient's complaint?
   a. Blood pressure
   b. Deep tendon reflex (DTR)
   c. Capillary glucose
   d. Skin color

18. To prevent damage to the developing neural tube of a fetus, it is important for women of childbearing age to have adequate daily intake of folate, which can be found in (Select all that apply.)
   a. asparagus.
   b. egg yolks.
   c. lentils.
   d. liver.
   e. meat.
   f. milk.
   g. oranges.
   h. spinach.
   i. whole wheat.
   j. yogurt.

19. A 56-year-old man is admitted with unexplained severe shortness of breath with minimal activity. Lung sounds are clear. Pulse is rapid. Abnormal lab results include low hemoglobin and hematocrit, elevated MCV, very high levels of ALT. The nurse reviews the patient's history, which reveals alcohol abuse. The patient's wife states that she does not know how he could be anemic. He takes iron and eats red meat every day. The basis of the nurse's response is alcohol abuse
   a. impairs the absorption of iron.
   b. increases urinary excretion of iron.
   c. interferes with enterohepatic recirculation.
   d. prevents the absorption of vitamin B_{12} (cyanocobalamin).

CASE STUDIES AND PATIENT TEACHING

(Use a separate piece of paper for your responses.)

Case Study 1

An 11-month-old, who drinks 8-ounce bottles of whole milk 5 to 6 times a day, is diagnosed with iron-deficiency anemia.

1. What can the nurse teach the parents about factors that could be contributing to the anemia and measures to change the factors that can be altered?

2. The pediatrician prescribes ferrous sulfate drops 25 mg twice a day. The child weighs 22 lb, and the recommended dose is 5 mg/kg/day. Is the dose safe and effective?

3. Ferrous sulfate drops are available as 75 mg in 0.6 mL. How much should the parents administer with each dose?

4. What should the nurse teach the parents about ferrous sulfate therapy?

Case Study 2

A 28-year-old female has gastric bypass surgery. She has lost 25 lb in the past 2 months. She comes to her primary care provider (PCP) with complaints of fatigue and glossitis (smooth, beefy, red tongue).

1. Because of a history of this surgery, the patient is at risk for what type of anemia? Why?

2. The patient is prescribed parenteral injections of vitamin B_{12} (30 mcg) and folic acid 200 mcg daily for 1 week. She then will receive oral cyanocobalamin 10,000 mcg/day and folic acid 400 mcg/day. The patient tells the nurse that she had learned that oral administration of cyanocobalamin is ineffective. How should the nurse respond?

3. The patient discusses concerns about taking "all of these pills" every day. The prescriber discontinues the oral cyclobalamin and prescribes intranasal cyclobalamin (Nascobal) one spray in one nostril once a week. What teaching will the nurse provide about intranasal administration of the drug?

4. The nurse teaches the patient to report which symptoms that suggest the uncommon, but significant, adverse effect of hypokalemia that is possible when taking cyanocobalamin (vitamin B_{12})?

5. Because this woman is of child-bearing age, the nurse teaches this patient that adequate daily consumption of folic acid is important. Why?

6. The patient states that she does not need a doctor, she does everything naturally. If she is tired, she will take megadoses of folic acid from the health food store when she is pregnant. How should the nurse respond?

Case Study 3

The nurse is preparing to administer intramuscular iron dextran to a patient who is hospitalized with severe blood loss associated with ulcerative colitis.

1. What special precautions should the nurse take when administering this drug?

55

Hematopoietic Growth Factors

Answers can be reviewed online at http://evolve.elsevier.com/Lehne/.

OBJECTIVES

See page 28 for the Objectives.

CRITICAL THINKING AND STUDY QUESTIONS

1. A patient with a history of diabetes mellitus (DM) type 2 and chronic renal failure (CRF) is receiving epoetin alpha (Procrit) because her failing kidneys do not produce adequate amounts of erythropoietin, and she has become anemic. Which of the following would be a reasonable goal for therapy?
   a. Hb 8 gm/dL; transferrin 25%; ferritin 150 ng/mL
   b. Hb 10 gm/dL: transferrin 20%; ferritin 125 ng/mL
   c. Hb 12 gm/dL: transferrin 10%; ferritin 80 ng/dL
   d. Hb 14 gm/dL: transferrin 15%; ferritin 100 ng/mL

2. Inhibiting the apoptotic mechanism maintains cellular integrity by
   a. forming new blood vessels.
   b. increasing blood cell formation.
   c. limiting the life of cells.
   d. preventing self-destruction of cells.

3. Benefits of administering epoetin alpha (Procrit) to a patient with DM type 2 may include
   a. increasing sensitivity of muscle and fat cells to insulin.
   b. limiting the release of glucose from the liver.
   c. preventing damage to kidneys.
   d. reducing the need for insulin therapy.

▸ 4. Which of these findings would be most significant if a patient was receiving darbepoetin alpha (Aranesp)?
   a. Blood pressure 170/120 mm Hg
   b. Pulse 104 beats/min
   c. Respirations 26
   d. Temperature 100.4 °F (38 °C)

5. A chemotherapy patient who has received three injections in the past week of epoetin alpha (Procrit) is due for the next dose. The patient's hemoglobin has not increased. The nurse should
   a. hold the next dose.
   b. administer the medication as ordered.
   c. consult the prescriber regarding assessing for renal failure.
   d. consult the prescriber regarding assessing for neutralizing antibodies.

▸ 6. Epoetin alpha (Procrit) 4000 units subcutaneous is ordered at 0900 pending endogenous erythropoietin levels for an anemic HIV-infected patient receiving zidovudine (AZT). Lab results arrived at 0830 including endogenous erythropoietin level of 578 milliunits/mL. The nurse should
   a. administer the epoetin alpha (Procrit) STAT.
   b. administer the epoetin alpha (Procrit) with the 0900 medications.
   c. hold the medication and consult the prescriber.
   d. hold the medication.

▸ 7. Nursing considerations regarding epoetin alfa (Procrit) include (Select all that apply.)
   a. Administer depot preparation intramuscularly for extended action.
   b. Assess for allergy to albumin.
   c. Check for dose adjustments.
   d. Dilute in 5 mL of bacteriostatic water for injection.
   e. Discard if preparation is discolored.
   f. Freeze for up to 1 month.
   g. Monitor hemoglobin results.
   h. Refrigerate until ready for use.
   i. Shake well to ensure that all particles have dissolved.

8. A patient in the United States asks a nurse about the advantages of the drug MPEG-epoetin beta (Micera) that she has heard is available in Canada. An advantage that the nurse could discuss is
   a. injections are given less often.
   b. it can be used in patients with myelogenous cancers.
   c. it has fewer adverse effects.
   d. it is more effective than other preparations.

9. Generally leukopoietic growth factor, filgrastim (Neupogen), is contraindicated in myelogenous cancers. Why is it being investigated for patients with acute myelogenous leukemia?

10. When administering filgrastim (Neupogen), how often should the nurse expect to review the WBC count?
    a. Once a week
    b. Twice a week
    c. Once a month
    d. Twice a month

▶ 11. Elevation of uric acid is an adverse effect of filgrastim (Neupogen) therapy. The most important assessment for the nurse to evaluate relating to possible elevations of uric acid is
    a. decreased urine output.
    b. elevated temperature.
    c. joint pain.
    d. joint tophi.

▶ 12. The nurse is teaching administration of filgrastim (Neupogen) to the mother of a child with congenital neutropenia who weighs 88 lb. The prescribed dose is 240 mcg (6 mcg/kg). The medication is available in a concentration of 300 mcg/mL in 1.6-mL vials. The nurse should teach the mother to administer
    a. 0.6 mL, discarding the vial after the first dose.
    b. 0.6 mL, obtaining 2 doses from each vial.
    c. 0.8 mL, discarding the vial after the first dose.
    d. 0.8 mL, obtaining 2 doses from each vial.

13. Administration directives for filgrastim (Neupogen) for a patient receiving chemotherapy include
    a. to administer after each dose of chemotherapy.
    b. to consult the prescriber once absolute neutrophil count has reached 10,000/mm^3.
    c. that it must be kept refrigerated at all times.
    d. wipe the rubber stopper with alcohol when re-entering vial.

14. Advantages of using pegfilgrastim (Neulasta) instead of filgrastim (Neupogen) include that
    a. it can be administered immediately before or after chemotherapy.
    b. the course of therapy is one injection lasting 2 weeks.
    c. it does not cause bone pain.
    d. there is less elevation of LDH, alkaline phosphatase, and uric acid.

15. Hematopoietic growth factors cannot be taken orally because

16. Which of the following would be a contraindication to administration of sargramostim (Leukine)?
    a. Allergy to chocolate
    b. Allergy to eggs
    c. Allergy to milk
    d. Allergy to yeast

▶ 17. Which of the following would be a symptom of a severe adverse reaction to sargramostim (Leukine)?
    a. Crackles (rales)
    b. Gurgles (rhonchi)
    c. Pleural friction rub
    d. Wheezes

18. If the final concentration of sargramostim (Leukine) is to be less than 10 mcg/mL, the drug should be diluted in 0.9%
    a. sodium chloride.
    b. sodium chloride with 20 mEq KCl.
    c. sodium chloride with 0.1% albumin.
    d. sodium chloride with 5% dextrose in water.

19. Oprelvekin (Neumega) (Select all that apply.)
    a. peaks in action in 24 hours.
    b. decreases count of abnormal platelets.
    c. increases production and maturity of megakaryocytes.
    d. is eliminated more rapidly in children than adults.
    e. is excreted in active form in the urine.
    f. is nearly identical in structure to human interleukin-11.

▸ 20. What assessments for adverse effects should be performed after the nurse administers oprelvekin (Neumega)? (Select all that apply.)
    a. Blurred vision
    b. Bone pain
    c. Dehydration
    d. Edema
    e. Palpitations
    f. Pulse for tachycardia and dysrhythmias
    g. Rash
    h. Red eyes
    i. Shortness of breath
    j. Tingling around the mouth

CASE STUDIES AND PATIENT TEACHING

(Use a separate piece of paper for your responses.)

Case Study 1

A 65-year-old patient has had DM for 40 years and chronic renal failure for 20 years. He has been maintained at home leading a relatively normal life. Recently, he has become more anemic, and a lack of erythrocyte production has been identified. He is prescribed epoetin alfa (Procrit) to help maintain his erythrocyte count. The prescriber has ordered baseline laboratory tests including BUN, creatinine, phosphorus, potassium, RBC indices, hemoglobin, transferring saturation, and ferritin. The patient is tired of "being jabbed" and asks the nurse why these tests have to be done.

1. Describe the rationale for each test in a way the patient can understand.
   a. Bun/creatinine
   b. Phosphorus
   c. Potassium
   d. Hemoglobin
   e. RBC indices
   f. Ferritin

2. What adverse effects should the nurse assess in this patient?

3. The prescriber has ordered 75 units/kg for maintenance therapy 3 times a week. The patient weighs 80 kg. How many units should the nurse administer in 1 dose?

4. The nurse is reviewing laboratory results for this patient. Hemoglobin is 13.5 gm/dL. What should the nurse do?

Case Study 2

A patient is prescribed Sargramostim (Leukine) 250 mcg/m² after a bone marrow transplant.

1. What is the rationale for this therapy?

2. What should the nurse do or not do if the patient experiences these adverse effects?
   a. Diarrhea
   b. Weakness
   c. Rash
   d. Bone pain

3. The patient weighs 50 kg and is 163 cm tall. The pharmacy delivers Sargramostim (Leukine) 500 mcg/mL, which the nurse dilutes to a concentration of 10 mcg/mL. How much Sargramostim (Leukine) should be administered?

4. The intravenous pumps are calibrated at mL/hour. The drug is to be infused over 4 hours. What rate should the nurse program into the pump?

56

Drugs for Diabetes Mellitus

Answers can be reviewed online at http://evolve.elsevier.com/Lehne/.

OBJECTIVES

See page 28 for the Objectives.

CRITICAL THINKING AND STUDY QUESTIONS

1. When assessing a patient who is receiving drugs for diabetes mellitus (DM), it is important to remember that the underlying cause of most chronic complications of DM is affects on which body system?
   a. Musculoskeletal
   b. Renal
   c. Respiratory
   d. Vascular

2. Which of the following antihypertensive drugs might be prescribed for a patient with DM who does not have the diagnosis of hypertension?
   a. Benazepril (Lotensin)
   b. Carvedilol (Coreg)
   c. Diltiazem (Cardizem)
   d. Furosemide (Lasix)

3. A goal of drug therapy with metoclopramide (Reglan) for a patient with DM is
   a. alert and oriented ×3.
   b. no adventitious lung sounds.
   c. palpable peripheral pulse.
   d. soft, nondistended abdomen.

4. Which of the following interventions would be most appropriate for a 23-year-old patient who, for the first time, has a fasting plasma glucose level of 145 mg/dL?
   a. Advise the patient to include 30 minutes of vigorous exercise in his daily activities.
   b. Discuss possible diet changes.
   c. Explain the need for oral antidiabetic medication.
   d. Teach the patient how to do a urine dip for glucose and ketones.

5. The nurse is developing a teaching plan for a 15-year-old female newly diagnosed as a type 1 diabetic. This teaching plan should include which of the following statements? (Select all that apply.)
   a. Blood sugar control will best be achieved if the patient follows a plan created by the healthcare providers.
   b. Clear insulin is always short acting.
   c. Insulin therapy with one long-acting agent that mimics the body's basal insulin secretion and another short-acting agent to cover eating is best.
   d. Once the patient's blood sugar is stabilized, she should be able to maintain control with oral drugs.
   e. Saturated fats should be limited to less than 10% of the total calories.
   f. Taking insulin and not eating can cause serious effects from the blood sugar going too low.
   g. Tight glucose control decreases the incidence of kidney failure.
   h. Treatment can be monitored by blood or urine.
   i. Weight loss is needed to decrease the patient's insulin requirements.

* 6. Whenever a patient's self-monitoring of blood glucose (SMBG) is within normal limits and the glycolated hemoglobin (HbA$_{1C}$) is above goal, the priority nursing intervention should be to
   a. assess the patient's technique of performing SMBG.
   b. check the expiration date on the insulin bottle.
   c. explain that the glycolated hemoglobin indicates that the blood sugar has been high.
   d. teach the patient to count carbohydrates and calculate insulin needs.

* 7. It would be a priority for the nurse to respond to which of the following symptoms if exhibited by a patient who is receiving insulin therapy for diabetes?
   a. Fatigue and blurred vision
   b. Perineal itching and copious urine
   c. Profuse sweating and difficult to arouse
   d. Thirst and constant hunger

156

Copyright © 2010, 2007, 2004, 2000, 1999 by Saunders, an imprint of Elsevier Inc. All rights reserved.

8. Which of these outcomes would be appropriate for a patient who is taking insulin glargine once a day?
   a. Premeal glucose level of 90 mg/dL
   b. Premeal glucose level of 140 mg/dL
   c. Premeal glucose level of 180 mg/dL
   d. Premeal glucose level less than 200 mg/dL

▶ 9. The nurse assesses for which of these symptoms of the electrolyte imbalance that is most likely when a patient is receiving large doses of insulin?
   a. Muscle weakness
   b. Restlessness
   c. Spasm of the wrist and fingers when circulation of the upper arm is constricted for several minutes
   d. Twitching of the facial nerve when the face is tapped over the nerve

▶ 10. The nurse is caring for a 62-year-old who has been a type 2 diabetic for 15 years. She is prescribed Humulin N 25 units in the AM. Recently the patient has experienced several hypoglycemic episodes despite maintaining her usual medication, diet, and exercise regimen. The patient's lab studies include C-peptide 1 ng/mL (normal 5 to 12 ng/mL). It would be most important for the nurse to assess this patient's
   a. calibration of her glucose meter.
   b. intake of carbohydrates.
   c. level of daily exercise.
   d. sight for administering the proper amount of insulin.

11. When teaching about the onset, peak, and duration of different insulins, the nurse explains that which of the following insulin types is most like the "natural" insulin produced by the body?
   a. Aspart (NovoLog)
   b. Lispro (Humalog)
   c. Regular (Humulin R)
   d. Neutral protamine Hagedorn (NPH) (Humulin N)

▶ 12. When obtaining a new vial of NPH insulin from refrigeration, the nurse notes that the suspension is partially frozen. The nurse should
   a. discard the vial and obtain a new one from the pharmacy.
   b. shake the vial vigorously to produce heat.
   c. warm the suspension in warm water.
   d. withdraw the unfrozen portion then discard the rest.

▶ 13. A patient is admitted in a state of diabetic ketoacidosis. Orders include insulin lispro 0.1 mg/kg/hr to be administered by intravenous (IV) drip. The nurse should
   a. calculate the insulin dose and mix it with 100 mL of normal saline.
   b. calculate the insulin dose and mix it with 100 mL of D$_5$W.
   c. calculate the insulin dose and infuse the solution prepared by the pharmacy.
   d. consult the prescriber STAT.

▶ 14. The nurse has done an initial assessment on assigned patients and is preparing to administer prescribed insulin. All patients are alert and oriented. It is 8:00 AM, and breakfast trays are scheduled to arrive at 8:20 AM. To which of the following patients should the nurse administer the insulin first?
   a. 7:00 AM SMBG 60 mg/dL; prescribed NPH insulin (Novolin N) 34 units
   b. 7:00 AM SMBG 90 mg/dL; prescribed regular insulin (Humulin R) 5 units
   c. 7:00 AM SMBG 130 mg/dL; prescribed insulin aspart (NovoLog) 5 units
   d. 7:00 AM SMBG 180 mg/dL; prescribed insulin glulisine (Apidra) 7 units

15. A patient has been prescribed 5 units of insulin aspart (NovoLog) and 25 units of insulin detemir (Levemir) to be administered at 0800. The nurse should
   a. draw up the two insulins in different syringes.
   b. draw up 5 units of aspart first, then 25 units of detemir insulin in the same syringe.
   c. draw up the clear insulin then the cloudy insulin in the same syringe.
   d. inject the insulins in a different subcutaneous site (abdomen versus arm versus thigh) than the previous morning.

16. What special administration techniques must the nurse use when administering NPH insulin?
   a. Never mix with another insulin.
   b. Only administer this insulin at bedtime.
   c. Roll the vial gently to mix particles in solution.
   d. When mixing with another insulin, draw the NPH into the syringe first.

17. A nursing student asks an emergency department (ED) nurse why premixed IV regular

insulin solutions are not available in the ED as a stock drug. The best explanation is
a. insulin can be absorbed into the plastic, altering the concentration.
b. insulin is affected by light, and IV bags are clear.
c. insulin rapidly biodegrades when mixed with a diluent.
d. the appropriate insulin diluent cannot be refrigerated.

18. A patient is prescribed 4 units of insulin aspart (NovoLog) based on a sliding scale relating to SMBG. Available syringes are marked 50 units in 0.5 mL or 100 units in 1 mL. The nurse chooses the 50 units in 0.5-mL syringe to administer this dose because it is
a. the only syringe that can accurately measure this dose.
b. the only syringe that has the correct needle for administering this dose.
c. easier to administer the insulin using this syringe.
d. easier to see the line indicating the 4 units on this syringe.

19. Which of the following laboratory test results might be treated with IV infusion of regular insulin?
a. Calcium 13 mg/dL
b. Magnesium 2.7 mg/dL
c. Potassium 6.2 mEq/L
d. Sodium 152 mEq/L

20. Research suggests that intensive insulin therapy (tight control) in type 1 and 2 diabetes is most effective in preventing
a. cerebral vascular accidents (CVAs).
b. neuropathic pain.
c. peripheral vascular disease requiring amputation.
d. visual damage.

✳ 21. When performing the initial morning assessment on a diabetic patient, the nurse notes that the patient is very difficult to arouse. The nurse checks the SMBG, which is 37 mg/dL. The priority assessment before administering the orange juice is
a. blood pressure.
b. deep tendon reflexes.
c. swallowing reflex.
d. temperature.

▸ 22. The nurse is reviewing the laboratory results of a patient who is prescribed metformin (Glucophage). Results include ALT 112 international units/L, BUN 38 mg/dL, creatinine 2.6 mg/dL, hemoglobin 11 gm/dL, and hematocrit 33%. The nurse assesses the patient. Which of the following would be of most concern to the nurse?
a. Dorsalis pedis pulse difficult to palpate
b. Respirations 32 breaths per minute and deep
c. Pulse 100 beats/min
d. Severe frontal headache

23. Which of the following dietary teachings can decrease adverse effects of metformin (Glucophage) related to vitamins?
a. Eat less meat
b. Eat more green, leafy vegetables
c. Eat less whole grains
d. Eat more dairy products

24. After teaching about the drug glipizide (Glucotrol), which of the following statements, if made by the patient would suggest the patient understood the teaching?
a. "I can eat what I want as long as I take enough of the drug."
b. "I need to notify my doctor if I have episodes of sweating and shakiness."
c. "I should not experience low blood sugar with this drug because it does not stimulate the release of insulin."
d. "This drug is less potent than the newer drugs."

25. The nurse teaches the diabetic patient who is prescribed tolbutamide (Orinase) and metoprolol that the metoprolol
a. can prevent the patient from feeling the symptoms of hypoglycemia.
b. is prescribed to prevent reflex tachycardia.
c. prevents cardiac toxicity caused by tolbutamide.
d. should be administered 1 hour after insulin administration.

▸ 26. Which of the following would warrant the nurse not administering repaglinide (Prandin) and consulting the prescriber?
a. Fasting blood glucose 95 mg/dL
b. Glycolated hemoglobin (HbA$_{1C}$) 5.5%
c. Patient is NPO for a colonoscopy
d. Patient is scheduled for hemodialysis at 1000

27. The nurse would consult the prescriber if a patient with type 2 DM was scheduled for a diagnostic test with contrast dye, Urografin, if the patient had taken which of the following drugs?
    a. Acarbose
    b. Insulin
    c. Metformin
    d. Pioglitazone

28. Which of the following laboratory test results increases the risk that a patient who is prescribed glimepiride (Amaryl) might experience hypoglycemia?
    a. ALP 142 international units/L
    b. BUN 24 mg/dL
    c. eGFR 42 mL/min
    d. G6PD 2.4 U/gm of hemoglobin

▶ 29. The nurse is preparing to perform the first assessment of the 3- to 11-shift at 3:30 PM (1530). Several assigned patients are diabetics. The patient receiving which of the following drugs should be assessed for hypoglycemia first?
    a. Acarbose (Precose) 50 mg 3 times a day with meals
    b. Glargine (Lispro) insulin units every evening plus insulin aspart (NovoLog) according to dietary intake and SMBG
    c. Metformin (Glucophage) 500 mg before breakfast and supper
    d. Neutral protamine Hagedorn (NPH) (Humulin N) 35 units every morning

✳ 30. The nurse is assessing a diabetic patient who is prescribed rosiglitazone (Avandia) and Novolin 70/30. The nurse notes the patient has become increasingly restless and short of breath with exertion. Which of the following is a priority for the nurse to assess and report to the prescriber?
    a. Change in weight
    b. LDL levels
    c. SMBG
    d. Temperature

31. Which of these nursing outcomes would be most appropriate for a patient who is prescribed acarbose (Precose)?
    a. Bedtime SMBG 160 mg/dL
    b. Fasting blood glucose less than 90 mg/dL
    c. Glycolated hemoglobin (HbA$_{1C}$) 7%
    d. Two-hour postprandial blood sugar less than 150 mg/dL

▶ 32. A blind, diabetic hospitalized patient is receiving acarbose (Precose) 50 mg 3 times a day with meals. The nurse plans interventions that include the fact that the patient is at risk for
    a. activity intolerance.
    b. ineffective coping.
    c. injury.
    d. powerlessness.

▶ 33. A diabetic patient who receives glipizide and miglitol (Glyset) is diaphoretic, tachycardic, and anxious. The SMBG is 43 mg/dL. Which of the following would be most effective to quickly raise the patient's blood sugar?
    a. Glucose tablet
    b. Honey
    c. Orange juice
    d. Sugar cube

34. The nurse is teaching a type 1 diabetic patient who has been prescribed pramlintide (Symlin). Which of the following information should be included? (Select all that apply.)
    a. A common adverse effect of pramlintide is nausea.
    b. Patients need to estimate calorie and carbohydrate content of meals to determine if pramlintide should be administered.
    c. Pramlintide can interfere with the absorption of oral drugs.
    d. Pramlintide decreases the need for insulin.
    e. Pramlintide increases the release of glucagon.
    f. Pramlintide is more effective if prescribed along with acarbose (Precose).
    g. Pramlintide is used in place of insulin.
    h. Pramlintide should be administered with the daily long-acting insulin dose.
    i. Pramlintide speeds gastric emptying.
    j. Risk for hypoglycemia is greatest within 3 hours of administration.

35. The nurse knows that the only drug recommended to treat type 2 diabetes during pregnancy and lactation is
    a. acarbose.
    b. insulin.
    c. metformin.
    d. pioglitazone.

36. After administration of glucagon for severe hypoglycemia, the nurse anticipates treatment to
    a. correct acidosis.
    b. correct cachexia.
    c. restore stores of glycogen in the liver.
    d. treat the adverse effect of diarrhea.

37. Matching possible drug interactions with insulin.

_____ a. Need less insulin   1. Alcohol binge
_____ b. Need more insulin   2. Beta blockers
                                         3. Glucocorticoids
                                         4. Meglitinides
                                         5. Pramlintide
                                         6. Sulfonylureas
                                         7. Thiazide diuretics

CASE STUDIES AND PATIENT TEACHING

(Use a separate piece of paper for your responses.)

CASE STUDY 1

A 28-year-old man, who is 5 feet 8 inches and 132 lb, is admitted to the hospital after experiencing nausea, vomiting, and increasing confusion. BP 90/50 mm Hg, apical pulse 112 beats/min, respirations 29 breaths per minute and deep with fruity odor. His skin is hot, dry, and flushed. Urine is pale in color and smells like rotting apples. The patient responds to verbal and tactile stimuli, but has become increasingly lethargic. According to a family member, the patient has had diabetes for 6 years and takes Humulin N 35 units and Humulin R 15 units every morning and Humulin N 17 units at dinnertime. He had stopped exercising this week and has not taken his insulin for 2 days because of having a "stomach flu."

Lab results include serum glucose 545 mg/dL; BUN 20 mg/dL; serum osmolarity 400 mOsm/kg; creatinine 2 mg/dL: urine + acetone, + sugar; potassium 3.3 mEq/L; sodium 139 mEq/L; WBC 18.3 × 10³/mcL. The prescriber orders:

- *Intravenous fluid infusion of 1000 mL of half-normal saline (0.45% NaCl) with 10 mEq of KCl to be infused in 1 hour followed by 1000 mL of 0.45% sodium chloride at a rate of 300 mL/hr.*
- *Regular insulin bolus of 0.15 units/kg.*
- *Intravenous infusion of regular insulin at 0.1 units/kg/hr.*
- *Bedside blood glucose level determination every 30 minutes.*
- *I&O every hour.*
- *Repeat serum osmolality, BUN, and creatinine in 4 hours.*
- *Once serum glucose reaches 250 mg/dL, change IV infusion to 1000 mL of 5% dextrose in water (D_5W) at a rate of 125 mL/hr.*

1. Why is it important for the nurse to initiate the IV solution first?

2. Based on the prescriber's orders, how much insulin should the nurse administer by bolus injection?

3. The insulin comes mixed as a solution of 25 units in 100 mL of normal saline. The IV pump calibration is in milliliters per hour. What rate should the nurse program for the continuous IV insulin drip?

4. The patient's wife asks why regular insulin is being infused instead of the patient's usual NPH. How should the nurse respond?

5. The patient is stabilized and transferred to the medical-surgical unit. The patient's wife is frightened that the patient will experience another episode. What teaching can the nurse provide to help prevent another episode like this one?

6. The patient states that he has been rotating injection sites. What information should the nurse provide about current recommendations for rotating insulin injection sites?

7. While in the hospital, the patient is on a sliding scale insulin program before meals and at bedtime. The patient admits to being afraid of administering insulin at bedtime because he is not eating during the night. How should the nurse respond?

The schedule is as follows:
- SMBG <150, give no insulin.
- SMBG 151 to 200, give 2 units regular insulin.
- SMBG 201 to 250, give 4 units regular insulin.
- SMBG 250 to 300, give 6 units regular insulin.
- SMBG >300, call the prscriber.

8. His Accucheck reading is 202. How much regular insulin should the nurse administer?

9. The prescriber has discussed changing the patient's insulin regimen to insulin glargine for once-a-day basal insulin needs and insulin lispro based on eating patterns. After meeting with a diabetic educator, the patient asks the nurse to explain again why he needs to count "carbs."

10. The patient is scheduled to come back to see the diabetes nurse educator in 1 week. Why should he do this even though he has had diabetes for some time and has been given additional information while in the hospital?

Case Study 2

A 46-year-old married construction worker with a history of hypertension has been admitted for testing after experiencing transient acute visual disturbances that caused a fall from a scaffold. The patient is a smoker, 5 feet 9 inches and weighs 203 lb and is often nonadherent with his antihypertensive medication. He has been generally healthy, except for noting that he has been urinating more frequently. Neurologic examination and laboratory results are within normal limits, except for the glycolated hemoglobin (HbA$_{1c}$) 6.8% and triglycerides 438 mg/dL. The healthcare provider has just reviewed the laboratory results with the patient and informed the patient that a 75-gm 2-hour oral glucose tolerance test (OGTT) has been scheduled for tomorrow. The nurse is instructed to explain the test procedure to the patient. After the healthcare provider leaves, the patient asks the nurse why he needs to have this test done if his fasting blood sugar is normal.

1. How should the nurse respond?

2. The patient asks how blood sugar could be related to visual changes. How should the nurse respond?

3. What factors in the patient's history suggest that this patient is developing type 2 diabetes?

4. Besides safety related to visual changes, why is it important to identify and treat if this patient is a diabetic?

5. The patient's 3-hour glucose tolerance test results are shown in the table below:

	Blood Glucose	Urine Glucose	Urine Ketones
Fasting	97 mg/dL	negative	negative
30 min	225 mg/dL	45 mg	negative
1 hr	283 mg/dL	111 mg	negative
2 hr	261 mg/dL	387 mg	negative

The healthcare provider explains the impairment of glucose tolerance to the patient. What teaching should the nurse provide to assist this patient with controlling his blood sugar and preventing complications?

Case Study 3

A 17-year-old high school sophomore is a type 1 diabetic. She has been attempting to maintain tight control of her serum glucose levels using intensive insulin therapy.

1. Why is it important to monitor this patient's weight?

2. Recently the teen has been experiencing frequent occurrences of hypoglycemia. After establishing rapport with the patient, what questions should the nurse ask in an attempt to identify factors that could be causing these episodes?

3. The patient is concerned about being different from her friends and has verbalized resentment that she must alter her diet or excuse herself from activities to take needed insulin. Her pediatric endocrinologist has recommended an insulin pump. The physician asks the diabetes nurse to explain how the pump works. What information should the nurse provide?

4. The patient asks if the pump can be removed when she wears something special, such as a prom gown. How should the nurse respond?

5. The patient confides in the nurse that she will not wear the pump to the prom. What is a possible solution to this problem?

Case Study 4

The diabetic nurse educator is presenting a seminar to nursing students on insulin. What would be the best response to these questions?

1. Why is regular insulin the only insulin administered intravenously?

2. If regular insulin is most like human insulin, why do doctors prescribe rapid-acting insulin such as insulin aspart (NovoLog) and insulin glulisine (Apidra)?

3. How is using detemir (Levemir) or glargine (Lantus) insulin better than using NPH insulin?

4. What is the disadvantage of using basal glargine (Lantus) insulin?

5. Some prescribers order basal glargine (Lantus) insulin in the morning rather than the evening as the literature recommends. Why would they do this?

6. Patients sometimes need both basal and bolus doses of insulin at the same time. What could happen if the basal detemir (Levemir) or glargine (Lantus) insulin is mixed with a bolus of insulin aspart (NovoLog) or other rapid or fast acting insulins?

7. What should the patient or nurse do if an insulin vial is cloudy?

57

Drugs for Thyroid Disorders

Answers can be reviewed online at http://evolve.elsevier.com/Lehne/.

OBJECTIVES

See page 28 for the Objectives.

CRITICAL THINKING AND STUDY QUESTIONS

1. A patient asks why thyroid hormone affects decline slowly. The basis of the nurse's response is that thyroid hormone
   a. contains iodine.
   b. is excreted by the kidneys.
   c. interacts with many other drugs.
   d. is primarily protein bound.

2. The primary function of tetraiodothyronine (T_4) in the body is
   a. catalyzing the oxidation of iodide to iodine.
   b. enzymatic conversion to thyroxine (T_3) in tissues.
   c. modulating gene transcription.
   d. producing proteins that promote thyroid hormone effects.

3. Which of the following best explains control of the release of thyroid hormone?
   a. High plasma levels of T_3 and T_4 signal the hypothalamus to decrease production of thyrotropin-releasing hormone (TRH).
   b. High plasma levels of T_3 and T_4 signal the hypothalamus to decrease production of thyrotropin (TSH).
   c. Low plasma levels of T_3 and T_4 signal the pituitary to increase production of TRH.
   d. Low plasma levels of T_3 and T_4 signal the hypothalamus to increase production of TSH.

4. The nurse is preparing to administer synthetic levothyroxine (Synthroid). Which of the following laboratory values, if significantly low, would be a reason for the nurse to withhold the medication and consult the prescriber?
   a. Free T_3
   b. Free T_4
   c. TSH
   d. T_3

5. Adequate maternal thyroid hormone replacement therapy during pregnancy is most important to the fetus during the
   a. first week of pregnancy.
   b. first trimester of pregnancy.
   c. second trimester of pregnancy.
   d. third trimester of pregnancy.

6. Which of the following statements, if made by a patient receiving the antithyroid drug propylthiouracil (PTU), would indicate a need for further teaching?
   a. "After this drug gets to a therapeutic level, it should help my heart to stop feeling like it is racing."
   b. "I should gain weight while eating less when I am on this drug."
   c. "This drug should help decrease the bulging appearance of my eyes."
   d. "This drug should stop the feeling that I am always too hot."

✶ 7. Which of the following assessment findings would be most critical for the nurse to report to the prescriber immediately if noted in a patient with urosepsis who has a history of Graves' disease treated by an antithyroid drugs?
   a. Blood pressure 150/88 mm Hg
   b. Pulse 90 beats/min
   c. Respirations 24 breaths per minute
   d. Temperature 104°F (40°C)

8. The nurse is caring for a patient who receives levothyroxine. Which of the following drugs, if also prescribed, should be separated by hours from the administration of levothyroxine?
   a. Carbazamepine (Tegretol)
   b. Ferrous sulfate (iron supplement)
   c. Rifampin (Rifadin)
   d. Sertraline (Zoloft)

▶ 9. Because of drug interactions, the nurse should monitor a patient who has been taking warfarin and has recently been prescribed levothyroxine for
   a. bleeding.
   b. dysrhythmias.
   c. insomnia.
   d. tachycardia.

10. Which of the following statements, if made by a patient who has type 1 diabetes mellitus and was recently diagnosed with hypothyroidism and prescribed levothyroxine (Synthroid), would indicate a need for further teaching?
    a. "I should check my blood sugar if I get really thirsty, hot, and feel flushed."
    b. "I will not need as much insulin when I am taking Synthroid."
    c. "It is very important to check my blood sugar before meals and at bedtime."
    d. "It will be weeks before the level of Synthroid levels off in my blood and my basal insulin dose can be adjusted accordingly."

11. A patient tells the nurse that for her insurance company to pay for prescription drugs her insurance requires that she use a generic drug if one is available. Up to now, she has been taking brand name Synthroid. The nurse should advise the patient to
    a. ask the pharmacist what is best.
    b. discuss this change with her prescriber.
    c. pay for the brand name.
    d. use the generic brand; there is no difference.

12. A patient has received instructions regarding administration of levothyroxine (Synthroid). Which of these statements made by the patient would indicate that the patient understood the directions?
    a. "I should take the drug in the morning with breakfast."
    b. "Stomach upset occurs if the drug is taken with an antacid."
    c. "Taking the drug on an empty stomach 30 minutes before breakfast increases drug absorption."
    d. "Taking the drug with orange juice increases drug absorption."

▶ 13. Because of the risk of agranulocytosis, the nurse should teach the patient who has been prescribed propylthiouracil (PTU) to report which of the following symptoms?
    a. Anorexia
    b. Bleeding gums
    c. Pale conjunctiva
    d. Sore throat

14. A 34-year-old female is prescribed Iodine[131] for toxic nodular goiter. Which statement, if made by this patient, would indicate a need for further teaching?
    a. "I can develop inadequate thyroid hormone secretion from this therapy."
    b. "I must stay at home during therapy to avoid exposing others to radiation."
    c. "I need to use two reliable methods of birth control."
    d. "This drug takes months before it is fully effective."

15. Which of these factors, if identified in a patient receiving Lugol's solution, would be a concern to the nurse?
    a. Decrease in free T_3
    b. Gain of 2 lb in 2 weeks
    c. States beverages have a brassy taste
    d. Takes the drug with grapefruit juice

CASE STUDIES AND PATIENT TEACHING

(Use a separate piece of paper for your responses.)

Case Study 1

A 30-year-old mother of two notices that she is gaining weight. She visits her family physician complaining that she has been experiencing unusual fatigue, lethargy, and intolerance to cold. At the visit her vital signs are BP 100/58 mm Hg, P 62, R 16, and T 97.8°F.

1. What thyroid disorder do these symptoms suggest?

2. What laboratory test results would the nurse expect to see on this patient if she is hypothyroid?

3. After appropriate history, physical examination, and laboratory studies, she is diagnosed with primary hypothyroidism and started on levothyroxine (Synthroid) 112 mcg once a day. What teaching should the nurse provide about expected timing for relief of symptoms?

4. What teaching should the nurse provide to this patient about administration of levothyroxine (Synthroid)?

5. The nurse should teach about possible adverse effects of levothyroxine. What adverse effects warrant notification of the prescriber?

6. The patient tells the nurse that her sister has asked for some of her thyroid pills to help her lose weight. She wants to know if this would be a problem. How should the nurse respond?

7. The patient returns for her 1-year checkup. She wonders if she still needs the medication because she sometimes forgets to take the drug and does not feel any different on those days. How should the nurse respond?

Case Study 2

Propranolol (Inderal) 10 mg and propylthiouracil (PTU) 100 mg 3 times a day are prescribed for a 25-year-old woman who was recently diagnosed with Graves' disease.

1. What laboratory results would the nurse expect to see when reviewing this patient's chart?

2. The patient asks the nurse why two drugs have been prescribed. What information should the nurse provide regarding the need for both drugs?

3. The drug methimazole (Tapazole) only needs to be taken once a day and PTU needs to be taken 3 times a day. What would be a reason why the prescriber chose PTU for this patient?

4. What assessments should the nurse teach the patient to monitor, and what findings should be reported to the prescriber?

5. Six months later, the patient's heart rate, blood pressure, TSH, and free T_3 levels are within normal limits. The prescriber provides a plan for gradual decrease, then discontinuation of propranolol (Inderal). Why was this drug dose tapered rather than discontinued if vital signs are normal?

Answers can be reviewed online at http://evolve.elsevier.com/Lehne/.

OBJECTIVES

See page 28 for the Objectives.

CRITICAL THINKING AND STUDY QUESTIONS

1. Match the following hormones (abbreviations) with their functions.

a. ACTH	1.	Inhibits the release of GH
b. ADH	2.	Stimulates adrenal cortex
c. FSH	3.	Stimulates development of
d. GH		structure within a ruptured ovarian
e. LH		follicle that secretes estrogen
f. Oxytocin		and progesterone
g. Prolactin	4.	Stimulates maturation of ova in
h. Somastatin		ovary
i. TSH	5.	Stimulates milk production
	6.	Stimulates tissue growth
	7.	Stimulates thyroid
	8.	Stimulates uterine contractions
	9.	Stimulates water resorption by
		the kidney

2. Which of the following findings would the nurse expect to find in a child who has a deficiency in secretion of growth hormone (GH)?
   a. Cognitive deficiency
   b. Long trunk and short extremities
   c. Profuse sweating
   d. Thin arms and legs

3. Which of the following laboratory results would the nurse expect in an otherwise healthy child who is receiving GH?
   a. Decrease in blood urea nitrogen
   b. Decrease in fasting blood sugar
   c. Increase in blood urea nitrogen
   d. Increase in fasting blood sugar

4. Which of these assessment findings, if identified in a patient who is receiving pegvisomant (Somavert), most likely suggests possible liver injury and should be reported to the prescriber?
   a. Headache
   b. Nasal congestion
   c. Malaise
   d. Tea-colored urine

5. The nurse is teaching a patient how to administer intranasal desmopressin. In order to prevent local injury, the nurse should teach the patient to administer the spray
   a. lying down with the head turned toward the side of administration.
   b. on arising in the morning.
   c. using the hand that is on the opposite side of the nostril.
   d. when inhaling.

6. A patient who was recently diagnosed with hypothalamic diabetes insipidus and prescribed vasopressin reports weight gain of 1 to 2 lb per day for the past week. The nurse should recognize that this may indicate
   a. failure to comply with directions for administration of the drug.
   b. failure to limit water intake.
   c. improper diagnosis.
   d. the drug dose is inadequate.

7. When administering vasopressin to a patient with diabetes insipidus, which of the following urine specific gravity results would indicate that therapy has achieved the desired effect?
   a. 1.0002
   b. 1.002
   c. 1.02
   d. 1.2

165

8. An adolescent girl with schizophrenia that is being treated with haloperidol (Haldol) is prescribed carbergoline (Dostinex). The patient's mother asks why this drug is being prescribed. The nurse explains that the drug counteracts which adverse effect of the antipsychotic drug?
   a. Breast tenderness
   b. Constipation
   c. Dry mouth
   d. Orthostatic hypotension

CASE STUDIES AND PATIENT TEACHING

(Use a separate piece of paper for your responses.)

Case Study 1

The nurse works in an endocrine clinic at a major pediatric center that sees children with short stature. When GH therapy with somatropin (Humatrope) is prescribed, the nurse must teach the patient and parents self-administration of the drug.

1. What should the nurse include in the teaching of the technique of subcutaneous injection of this drug?

2. What will the nurse include when explaining the importance of monitoring weight while on this drug?

3. A patient is prescribed somatropin (Humatrope) 0.18 mg/kg/wk to be divided into three doses administered on Monday, Wednesday, and Friday. The nurse teaches the parents of the child who weighs 28 kg to administer how much somatropin (Humatrope) at each dose?

4. Some parents want therapy with GH for their child, but the prescriber decides that risks are greater than benefits. What information can the nurse provide to reinforce prescriber teaching about why therapy with GH may not be advisable for children with the following conditions?
   a. Prader-Willi syndrome

   b. Diabetes mellitus

   c. Uncontrolled asthma

Case Study 2

Intramuscular vasopressin 5 units now and 5 units every 4 hours as needed are prescribed for a patient with postoperative abdominal distention.

1. What should the nurse assess before administering this drug?

2. What assessment findings would be a reason to withhold the drug and contact the prescriber?

Case Study 3

A child who has become unresponsive to somatropin (Humatrope) has been prescribed mecasermin (insulin-like growth factor-1). The nurse is teaching the patient and parent about possible adverse effects and management.

1. What would the nurse include in teaching about the following?
   a. Hypoglycemia
   b. Tonsilar hypertrophy
   c. Local and systemic allergic reactions

4. Antibodies are also known as (Select all that apply.)
   a. B lymphocytes.
   b. dendritic cells.
   c. gamma globulins.
   d. immunoglobulins.
   e. macrophages.
   f. monophils.

5. Match the following immunoglobulins and descriptors:

   _____ a. IgA
   _____ b. IgD
   _____ c. IgE
   _____ d. IgG
   _____ e. IgM

   1. Elevated in allergic reactions with histamine release
   2. First antibody produced in response to an antigen
   3. First line of defense in gastro-intestinal (GI) tract and lungs
   4. Most abundant antibody
   5. Only found on the surface of B cells

6. Salk developed an injected vaccine for polio. When Sabin developed an oral vaccine, people who already had received the Salk vaccine were revaccinated with the Sabin vaccine. Based on the fact that polio is transmitted via the oral-fecal route, the rationale for these mass revaccinations is the
   a. Sabin vaccine did not involve the pain of an injection.
   b. Sabin vaccine sensitized the GI mucosa to prevent the polio microbe from entering the bloodstream.
   c. Salk vaccine only stimulated the production of IgM.
   d. Salk vaccine did not cause adequate production of IgM on the surface of mature B cells.

7. Breast-feeding
   a. does not affect the infant's immunity.
   b. produces life-long immunity for the diseases for which the mother has immunity.
   c. transfers maternal IgA to the infant's GI tract.
   d. triggers the release of mediators from mast cells.

8. The ability of the immune system to identify different antigens is a result of

9. Autoimmune diseases occur when
   a. a new antigen is introduced to the body, and the immune system does not recognize the antigen.
   b. a person has an inflammatory reaction to an antigen.
   c. an antigen is introduced, and the immune response fades too quickly.
   d. there is a failure in major histocompatibility complex (MHC) molecules' ability to identify self.

10. A person who is allergic to penicillin would expect a more severe reaction with exposure to penicillin in the future because
    a. helper T cells attack the penicillin molecule.
    b. higher doses of penicillin would have to be used.
    c. memory cells that identified the penicillin as an antigen allow for a more rapid, intense, and prolonged response.
    d. the immune system cannot eliminate the penicillin.

11. An immunologic reason for the fact that red blood cells (RBC) can be transfused from one person to another is
    a. human RBC do not have class I MHC molecules.
    b. human blood is exactly the same in all individuals.
    c. human blood does not respond to class II MHC molecules.
    d. nonexistent because the above statement is not true.

12. The nurse is reviewing the laboratory tests for a patient who is jaundiced. Laboratory results include an elevated tumor necrosis factor (TNF). This suggests the patient has
    a. cirrhosis or hepatitis.
    b. diabetes mellitus or insipidus.
    c. inflammation or a tumor.
    d. kidney cancer or renal failure.

13. Cells that provide signals to regulate cell proliferation and function during immune responses are called
    a. antigen-presenting cells.
    b. cytokines.
    c. MHC molecules.
    d. opsonins.

14. Activation of the complement pathway occurs when the first component of the complement system (C1) encounters
    a. a free antibody.
    b. a free antigen.
    c. an antibody-antigen complex.

15. How do antibodies neutralize viruses?

16. A 45-year-old patient has been infected with *Mycobacterium tuberculosis*. What kind of immunity response has been activated?
    a. Activation of cytolytic T cells by recognizing *Mycobacterium tuberculosis* bound to a class I MHC molecule
    b. DTH where macrophage activates CD4 helper cells, which activate macrophages, allowing it to kill the bacteria residing within the macrophage

17. Macrophages increase production of lysosome and reactive oxygen to kill bacteria within the macrophage in response to
    a. granulocyte-macrophage colony-stimulating factor.
    b. interferon gamma.
    c. interleukins.
    d. TNF.

18. The principle job of cytolytic T lymphocytes is to kill self cells that are infected with
    a. bacteria.
    b. fungi.
    c. helminths.
    d. viruses.

CASE STUDIES AND PATIENT TEACHING

(Use a separate piece of paper for your responses.)

Case Study 1

The nurse is preparing to perform intradermal injection of house dust, molds, foods, and other common allergens.

1. Why are injected extracts called antigens?

2. The allergic reaction causes degranulation of mast cells. What cells respond in the skin, what do they release, and what dermal symptoms will the patient have if allergic to the antigen?

3. The patient is required to remain in the office for 20 minutes after injection of any antigen because that is the usual time frame for an immediate hypersensitivity reaction. What symptom is most important for the nurse to tell the patient to report?
    a. Itching
    b. Redness
    c. Rhinorrhea
    d. Tingling around the mouth

4. Why is it important to teach this patient about possible anaphylaxis?

67
Childhood Immunization

Answers can be reviewed online at http://evolve.elsevier.com/Lehne/.

OBJECTIVES

See page 28 for the Objectives.

CRITICAL THINKING AND STUDY QUESTIONS

1. The nurse has volunteered to work triaging people who have been trapped in their homes during a flood. To be protected from contracting disease from contaminated areas in the early days of this work, the nurse should obtain what type of immunization?
   a. Live attenuated vaccine
   b. Killed vaccine
   c. Pooled immunoglobulins
   d. Specific immunoglobulins

2. The pediatric office nurse is responsible for obtaining vaccine information sheets to be provided to parents before they consent to vaccinations for their children. The best source of this information is
   a. www.cdc.gov.
   b. www.immunize.org.
   c. pubmedcentral.nih.gov.
   d. www.webmd.com.

3. If smallpox has been eradicated from the planet earth, why has the Centers for Disease Control and Prevention (CDC) of the U.S. government recommended that certain healthcare providers consider vaccination against smallpox?

4. The nurse must be prepared for anaphylactic reactions after administering immunizations. The highest incidence of this type of reaction occurs with
   a. diphtheria, tetanus, acellular pertussis (DTaP).
   b. *Haemophilus influenzae* type b vaccine (Hib).
   c. measles, mumps, and rubella (MMR).
   d. oral poliovirus vaccine (OPV).

5. A 17-month-old child is not on schedule for receiving DTaP, MMR, varicella, and pneumococcal conjugate immunizations. The parent has brought the child to the pediatrician because she has been fussy, lethargic, and not eating. The child has a temperature of 100.1°F and is diagnosed with streptococcal pharyngitis. Amoxicillin is prescribed. The nurse expects that the immunizations that would bring this child up to date will
   a. be administered.
   b. be administered at the next scheduled well-child visit.
   c. not be administered until the child is afebrile.
   d. not be administered until the child has finished the antibiotic.

6. Research suggests that the most common serious adverse reaction that has been associated with the DTaP immunization is
   a. anaphylaxis.
   b. autism.
   c. encephalitis.
   d. Guillain-Barré syndrome.

7. Match the communicable diseases or microbes to the major concerns for each.

   _____ a. Diphtheria
   _____ b. Hepatitis
   _____ c. Hib
   _____ d. HPV
   _____ e. Measles
   _____ f. Meningococcal meningitis
   _____ g. Mumps
   _____ h. Pertussis
   _____ i. Pneumococcal
   _____ j. Poliomyelitis
   _____ k. Rotavirus
   _____ l. Rubella
   _____ m. Tetanus
   _____ n. Varicella

   1. Cerebellar ataxia and Reye's syndrome
   2. Cervical and anal cancer
   3. Congenital defects including deafness
   4. One hundred-day cough
   5. Encephalitis
   6. Liver damage
   7. Neurologic disability or death
   8. Obstructed airway
   9. Orchiditis and possible sterility
   10. Otitis media
   11. Pediatric dehydration
   12. Pneumonia and meningitis
   13. Skeletal muscle paralysis
   14. Skeletal muscle spasm

▶✳ 8. The literature states that wild-type polio has been eliminated from the Western Hemisphere. What type of polio is still present in the Western Hemisphere, and how could a person contract this type of polio?

▶✳ 9. The nurse would consult with the prescriber if which of the following immunizations was prescribed for a child who is receiving chronic high doses of prednisolone? (Select all that apply.)
   a. DTaP
   b. HAV
   c. HBV
   d. Hib
   e. IPV
   f. MCV4
   g. MMR
   h. Rota virus
   i. Varicella vaccine

▶ 10. Foster parents bring a 14-month-old child in for the first visit at the pediatrician's office. The child protective agency has been unable to obtain any immunization records. The office nurse would expect to
   a. administer the immunizations scheduled for 12 to 14 months.
   b. assist the pediatrician with reviewing the child's known medical history to determine which immunizations can be safely administered.
   c. delay immunizations until records can be found.
   d. immunize the child with the immunizations scheduled for 2 months of age.

▶ 11. The nurse knows that the MMR vaccine should not be administered to a child who
   a. has a mother receiving chemotherapy for breast cancer.
   b. has been diagnosed with leukemia.
   c. has had a positive Monospot test (EBV infection).
   d. is asymptomatic, but HIV positive.

▶ 12. The nurse is preparing to immunize an 18-year-old college-bound female. The nurse tells the patient "You cannot get pregnant for 2 months if I give you this shot." Why is this not a good statement for the nurse to make to this adolescent?
   a. Pregnancy is not contraindicated after MMR vaccination.
   b. The statement assumes that the teen is sexually active.
   c. The statement is a communication blocker.
   d. The teen may interpret the statement as the injection prevents pregnancy.

13. Which of the following would be critical to include when the office nurse is discussing a scheduled MMR vaccination with the parents of a 12-month-old boy? (Select all that apply.)
   a. Does your child have allergies to gelatin?
   b. Any adverse effects that occur from this vaccine should occur within 48 hours of receiving the vaccination.
   c. Has your child received any blood or blood products in the past 6 months?
   d. Is your child taking an antibiotic?
   e. Contact the office if you notice the child having any unusual bleeding or bruising.
   f. The child should not have close contact with anyone who is pregnant for 3 weeks after receiving the vaccine.
   g. There is a small risk that your child can experience seizures relating to a high fever.
   h. Vomiting and diarrhea are common adverse effects of this vaccine.

14. When choosing a site for vaccinations, the nurse is aware that it is generally recommended that live vaccinations be administered
   a. intradermally.
   b. intramuscularly.
   c. orally.
   d. subcutaneously.

▶ 15. The triage nurse receives a call from a mother who is concerned about her 2-month-old son who received the first DTaP vaccination 5 days ago. Which of the following, if reported by the mother, would be of most concern to the nurse?
   a. Crying inconsolably for the past 2 days
   b. Only nursing for 10 minutes every 4 or 5 hours
   c. Redness and swelling at the injection site
   d. Temperature of 103°F

16. The CDC currently recommends the inactivated poliovirus vaccine (IPV or Salk) instead of the oral polio vaccine (OPV or Sabin) because
    a. immune compromised people can contract polio from OPV.
    b. IPV causes less adverse effects than OPV.
    c. IPV is less expensive than OPV.
    d. OPV is less effective than IPV.

17. Which of the following, if elicited by the nurse from the parent of a 15-month-old who is scheduled to receive the varicella vaccine, would be a reason to withhold administering the vaccine and consulting the prescriber?
    a. The child had a severe reaction to the MMR vaccine.
    b. The child is allergic to eggs.
    c. The mother's sister and her newborn are temporarily staying with the family.
    d. The office has used all of the syringes with 1-inch needles.

18. The triage office nurse receives a call from the father of a 16-year-old who received a varicella vaccine 10 days ago. The teen experienced a fever after the injection, which was treated with aspirin. Yesterday the teen stayed home from school with stomach flu. He has not vomited today, but the father is having difficulty awakening him. The nurse should direct the father to
    a. allow the teen to rest and call back tomorrow morning.
    b. make an appointment to be seen in the office.
    c. reassess the teen's temperature.
    d. seek medical care immediately.

19. The nurse would expect to administer a booster dose of varicella vaccine one month after the first dose to a child who is (has)
    a. not gotten a fever from the first dose.
    b. older than 12 years at the time of the first dose and has not had chickenpox.
    c. 13 years old at the time of the first dose and has had chicken pox.
    d. younger than 18 months.

20. The nursery nurse would expect to administer which of the following vaccinations to the neonate if the mother of the neonate is HBsAg-positive? (Select all that apply.)
    a. Hepatitis B immunoglobulin (HBIG)
    b. Havrix

c. Influenza vaccine
d. Pneumovax
e. Recombivax HB
f. Twinrix

21. The nurse would consult the prescriber before administering vaccinations if a patient who has a history of Guillain-Barré syndrome is scheduled to receive which of the following vaccinations? (Select all that apply.)
    a. DTaP
    b. HBV
    c. Hib
    d. HPV
    e. Influenza vaccine
    f. IPV
    g. MCV
    h. MMR
    i. Varicella

22. A patient who has had a splenectomy asks why he needs to get a meningitis vaccine. The basis of the nurse's response is that the spleen
    a. destroys old red blood cells.
    b. forms blood cells.
    c. is a critical defense whenever a patient has a fever.
    d. removes encapsulated bacteria from the bloodstream.

CASE STUDIES AND PATIENT TEACHING

(Use a separate piece of paper for your responses.)

Case Study 1

A mother brings her 7-month-old child to the clinic. She states that she was told by the emergency department (ED) physician of the local hospital to bring the child in for "baby shots." The mother is concerned, stating that she has heard children die from these "baby shots."

1. What teaching can the nurse provide about the safety and benefits of the immunizations?

2. The mother has difficulty understanding complex concepts. How can the nurse explain reactions to immunizations?

3. How would the nurse explain laws requiring children to have immunizations before they can attend school and, in some cases, day care?

4. What information does the mother need to collect when a child is scheduled for an immunization?

Case Study 2

Parents of an elementary school child in western Pennsylvania have verbalized to the school nurse that their children have never been "contaminated" with immunizations. The parent cites that her unimmunized child has not contracted the measles, mumps, diphtheria, or other illness for which immunizations are routinely administered.

1. How should the school nurse respond?

2. The parents state that they are particularly concerned about MMR because of its association with autism. What has research suggested about the association of MMR and autism?

3. The school nurse is aware that exposure to certain populations or situations put unvaccinated children at risk for contracting vaccine-preventable disease. What are possible populations and situations that would put children at risk in this school and geographic area?

Case Study 3

1. In addition to documenting the required information regarding vaccinations on the patient's chart, what procedure could the pediatric office nurse use to expedite identifying patients who have received specific vaccines in case of future issues with specific manufacturers?

Case Study 4

During pharmacology class, a nursing student remarks that she would not have her 11-year-old daughter vaccinated with Gardasil because "she is a good girl."

1. What should be included in the discussion about this parental reaction?

2. The concerned parent nursing student agrees with the explanation but states that her daughter has heard that the injection is painful. What might the nurse discuss with the pediatrician about this concern?

3. The literature reports a number of adolescent patients fainting when given the human papilloma virus (HPV) vaccine. What might contribute to this reaction, and what can the office nurse do to prepare for this possible reaction?

Answers can be reviewed online at http://evolve.elsevier.com/Lehne/.

OBJECTIVES

See page 28 for the Objectives.

CRITICAL THINKING AND STUDY QUESTIONS

✳ 1. The nurse is doing postoperative teaching for a patient who has had carpal tunnel release surgery and who is receiving immunosuppressant therapy for rheumatoid arthritis. Based on the surgery and medication, the priority nursing concern would be preventing
   a. airway constriction.
   b. infection.
   c. pain.
   d. impaired tissue perfusion.

2. The nurse teaches a patient who has been prescribed immunosuppressant drugs to report early signs of infection, such as
   a. chills and rigor.
   b. cough.
   c. rash.
   d. sore throat.

3. The nurse is administering intravenous (IV) cyclosporine (Sandimmune). Within 15 minutes after beginning the infusion, the patient complains of feeling hot. Her skin is flushed. The nurse assesses vital signs. Her blood pressure is 80/55 mm Hg, pulse is 108 beats/min, and respirations are 25 breaths per minute. The nurse should discontinue the infusion and administer prescribed as needed
   a. acetaminophen (Tylenol).
   b. epinephrine (Adrenalin).
   c. lorazepam (Ativan).
   d. ondansetron (Zofran).

4. A sexually active female patient is prescribed cyclosporine to prevent rejection of her kidney transplant. It is important for the nurse to teach the patient about the drug's possible effects on a developing fetus and that current contraceptive recommendations include use of which type of birth control
   a. barrier, such as a latex condom.
   b. contraceptive patch containing norelgestromin and estradiol.
   c. oral contraceptive containing estradiol.
   d. oral contraceptive containing mestranol.

▶ 5. When reviewing the laboratory results of patients receiving cyclosporine (Sandimmune) and tacrolimus (Prograf), which of the following results would be a reason to contact the prescriber? (Select all that apply.)
   a. ALT   28 international units
   b. Bilirubin, direct   2 mg/dL
   c. BUN   17 mg/dL
   d. Creatinine   3.2 mg/dL
   e. Potassium   5.4 mEq/L
   f. WBC   7000/mm^3

6. A patient asks why he is prescribed ketoconazole in addition to cyclosporine. The nurse explains that the main reason these two drugs are administered concurrently is to
   a. decrease adverse effects of cyclosporine while maintaining therapeutic blood levels.
   b. decrease cyclosporine levels to prevent nephrotoxicity.
   c. increase cyclosporine levels to therapeutic levels.
   d. lower doses and costs of cyclosporine while maintaining therapeutic blood levels.

7. When should the nurse draw cyclosporine trough levels?
   a. Just after administering a dose
   b. Just before the next dose
   c. One-half hour after administering a dose
   d. One-half hour before administering a dose

191

8. The nurse is providing discharge teaching to a patient and his significant others regarding being prescribed oral cyclosporine to prevent rejection of a transplanted kidney. Which of the following statements, if made by the patient, suggests understanding of the teaching? (Select all that apply.)
   a. "I should make an appointment to see the doctor if I have episodes of nausea and abdominal pain or if my BM changes color."
   b. "I should use the same pharmacy for all of my prescriptions."
   c. I should be careful when I stand up because this drug commonly makes people feel dizzy."
   d. "If I'm not peeing as much as usual, it is probably due to the drug, not failure of the new kidney."
   e. "It is important to see my dentist regularly."
   f. "This drug is known to cause life-threatening allergic reactions so I need to call 911 if I feel flushed or feel my heart beating when I take this drug."

9. A renal transplant patient's orders include discontinuation of IV tacrolimus (Prograf) and starting oral tacrolimus. The last IV dose was administered at 10:00 AM. The first oral dose should be administered no sooner than
   a. 2:00 PM.
   b. 4:00 PM.
   c. 6:00 PM.
   d. 8:00 PM.

▶ 10. A liver transplant patient who takes tacrolimus reveals that he has been drinking grapefruit juice, but he has made sure it has been at least 4 hours between the juice and the medication. Which of the following suggests a drug-food interaction?
   a. Blood pressure 88/47 mm Hg
   b. Fasting blood sugar 235 mg/dL
   c. Temperature 102°F
   d. Urine output 100 mL/4 hr

11. A 16-month-old child receives a heart-lung transplant. What teaching should the nurse provide about immunizations relating to immunosuppressant therapy? (Select all that apply.)
   a. The child may need more than the usual recommended doses of inactivated vaccines.
   b. The child may need more than the usual recommended doses of live vaccines.
   c. The child should not receive any inactivated vaccines.
   d. The child should not receive any live vaccines.
   e. The child should not receive any vaccines.

12. Body image is developmentally important to many patients. It is important for the nurse to discuss body image when cyclosporine has been prescribed to a young woman because the drug can cause
   a. acne.
   b. facial hair.
   c. rash.
   d. weight gain.

13. The main reason why tacrolimus therapy is discontinued is toxicity. Which of the following drugs, if taken with tacrolimus, is most likely to cause toxicity?
   a. Erythromycin
   b. Phenobarbital
   c. Phenytoin
   d. Rifamycin

▶ 14. Trough levels of tacrolimus are 10 ng/mL. The nurse should
   a. administer the medication.
   b. hold the medication.

15. Match the following drugs and adverse effects. (Answer may be used more than once.)
   _____ a. Azathioprine   1. Decreased bone density
   _____ b. Cyclosporine   2. Hyperglycemia
   _____ c. Prednisone   3. Hypercholesterolemia
   _____ d. Sirolimus   and hypertriglyceridemia
   _____ e. Tacrolimus   4. Tremor
                              5. Unexplained bleeding

16. Because sirolimus has a half-life of 2.5 days and it is categorized as pregnancy category C, the nurse teaches women of child-bearing years to continue using birth control for what period of time after discontinuing use of sirolimus?
   a. 1 week
   b. 4 weeks
   c. 8 weeks
   d. 12 weeks

17. The nurse should teach patients who take sirolimus to take the medication
   a. consistently with or consistently without food.
   b. on an empty stomach.
   c. with food.
   d. with 8 ounces of water.

18. A patient receiving azathioprine develops gout and is prescribed allopurinol. In addition to monitoring renal functioning because of possible damage to the kidneys by the elevated uric acid, the nurse would expect the prescriber to
    a. decrease the dose of allopurinol.
    b. increase the dose of allopurinol.
    c. decrease the dose of azathioprine.
    d. increase the dose of azathioprine.

19. The nurse is providing discharge instructions for a patient who is prescribed mycophenolate mofetil (CellCept). Which of the following over-the-counter drugs can prevent mycophenolate mofetil from reaching therapeutic concentrations in the blood?
    a. Acetaminophen (Tylenol)
    b. Antacids
    c. Diphenhydramine (Benadryl)
    d. NSAIDs

20. Which of the following should be employed when administering antilymphocyte globulin (Atgam)? (Select all that apply.)
    a. Administer using an in-line filter.
    b. Assess for flushing, dyspnea, and generalized anxiety.
    c. Do not take aluminum or magnesium antacids because they decrease absorption of the drug.
    d. Infuse slowly—over 4 hours or more.
    e. Premedicate with a glucocorticoid to prevent adverse effects.
    f. Administer via a central line.
    g. Instruct the patient not to drink grapefruit juice.

21. A neonate is Rh negative. The nurse would expect to administer Rh$_o$(D) immune globulin to
    a. the mother if she is Rh negative.
    b. the mother if she is Rh positive.
    c. the mother if she is Rh positive or negative.
    d. the neonate.

CASE STUDIES AND PATIENT TEACHING

(Use a separate piece of paper for your responses.)

Case Study 1

A 4-year-old girl received an allogenic heart transplant at age 16 months for transposition of the great vessels and only one ventricle, which resulted in cardiac failure.

1. What is an allogenic transplant?

The patient was discharged on cyclosporine, azathioprine (Imuran), and prednisone. She is brought back to the transplant site monthly for blood work to monitor rejection status and performance of her new heart. During the past year, she has shown no sign of rejection or limitation of her activities. Her growth has more closely followed normal growth charts and outwardly she appears to be a healthy 4-year-old. Recently, following a trip to a national park, she developed fatigue and appeared tired. Blood work indicated evidence of macrophages and monocytes beginning the rejection process. She was hospitalized and diagnosed with evidence of transplant rejection.

2. What are nursing priorities for this patient?

3. Intravenous muromonab-CD3 is added to the patient's medication regimen to prevent rejection of the transplanted heart. What actions should the nurse take in the hospital to prevent the patient from contracting an infection?

4. What special steps must be taken when administering this drug IV?

5. Four hours after receiving the first dose of muromonab-CD3 the mother tells the nurse that the patient is shivering. Her temperature is 102.6°F. These symptoms could be indicative of further organ rejection or adverse effects to the drug. What should the nurse do?

Case Study 2

A 38-year-old female kidney transplant recipient is prescribed immunosuppressant therapy with IV cyclosporine (Sandimmune), prednisone, and ketoconazole.

1. What teaching should the nurse provide relating to the adverse effect of increased risk of neoplasms from taking cyclosporine?

2. The patient has a history of knee pain and a seizure disorder. What should be included in the plan of nursing care relating to immunosuppressant therapy that she is receiving and her medical history?

3. Intravenous cyclosporine is discontinued, and the patient is started on oral cyclosporine (Gengraf) 9 mg/kg/day divided into 2 doses 12 hours apart. The patient weighs 132 lb, and the medication is available as a solution of 100 mg/mL. What is the prescribed dose in mg?

4. How much medication should the nurse administer?

5. How should the nurse teach the patient to administer this dose of medication?

6. The hospital pharmacy sends the Sandimmune formulation (100 mg/mL). What should the nurse do?

69
Antihistamines

Answers can be reviewed online at http://evolve.elsevier.com/Lehne/.

OBJECTIVES

See page 28 for the Objectives.

CRITICAL THINKING AND STUDY QUESTIONS

1. A patient is scheduled to receive a radiocontrast media for a CAT scan. The patient has never received any radiocontrast media. The radiology nurse must carefully assess for an allergic reaction because allergic reactions
   a. are common because patients often are unaware if they have had radiocontrast media in the past.
   b. are very likely to occur.
   c. can occur even without prior exposure to radiocontrast media.
   d. to contrast media are usually asymptomatic until anaphylaxis occurs.

2. The mother of a 3-year-old child who was recently diagnosed with asthma calls during phone hour at the pediatrician's office. Her child has a cold, which often triggers an asthma attack. She has forgotten which drug she should give him if he starts wheezing. Which of the following drugs would be safe and effective?
   a. Diphenhydramine (Benadryl)—first-generation H_1 antagonist
   b. Loratadine (Claritin)— second-generation H_1 antagonist
   c. Fexofenadine (Allegra)—second-generation H_1 antagonist
   d. No antihistamines are safe and effective for wheezing

3. It is important to teach patients to be sensitive for allergic reactions every time they take a drug because allergic reactions
   a. are common.
   b. are most likely to occur on the third or fourth day of taking a drug.

c. frequently occur even if a patient has never been exposed to the drug or its components.

d. usually occur after previous exposure to a drug or its components.

4. H_1 blocking drugs for allergic reactions (Select all that apply.)

a. are the active ingredient in most over-the-counter (OTC) drugs to induce sleep.

b. can cause excitement, nervousness, and tremors.

c. can cause urinary retention.

d. cause the skin to become red and warm.

e. decrease release of histamine present in high levels in the skin and lungs tract.

f. decrease pruritus.

g. elevate the pH of stomach secretions.

h. have sedation as the most common adverse effect.

i. prevent local edema.

j. prevent the release of histamine from mast cells and basophils.

5. On admission, the nurse is reviewing all of the drugs that a 78-year-old patient takes at home. The patient has a history of hypertension and diabetes. The patient takes OTC diphenhydramine (Benadryl) when she has a cold. That nurse explains the effect of first-generation drugs on the body and on a cold. Which of the following statements, if made by the patient after the teaching, suggests a need for additional teaching?

a. "Benadryl does not prevent colds but it can make my cold get better faster."

b. "Benadryl can make mucus from a cold hard to expel because it thickens the mucus."

c. "Benadryl can make my constipation worse."

d. "My 3-year-old grandson could have convulsions if he would take some of my Benadryl from my purse."

6. The term "antihistamine" is commonly used to refer to drugs that block

a. H_1 receptors.

b. H_2 receptors.

c. H_1 and H_2 receptors.

7. Second-generation H_1 blockers cause less sedation than first-generation H_1 blockers because they

a. are less potent.

b. bind reversibly to histamine receptors.

c. do not cross the blood-brain barrier.

d. are rapidly metabolized.

▶ 8. Which of these assessment findings, if identified by the delivery room nurse in a full-term neonate whose mother has taken diphenhydramine (Benadryl) just before going into labor should be reported to the pediatrician immediately?

a. Systolic BP 60 mm Hg

b. Temperature 39.2°C

c. Pulse 180 beats/min

d. Respirations 37 breaths per minute

9. The nurse is teaching a patient who has a history of benign prostatic hypertrophy (BPH) and allergic rhinitis about taking desloratadine (Clarinex). Teaching should include (Select all that apply.)

a. to avoid alcohol and other CNS depressants.

b. to avoid any activity that requires coordination or alertness.

c. that high doses are more likely to cause sedation.

d. that many patients find hard candy relieves the adverse effect of dry mouth.

e. that monitoring of an ECG for long QT syndrome should be done after starting the drug.

f. that taking doses higher than recommended does not help the drug work better.

g. that the drug may aggravate urinary retention from the enlarged prostate.

▶ 10. The nurse is administering 6 AM medications, including chlorpheniramine (Chlor-Trimeton) 4 mg every 6 hours for urticaria. The patient complains of nausea associated with the medication. The nurse should

a. change the timing of the medication to 8 AM (0800), 12 noon (1200), 4 PM (1600), and 8 PM (2000) to correspond to meals and bedtime snack.

b. decrease the dose of the medication.

c. hold the medication and consult the prescriber.

d. provide a snack with each dose of medication.

▶ 11. A 3-year-old child is brought into the emergency department (ED) after ingesting an unknown quantity of his grandmother's cetirizine (Zyrtec). The child is restless, incoherent, skin is flushed and hot, pulse is 70 beats/min, BP is 70/42 mm Hg, and respirations are 35 breaths per minute. The nurse should be prepared to

a. assess for abnormal movements.

b. administer an antidote.

c. monitor for hypertension.

d. warm the patient.

12. Which of the following H₁ blockers is most likely to cause a sore throat?
    a. Azelastine (Astelin)
    b. Diphenhydramine (Benadryl)
    c. Fexofenadine (Allegra)
    d. Loratadine (Claritin)

CASE STUDIES AND PATIENT TEACHING

(Use a separate piece of paper for your responses.)

Case Study 1

A 25-year-old truck driver has come to his healthcare provider to obtain information and help for his "hay fever." He says he doesn't know what to take because OTC drugs seem so confusing. His condition is diagnosed as allergic rhinitis and is seasonal with reactions lasting from May until the end of June each year. He also says that he is occasionally bothered by dust during the rest of the year. He complains of headache; congestion; sneezing; rhinorrhea (runny nose); and itchy, burning, and watery eyes.

1. What is the physiology involved in this allergic response?

2. What are the disadvantages to antihistamines for those who drive or use heavy equipment at work?

3. The patient is concerned about cost. He asks if prescription antihistamines are more effective than OTC diphenhydramine (Benadryl). How should the nurse respond?

4. How do second-generation antihistamines work but not cause sedation?

5. The prescriber orders azelastine (Astelin) 2 sprays of 250 micrograms in each nostril twice a day. Why is this medication ordered specifically for this patient?

6. What suggestions can the nurse make if the patient chooses to use one of the antihistamines that cause sedation?

70

Cyclooxygenase Inhibitors: Nonsteroidal Anti-inflammatory Drugs and Acetaminophen

Answers can be reviewed online at http://evolve.elsevier.com/Lehne/.

OBJECTIVES

See page 28 for the Objectives.

CRITICAL THINKING AND STUDY QUESTIONS

1. The nurse is administering celecoxib (Celebrex) 100 mg to an 82-year-old patient with osteoarthritis (degenerative joint disease, DJD). Which of the following adverse effects, if present, would be of most concern to the nurse?
   a. Edema
   b. Flatulence
   c. Headache
   d. Nausea

▶ 2. The following information was included in the change of shift report on patients who are prescribed aspirin for its anticoagulant effects. Which of the following patient symptoms, if present, would be most important for the nurse to report to the attending physician?
   a. Abdominal bloating
   b. Coffee ground emesis
   c. Heartburn when recumbent
   d. Two liquid stools in the past 24 hours

▶ 3. Which of the following would not be an appropriate reason for the nurse to administer aspirin 650 mg by mouth that has been ordered every 4 hours as needed?
   a. Hand pain and stiffness when arising
   b. Knee pain with ambulation

    c. Right temporal headache associated with a tense neck

    d. Right upper quadrant pain that intensifies with deep inspiration

4. A 13-year-old girl has been prescribed ibuprofen 600 mg, 1 tablet every 6 hours as needed for severe cramping menstrual pain. Her mother contacts the telephone advice nurse and asks if she can give her over-the-counter (OTC) ibuprofen instead because it is less expensive and she does not have prescription insurance coverage. What information is most accurate for the nurse to include in her response?

    a. Aspirin is just as effective as ibuprofen at relieving menstrual cramps.

    b. Aspirin is ineffective in relieving menstrual pain, even at high doses.

    c. Brand-name preparations of ibuprofen are more effective than generic products.

    d. Three 200-mg generic over-the-counter ibuprofen tablets are equivalent to 600-mg prescription strength ibuprofen.

5. A patient is scheduled for a total knee replacement. Preoperative teaching by the nurse should include that the patient should discontinue high-dose aspirin therapy prescribed for joint pain for what period of time before surgery?

    a. One hour

    b. One day

    c. One week

    d. One month

6. A 52-year-old nurse has just read the results of the Women's Health Initiative (WHI) study published in 2005. Based on this research, it would be appropriate for the nurse to discuss which of the following aspirin therapy regimens with her primary care practitioner (PCP)?

    a. 81 mg once a day

    b. 100 mg every other day

    c. 325 mg once a day

    d. 650 mg once every other day

7. Research suggests that long-term low-dose aspirin use has been shown to prevent

    a. Alzheimer's disease progression.

    b. colon cancer.

    c. hemorrhagic stroke.

    d. myocardial infarction (MI).

▶ 8. To prevent the most common adverse effect of long-term aspirin therapy, the nurse should

    a. administer the drug with food.

    b. assess lung sounds for wheezing before administering the drug.

    c. monitor urine output.

    d. teach the patient to report tarry colored stool.

9. Which of the following statements, if made by a patient who is receiving aspirin therapy for rheumatoid arthritis, suggests that the patient needs further teaching?

    a. "Drinking a full glass of water with my aspirin can help prevent the pill particles from getting trapped in the inside folds of my stomach."

    b. "I will know if aspirin is causing ulcers because it will cause abdominal pain."

    c. "If I drink alcohol, it can irritate my stomach and make it easier for aspirin to cause it to bleed."

    d. "I should stop taking aspirin and consult with my physician if I experience sudden watery runny nose and chest tightness."

▶ 10. It would be extremely important for the nurse to communicate self-prescribed aspirin use to the primary care provider for which of the following patients? (Select all that apply.)

    a. Abuses cocaine

    b. Admitted with status asthmaticus

    c. Has genetic hypercoagulability disorder

    d. History of hemorrhagic cerebral vascular accident (CVA, stroke)

    e. History of hypertension and diabetes mellitus type 2

    f. Sexually active woman using aspirin for dysmenorrhea and not using any form of birth control

    g. Smokes two packs of cigarettes per day

11. How many regular strength aspirin (325 mg) tablets are equivalent to the lowest dose of aspirin that is known to be potentially fatal?

    a. 12

    b. 16

    c. 20

    d. 24

12. The nurse should instruct patients to dispose of aspirin tablets if they develop an odor that smells like

    a. ammonia.

    b. alcohol.

    c. vanilla.

    d. vinegar.

✱ 13. A patient brought into the emergency department (ED) after taking aspirin for a headache exhibits the following symptoms. Which symptom would be a priority for the nurse to address?
a. Bronchospasm
b. Profuse watery nasal discharge
c. Tachycardia
d. Urticaria

▸ 14. The nurse notes a respiratory rate of 41 breaths per minute when assessing an 18-month-old child with suspected salicylate poisoning. Which of the following laboratory results support this diagnosis?
a. pH 7.32; $PaCO_2$ 40 mm Hg; HCO_3^- 24 mEq/L
b. pH 7.35; $PaCO_2$ 37 mm Hg; HCO_3^- 22 mEq/L
c. pH 7.41; $PaCO_2$ 35 mm Hg; HCO_3^- 20 mEq/L
d. pH 7.46; $PaCO_2$ 31 mm Hg; HCO_3^- 18 mEq/L

15. A patient has been prescribed aspirin 81 mg once a day after angioplasty. It is important for the nurse to teach this patient to avoid using which of the following over-the-counter (OTC) medications?
a. Acetaminophen (Tylenol)
b. Calcium carbonate (TUMS)
c. Guaifenesin (Robitussin)
d. Ibuprofen (Motrin, Advil)

16. A post-MI patient with a history of diabetes mellitus and hypertension is advised by his primary care provider to take 325-mg aspirin each day for antiplatelet effects. He asks the nurse which preparation would provide the best results for him and not irritate his stomach. The best response is
a. buffered aspirin solution.
b. enteric-coated aspirin.
c. four chewable children's aspirin.
d. timed-release aspirin.

17. The daughter of a cardiac patient asks why her father has been instructed to take 1 baby aspirin every day. The basis of the nurse's response should be that low-dose aspirin
a. dissolves blood clots.
b. is less irritating to the stomach.
c. prevents platelets from sticking together.
d. relieves chest pain.

18. The nurse instructs a preoperative coronary bypass patient to not take any nonaspirin traditional nonsteroidal anti-inflammatory drugs (NSAIDs) for 14 days before surgery because these drugs
a. cause irreversible inhibition of cyclooxygenase so anticoagulant effects are long lasting.
b. increase the risk of bleeding during surgery.
c. increase the risk of developing a blood clot.
d. increase the risk that the graft will not improve coronary blood flow.

▸ 19. When obtaining a history from a patient, the nurse questions the patient on use of over-the-counter (OTC), herbal, and natural medications. The patient reports regular use of sodium salicylate for joint pain. The nurse would be most concerned about use of this OTC product if the patient has a history of
a. chronic obstructive pulmonary disease.
b. heart failure.
c. diabetes mellitus.
d. excessive bleeding with dental procedures.

▸ 20. The nurse is teaching a patient who has just been prescribed OTC ibuprofen (Advil, Motrin). Which of the following is a symptom of a minor adverse effect that would not need to be immediately reported to the prescriber?
a. Black, sticky stool
b. Chest pain
c. Frontal headache
d. Vesicular rash

21. A patient has been prescribed naproxen plus lansoprazole (Prevacid NapraPAC). Teaching regarding administration of this drug has been successful if the patient states
a. "I should take 1 naproxen and 1 lansoprazole before breakfast and 1 naproxen 12 hours later."
b. "I should take 1 naproxen and 1 lansoprazole before breakfast and again 12 hours later."
c. "I should take 1 lansoprazole before breakfast and 2 naproxen 12 hours later."
d. "I should take 1 combination pill with naproxen and 1 lansoprazole with breakfast."

22. A hospitalized patient is prescribed diclofenac plus misoprostol (Arthrotec) for knee pain associated with osteoarthritis. He had been taking ibuprofen at home. He asks the nurse how this drug differs from ibuprofen. When describing

the misoprostol component of Arthrotec, the nurse explains that this drug prevents GI distress associated with NSAIDs by
a. decreasing stomach acid production.
b. decreasing stomach acid production and promoting gastric mucous production.
c. preventing gastric reflux and promoting gastric mucous production.
d. promoting gastric mucous and acid production.

23. The parents of a premature neonate ask the nurse to explain the medications that are prescribed for their baby. The most logical explanation for indomethacin (Indocin) being prescribed for this neonate is to promote closure of the duct between the
a. inner ear and cochlea.
b. liver and the duodenum.
c. pulmonary artery and the aorta.
d. umbilical vein and the neonate's abdomen.

24. It is most important for the nurse to know how long a patient has been prescribed
a. ketorolac (Toradol).
b. nabumetone (Relafen).
c. piroxicam (Feldene).
d. sulindac (Clinoril).

▸ 25. The nurse works in a large university teaching hospital. A medical resident has prescribed ketorolac (Toradol) 15 mg IM for a woman who is requesting pain relief during labor. The nurse should
a. assess the patient's stage of labor and question the order if the patient is in transition.
b. question administering an intramuscular (IM) injection for a woman in labor.
c. monitor the neonate's respirations for depression after delivery.
d. withhold the drug and question the prescriber.

▸ 26. The prescriber orders celecoxib (Celebrex) 100 mg to be administered twice a day. The nurse would withhold this drug and consult the prescriber if a patient is allergic to
a. amoxicillin.
b. bactrim.
c. ceftin.
d. zithromax.

27. Which of the following assessment findings would be a priority for the nurse to report if a patient was receiving celecoxib (Celebrex)?
a. Bruising of arms and shins
b. A weight gain of 1 lb each day for 3 days
c. Heartburn at night
d. Inadequate joint pain relief after taking for 1 week

▸ 28. The only pain relief order on admission for a new patient is the routine order of acetaminophen 650 mg every 4 hours as needed. The nurse should consult the prescriber regarding possible prescription of an NSAID if the nurse identified that the patient was experiencing
a. muscle cramping.
b. stress headache.
c. swollen, painful joints.
d. temperature greater than 102°F.

▸ 29. A patient is prescribed oxycodone-acetaminophen (Percocet) for postoperative pain. Based on the drug containing acetaminophen, it would be most important for the nurse to consult the prescriber before administering the drug if the patient developed
a. bleeding gums.
b. dyspepsia.
c. jaundice.
d. peripheral edema.

30. Based on the Women's Health Initiative Study, the nurse should teach women who take acetaminophen on a regular basis the importance of frequent assessment of their
a. blood glucose.
b. blood pressure.
c. pulse.
d. serum lipids.

▸ 31. A patient with a known history of chronic obstructive pulmonary disease (COPD) is admitted to an extended-care facility for rehabilitation after an open reduction and internal fixation (ORIF) of a hip fracture. The patient requests acetaminophen 325 mg-oxycodone 5 mg (Percocet) 1 tablet, ordered every 4 hours as needed, before going to physical therapy. The patient states that her pain is 3 of 10 currently, but she experiences unbearable pain if

she does not take the Percocet before therapy. The patient has not received a dose of this drug in the last 4 hours. The nurse should
a. administer the drug.
b. encourage the patient to wait until after therapy to take the drug so that it is longer between doses.
c. withhold the drug and question the prescriber because a patient with liver disease should never take acetaminophen.
d. withhold the drug because the patient's pain does not warrant administration of a narcotic.

▶ 32. The mother of a child calls the pediatrician's office stating that her 15-month-old child just ate an unknown quantity of children's chewable Tylenol tablets while she was busy preparing breakfast. The nurse should
a. assess for the presence of nausea, vomiting, abdominal pain, or diaphoresis.
b. direct the mother to seek medical care for the child immediately.
c. make an appointment for the child to be seen as soon as possible.
d. take the opportunity to teach the mother about child proofing her home.

▶ 33. Acetylcysteine (Acetadote) 2250 mg intravenous to be infused over 30 minutes is prescribed for a 33-lb child who drank Tylenol extra strength liquid. The drug is diluted in 200 mL of 5% dextrose. The infusion pump is calibrated in mL/hr. What rate should the nurse enter as the infusion rate?
a. 100 mL
b. 200 mL
c. 300 mL
d. 400 mL

▶ 34. While infusing acetylcysteine (Acetadote) for acetaminophen overdose, the nurse notes that the patient is scratching her arms. The initial response of the nurse should be to
a. assess respirations, breath sounds, and vital signs.
b. consult the prescriber regarding slowing of the infusion.
c. report the itching to the prescriber.
d. stop the infusion and contact the prescriber STAT.

▶ 35. The pediatric nurse practitioner asks the office nurse to give a parent of a 13-month-old, who has just received an MMR vaccine, a sample of acetaminophen drops (80 mg/0.8 mL) and to explain the age-appropriate dose. The nurse teaches the mother to use the dropper to administer how many mL of the acetaminophen per dose?
a. 0.8 mL
b. 1.2 mL
c. 1.6 mL
d. 2.4 mL

▶ 36. A 3-year-old child is brought to the ED. Nursing triage assessment reveals a lethargic child who does not resist examination. The child's mother states that he had a runny nose, cough, and fever over a week ago. He vomited several times last night. This morning he was so drowsy that she could not arouse him, so she brought him in to the hospital. It is important for the nurse to ask the mother if she administered which of the following products to her child during his illness?
a. Robitussin cough syrup
b. Sudafed decongestant
c. St. Joseph's baby aspirin
d. Tylenol elixir

CASE STUDIES AND PATIENT TEACHING

(Use a separate piece of paper for your responses.)

Case Study 1

The nurse is assisting an obese 58-year-old science teacher who is postoperative total abdominal hysterectomy and bilateral salpingoophorectomy (TAH-BSO) with ambulating in the hallway when the patient complains of knee pain and stiffness. The patient has a history of hypertension, impaired glucose tolerance, and osteoarthritis (degenerative joint disease, DJD). The patient was prescribed the cyclooxygenase-2 (COX-2) enzyme inhibitor rofecoxib (Vioxx) several years ago. She tells the nurse that the drug really helped her knee pain and did not cause stomach distress like other NSAID drugs. She asks the nurse what the difference is between rofecoxib (Vioxx) and other drugs used for mild-to-moderate pain.

1. What could the nurse include in her explanation?

2. The patient asks why rofecoxib (Vioxx) was removed from the market. What information can the nurse share with this patient?

3. The patient asks the nurse if this means she should not take celecoxib (Celebrex). How should the nurse respond?

4. The patient says "I am glad there is still one drug that I can take for my arthritis that does not cause side effects." How should the nurse respond?

5. What nonpharmacologic teaching can the nurse provide this patient?

Case Study 2

A 21-year-old female comes to the family planning clinic to determine what she can do for relief of moderate dysmenorrhea. She states that the pain is not incapacitating, but creates discomfort during the first day of her menses. She says she does not want anything that makes her sleepy and that she has tried acetaminophen without relief. After further assessment, the nurse practitioner suggests that she try ibuprofen as a beginning drug to see how she responds. She is told to take 2 ibuprofen (200 mg tablets) every 4 hours for the first 2 to 3 days of her menstrual period, starting with the first symptom of menses or cramping.

1. Why is this schedule appropriate in this situation?

2. What information should be provided to this patient about possible adverse effects of this drug therapy?

3. Based on the developmental stage of this patient, what teaching should the nurse provide about use of ibuprofen and other over-the-counter NSAID drugs?

Case Study 3

1. What should be included in the discharge teaching of a patient who is prescribed oxycodone/acetaminophen (Percocet) for postoperative pain relating to the non-narcotic component of the drug?

71

Glucocorticoids in Nonendocrine Diseases

Answers can be reviewed online at http://evolve.elsevier.com/Lehne/.

OBJECTIVES

See page 28 for the Objectives.

CRITICAL THINKING AND STUDY QUESTIONS

1. A patient with adrenocortical insufficiency verbalizes concern that she will loose muscle mass, gain weight, get a buffalo hump, and moon face if she takes the prescribed glucocorticoid. The nurse's response should be based on the fact that

   a. doses to treat adrenocortical insufficiency are similar to amounts produced normally by the body and should not cause these adverse effects.

   b. drug therapy is necessary to sustain life so the patient will have to deal with these adverse effects.

   c. these adverse effects are caused by mineralocorticoids, not glucocorticoids.

   d. these adverse effects can be minimized with proper diet and exercise.

▶ 2. An appropriate teaching for a patient who has been and is receiving a long-term pharmacologic dose of a glucocorticoid is
   a. apply alternating ice and heat to joints to relieve pain.
   b. be cautious when arising from a sitting or lying position because dizziness may occur.
   c. keep hallways and stairs well lit and free of clutter and throw rugs.
   d. low blood sugar is an adverse effect so always be prepared with a small snack.

▶ 3. The most appropriate nursing outcome for a patient who is receiving a glucocorticoid to treat rheumatoid arthritis is the patient will
   a. include rest periods in a moderate activity plan even if pain is not present.
   b. have full range of motion of arthritic joints when participating in desired activities.
   c. not experience inflammation when performing desired activities.
   d. take the drug as prescribed in order to cure the disease.

＊ 4. Which of the following laboratory test results would be of most concern to the nurse if a patient is receiving therapeutic doses of glucocorticoids?
   a. ALT 30 international units/L
   b. BUN 20 mg/dL
   c. HbA_{1C} 5.9%
   d. WBC 2000/mm³

▶ 5. The school nurse would notify the parents of a 4th grade child who is receiving oral glucocorticoids to control asthma symptoms if height and weight screening findings included
   a. a change from the 35th to 75th percentile in height.
   b. a change from the 75th to 35th percentile in height.
   c. a gain of 2 pounds in the last year.
   d. a gain of 5 pounds in the last year.

6. The nurse should be especially vigilant in assessing for adverse systemic effects of a topical glucocorticoid therapy when administering the preparation (Select all that apply.)
   a. as a cream.
   b. as an ointment.
   c. to dry cracked skin.
   d. on inflamed skin.
   e. to intertriginous areas.
   f. to mucous membranes.

   g. to well-hydrated skin.
   h. to infants.
   i. under an occlusive barrier.

▶ 7. Which of the following recommended immunizations for a 5-year-old child should not be administered by the nurse if the child is receiving glucocorticoid therapy? (Select all that apply.)
   a. Hepatitis A (Hep A)
   b. Diphtheria, tetanus, and acellular pertussis (DTaP)
   c. Inhaled influenza
   d. Injected influenza
   e. Injected polio vaccine (IPV)
   f. Measles, mumps, and rubella (MMR)
   g. Pneumococcal
   h. Varicella

▶ 8. Patients on chronic glucocorticoid therapy may minimize complications by having adequate servings of which of the following in their diet?
   a. Broccoli and cauliflower
   b. Dairy products
   c. Legumes
   d. Whole grains

9. Which of the following are common symptoms of hypokalemia caused by glucocorticoids with high mineralocorticoid activity?
   a. Anxiety and flushed skin
   b. Hypotension and cool, clammy skin
   c. Muscle weakness and abdominal distention
   d. Tingling around the mouth and fingers

10. Alternate day glucocorticoid therapy is most appropriate for a patient who is
   a. 9 years old.
   b. 29 years old.
   c. 45 years old.
   d. 65 years old.

11. Match the possible glucocorticoid-drug interactions.

   _____ a. Bisphosphonates   1. May need higher
   _____ b. Insulin   dose
   _____ c. Loop diuretics   2. Increase potassium
   _____ d. NSAIDs   loss from drug
   _____ e. Tetanus toxoid   3. Do not develop
                                     antibody response
                                  4. Increase risk of
                                     gastrointestinal (GI)
                                     bleeding
                                  5. Prevent osteoporosis

▸ 12. A patient who has been receiving glucocorticoid therapy for 2 months is being tapered off the glucocorticoids. Which of the following symptoms suggest a withdrawal syndrome?
   a. BP 84/47 mm Hg
   b. Fasting glucose 255 mg/dL
   c. Potassium 3.5 mEq/L
   d. Pulse 55 beats/min

▸ 13. A patient is taking dexamethasone for chronic obstructive pulmonary disease (COPD) and digoxin for heart failure (HF). The nurse should assess for (Select all that apply.)
   a. anorexia.
   b. positive Chvostek's sign.
   c. diarrhea.
   d. fever.
   e. flushed skin.
   f. irregular pulse.
   g. muscle weakness.
   h. visual halos.

CASE STUDIES AND PATIENT TEACHING

(Use a separate piece of paper for your responses.)

Case Study 1

A 35-year-old female was diagnosed with systemic lupus erythematosus (SLE) 2 years ago and has been in remission for more than 6 months. Lupus is a progressive, relapsing-remitting connective tissue disease. It appears to be an autoimmune process in which abnormal antibodies are produced and then react with the person's own tissue. She is seen today with complaints of joint pain, fever, generalized weakness, and fatigue. She is afraid that she is experiencing an exacerbation. Glucocorticoid therapy is prescribed. The patient is reluctant to take the medication because she has heard that glucocorticoids cause diabetes.

1. How should the nurse respond?

2. What data would the office nurse collect when initiating return healthcare visits?

3. The patient has been tapered from glucocorticoid therapy. What should the nurse teach the patient relating to the need for supplemental doses of glucocorticoids during times of stress for a period after the drug is discontinued?

4. Why is it important for the nurse to teach the patient symptoms of the disease that are important to report to the physician?

5. A nursing intervention for patients diagnosed with SLE is to enhance drug therapy. What type of environmental conditions and activities can trigger exacerbations and what realistic interventions can the nurse suggest?

6. The patient states she is planning to get pregnant. What counseling might she require?

Case Study 2

A 43-year-old man with severe persistent asthma is admitted with an acute exacerbation. After the crisis is averted, the patient is prescribed dexamethasone sodium succinate 4 mg IV push. The pharmacy sends dexamethasone acetate 16 mg/mL.

1. How much should the nurse administer?

2. The patient is switched to oral glucocorticoid therapy. Because of the severity of the patient's asthma, the prescriber explains that long-term oral glucocorticoids will probably be necessary in addition to an inhaled glucocorticoid and bronchodilators. What instructions should the nurse provide this patient regarding minimizing the following adverse effects of glucocorticoid therapy?
   a. Adrenal insufficiency
   b. Osteoporosis
   c. Infection: suppresses immune response and phagocytic activity of neutrophils and macrophages
   d. Glucose intolerance
   e. Myopathy
   f. Edema, hypernatremia, and hypokalemia
   g. Mood
   h. Cataracts and glaucoma
   i. Peptic ulcer disease

72
Drug Therapy of Rheumatoid Arthritis

Answers can be reviewed online at http://evolve.elsevier.com/Lehne/.

OBJECTIVES

See page 28 for the Objectives.

CRITICAL THINKING AND STUDY QUESTIONS

1. When planning the care of a patient with rheumatoid arthritis (RA) the nurse considers that this is a
   a. complication of a joint infection.
   b. disease that primarily affects weight-bearing joints.
   c. reaction of joints to deposit of urate crystals.
   d. systemic inflammatory disorder.

2. The nurse is teaching a patient who has been diagnosed with RA. The patient asks why her joints are so painful and stiff. The nurse could include in the explanation that
   a. an overgrowth of cartilage releases chemicals that damage the bone.
   b. the pain and swelling are due to overuse of the joint.
   c. her body is producing substances that damage the joint.
   d. the swelling and warmth are due to an infection.

3. The nurse is discussing with the patient interventions to protect joints affected by RA. The nurse determines that the patient does not understand the effect of activity on RA-afflicted joints if the patient states
   a. "I can use tools that make it easier for me to keep using the joint."
   b. "I need to quit walking with my co-worker at lunchtime because activity will make my pain worse."
   c. "I should try to alternate activities that involve painful joints with those that rest the joint rather than do the same thing for a long period of time."
   d. "Warm tub baths in the morning will help me get moving with less pain."

4. A housewife recently diagnosed with RA tells the nurse that she is concerned about her ability to perform household chores. Referral to which of the following specialists would be most appropriate for developing strategies to allow the patient to continue in this role but still protect her joints?
   a. Physical therapist
   b. Occupational therapist
   c. Social worker
   d. Specialist in vocational rehabilitation

5. Which of the following use of drugs for RA follows current guidelines?
   a. Do not discontinue glucocorticoid therapy once started because this will cause "flares."
   b. If symptoms cannot be controlled by a nonsteroidal anti-inflammatory drug (NSAID), add a disease-modifying antirheumatic drug (DMARD).
   c. Start with a DMARD within 3 months of diagnosis.
   d. Start with an NSAID and use glucocorticoids for "flares."

6. A patient has been prescribed methotrexate (DMARD) immediately after being diagnosed with RA. The patient has heard that these drugs can be dangerous and asks the nurse why the prescriber has not ordered a prescription-strength NSAID. The best response by the nurse should include
   a. methotrexate delays joint degeneration.
   b. methotrexate has fewer adverse effects than prescription-strength NSAIDs.
   c. methotrexate works faster than NSAIDs.
   d. prescription-strength NSAIDs can cause peptic ulcers; methotrexate does not.

7. A patient who is unwilling to take other drugs for his RA has been prescribed aspirin 975 mg (3 tablets) every 6 hours. Which of the following symptoms, if experienced by this patient, suggests aspirin toxicity?
   a. Bruising
   b. Epigastric pain
   c. Jaundice
   d. Ringing in the ears

8. A patient with RA is being treated with oral prednisolone for a flare of RA. Which of the following, if stated by the patient, would suggest to the nurse that this patient needs more teaching?
   a. "If I stop taking this drug suddenly, my body may not be able to deal with infection, healing, and stress."
   b. "It is important to keep active if I need to take this drug because it can make my bones weak."
   c. "I should not stop taking this drug without guidance from my doctor."
   d. "Taking this drug with food will prevent me from having any bad effects."

▶ 9. A 16-year-old female takes methotrexate once a week for juvenile RA. Which of the following laboratory test results for this patient would be of most concern to the nurse?
   a. Blood urea nitrogen (BUN) 20 mg/dL
   b. Erythrocyte sedimentation rate (ESR) 30 mm/hr
   c. Urine hCG positive
   d. White blood cell count 11,000/mm³

✳ 10. When a woman is prescribed hydroxychloroquine for RA, it is important for the nurse to assess the patient's adherence with follow-up care with a/an
   a. endocrinologist.
   b. gastroenterologist.
   c. gynecologist.
   d. ophthalmologist.

11. Which of these laboratory test results would be most important for the nurse to monitor when a patient is receiving sulfasalazine (Azulfidine) for RA?
   a. CBC
   b. Electrolytes
   c. SMBG
   d. Urine specific gravity

▶ 12. Which of these assessment findings, if identified in a patient who is receiving a DMARD II-biologic agent, should the nurse report to the prescriber immediately?
   a. Dizziness
   b. Fever
   c. Headache
   d. Injection-site erythema

▶ 13. The pediatric office nurse is preparing a referral to a rheumatologist for a child who has juvenile RA that has been unresponsive to methotrexate. It would be most important for the nurse to identify whether the child has received which of the following immunizations, if scheduled to be administered in the near future, before the child sees the specialist?
   a. DTaP
   b. IPV
   c. Influenza
   d. Varicella

14. A patient has returned to the office for reading of the PPD tuberculin test administered 50 hours ago before initiation of treatment for RA with adalimumab (Humira). The nurse would document the test results as positive and consult the prescriber if the skin reaction was greater than
   a. 5 mm of erythema.
   b. 5 mm of induration.
   c. 5 cm of erythema.
   d. 5 cm of induration.

▶ 15. When performing a nursing assessment on a patient receiving leflunomide (Arava), which of the following observations would be a reason for the nurse to hold the medication and contact the prescriber?
   a. Abdominal pain and dark urine
   b. Alopecia and skin rash
   c. Nausea and diarrhea
   d. Rhinorrhea and sneezing

16. It is most important for the nurse to counsel a male patient who has been receiving which of the following DMARDs about the need for a specific procedure to clear the body of the drug before attempting to impregnate his spouse?
   a. Adalimumab (Humira)
   b. Anakinra (Kineret)
   c. Infliximab (Remicade)
   d. Leflunomide (Arava)

✳ 17. The priority nursing concern when administering intravenous rituximab (Rituxin) is
   a. airway.
   b. hydration.
   c. infection.
   d,. infiltration.

▸ 18. Because of common adverse effects of gold therapy for RA, the nurse would assess for symptoms suggesting the need for which of the following nursing diagnoses?
   a. Activity intolerance
   b. Excess fluid volume
   c. Fatigue
   d. Impaired oral mucous membrane

CASE STUDIES AND PATIENT TEACHING

(Use a separate piece of paper for your responses.)

Case Study 1

A 34-year-old single mother who works as a grocery store clerk has been diagnosed with RA after seeking care for carpal tunnel syndrome.

1. The patient asks how she got the disease from carpal tunnel syndrome. How should the nurse respond?

2. The patient's physician has recommended that she see a vocational rehabilitation counselor. The patient asks the nurse "What type of job should I be thinking about?" What guidance can the nurse provide?

3. When developing a long-range plan of care for this patient, what interventions might the nurse include to address the four goals of RA therapy?
   a. Relieving symptoms
   b. Maintaining joint function
   c. Minimizing systemic joint involvement
   d. Delaying disease progression

4. The rheumatologist has recommended that the patient start a drug regimen including NSAIDs and methotrexate (Rheumatrex). Based on the developmental stage of this patient, what teaching would be especially important for the nurse to provide to this patient?

5. What symptoms of methotrexate toxicity to these organs should the nurse teach the patient to report to her prescriber?
   a. Liver
   b. Kidney
   c. Bone marrow
   d. GI

Case Study 2

The nurse is caring for a 47-year-old female patient who has a history of RA and hypertension controlled with 80 mg of valsartan (Diovan) who has undergone surgery to repair a ruptured Achilles tendon. She was diagnosed with RA 10 years ago and has been taking monthly injections of methotrexate but has been reluctant to treat her disease with DMARD II due to possible adverse effects. The patient is a prison guard at a state penitentiary.

1. Why would this patient be a greater risk for a life-threatening adverse effect than the general population?

2. If this patient had to resign from her job, what would be a primary obstacle to treatment with a DMARD II?

3. The patient has been notified that she is eligible for disability and has been prescribed etanercept (Enbrel) 50 mg subcutaneously once a week. What sites would the nurse instruct the patient to use when administering this drug?

4. The nurse is teaching about possible dermatologic adverse effects. The nurse teaches the patient that serious effects are most likely to occur during what period after initiation of therapy?

5. What are the symptoms that the nurse should teach the patient to report of these potentially dangerous adverse skin reactions?

73
Drug Therapy of Gout

Answers can be reviewed online at http://evolve.elsevier.com/Lehne/.

OBJECTIVES

See page 28 for the Objectives.

CRITICAL THINKING AND STUDY QUESTIONS

1. A patient who experiences an attack of gout once every one or two years has been self-treating with over-the-counter (OTC) drugs. Which of the following would the nurse expect to provide the least relief of gout pain?
   a. Acetaminophen (Tylenol)
   b. Aspirin (Bayer Aspirin)
   c. Ibuprofen (Advil, Motrin)
   d. Naproxen (Aleve)

▶ 2. A patient on the Atkins diet develops an acute gouty attack of the left first toe, impairing mobility. He is prescribed colchicine and is able to walk and return to work in 48 hours. The patient's wife calls the prescriber stating that her husband reported experiencing nausea, abdominal pain, and vomiting. She wants to know what he should do. The telephone triage nurse should advise the patient to
   a. stop taking the medication.
   b. take the medication in the evening before going to bed.
   c. take the medication with food.
   d. take the medication with milk.

▶ 3. A male patient has been prescribed allopurinol (Zyloprim) for chronic tophaceous gout. Which of the following laboratory test results should be reported immediately to the prescriber?
   a. BUN 22 mg/dL
   b. Creatinine 3.8 mg/dL
   c. ESR 28 mm/hr
   d. Uric acid 9 mg/dL

4. The nurse should withhold allopurinol (Zyloprim) if the patient experiences
   a. diarrhea.
   b. drowsiness.
   c. fever.
   d. headache.

5. The nurse is administering allopurinol to a patient who also receives warfarin. Which of the following laboratory test results would the nurse monitor to assess for allopurinol-warfarin drug interaction?
   a. BUN
   b. INR
   c. Platelets
   d. WBC

6. An important nursing action to prevent complications when administering drugs, such as probenecid, for gouty arthritis is to
   a. avoid taking BP or drawing blood from the affected extremity.
   b. increase fluid intake to 2500 to 3000 mL/day.
   c. elevate the affected extremity.
   d. measure intake and output.

7. It is important for the nurse to teach a patient who is prescribed sulfinpyrazone (Anturane) for chronic gout to avoid which of the following over-the-counter (OTC) medications?
   a. Aspirin
   b. Docusate
   c. Milk of Magnesia
   d. Naproxen (Aleve)

CASE STUDIES AND PATIENT TEACHING

(Use a separate piece of paper for your responses.)

Case Study 1

A 5-year-old child who is scheduled to start chemotherapy in 2 weeks for acute leukemia is prescribed allopurinol 150 mg once a day. His mother researched this drug on the Internet and asks the nurse why it is being prescribed when her son does not have gout.

1. How should the nurse respond?

2. The patient's mother does not like to give drugs to her children. What protective effects of allopurinol would be most important for the nurse to include in an explanation of why this drug is prescribed?

3. The child continues to take the allopurinol and is prescribed mercaptopurine 15 mg. The child weighs 38 pounds. The drug handbook states that the pediatric dose of mercaptopurine is 2.5 mg/kg. What is the dose for this child based on body weight?

4. Why would this child's dose be significantly lower than the recommended dose of mercaptopurine?

74

Drugs Affecting Calcium Levels and Bone Mineralization

Answers can be reviewed online at http://evolve.elsevier.com/Lehne/.

OBJECTIVES

See page 28 for the Objectives.

CRITICAL THINKING AND STUDY QUESTIONS

✳ 1. The nurse is caring for a patient whose lab results include calcium 12 mg/dL. The priority nursing is
   a. administering medications on time.
   b. adequate hydration.
   c. preventing falls.
   d. supporting respirations.

2. A 62-year-old woman is receiving chemotherapy for metastatic breast cancer. Which laboratory results would likely increase the risk that this patient will experience hypercalcemia?
   a. Creatinine 3.2 mg/dL
   b. H/H 11 g/dL/33%
   c. HDL 35 mg/dL
   d. SMBG 145 mg/dL

▶ 3. The plan of nursing care for a patient with bone cancer should include teaching to avoid which foods in the diet?
   a. Bran
   b. Canned sardines
   c. Spinach
   d. Whole-grain cereal

✳ 4. When taking a history from the parents of a 7-year-old who has been diagnosed with rickets, which question would be most important for the nurse to ask?
   a. "Does the child have any difficulties in school?"
   b. "Has your child ever had a kidney infection?"
   c. "Have you noticed a change in your child's energy level?"
   d. "How many hours a day does the child watch television?"

✳ 5. A priority nursing outcome for an asymptomatic patient with a history of Paget's disease is
   a. the ability to work a full 8-hour shift without fatigue.
   b. consumption of 32 ounces of milk each day.
   c. not to experience a fall.
   d. the ability to perform activities of daily living independently.

▶ 6. The nurse is assessing a postoperative thyroidectomy patient. Which assessments suggest that the parathyroid glands may have been damaged or removed during the surgery? (Select all that apply.)
   a. Dorsiflexion of the first toe and fanning of the other toes when the sole of the foot is stroked with a blunt object from lateral heel to medial toes
   b. Inflation of a BP cuff for 3 minutes produces involuntary spasms of the wrist

c. Involuntary flexion of the hips when the neck is flexed

d. Loss of balance when standing with the eyes closed, arms at sides, and legs together

e. Resistance to extension of the knee when the hip is flexed

f. Sharp calf pain with dorsiflexion of the foot

g. Twitching of facial muscles when the facial nerve is tapped

7. A 58-year-old woman is at risk for osteoporosis caused by a history of hypothyroidism treated with levothyroxine (Synthroid) 0.1 mg every morning. She has been instructed to take supplemental calcium. She is considering taking calcium carbonate (TUMS) with 400 mg of elemental calcium. Which statement, if made by the patient, would indicate a need for further teaching?

a. "I can take TUMS with food, but it will not be as well absorbed if I take it with bran cereal."

b. "I should take the TUMS with a large glass of water."

c. "The calcium will be better absorbed if I take each tablet at separate times throughout the day."

d. "TUMS are not as good of a source of calcium as oyster shell calcium, but they are less expensive."

8. The pediatric nurse is providing anticipatory guidance for parents of a toddler. During the discussion, the parents question why vitamins need to be kept out of the reach of children. The nurse's explanation includes effects from vitamin D toxicity, which include (Select all that apply.)

a. diarrhea.

b. growth suppression.

c. hyperactive deep tendon reflexes (DTRs).

d. kidney stones.

e. loss of calcium from bones.

f. nausea.

g. tetany.

h. vomiting.

9. Research suggests that adequate intake of vitamin D may protect against (Select all that apply.)

a. inflammatory bowel disease (IBD).

b. type 1 diabetes mellitus (DM).

c. multiple sclerosis (MS).

d. osteoporosis.

e. rheumatoid arthritis (RA).

10. Patients with which chronic disorders are at greater risk for vitamin D deficiency? (Select all that apply.)

a. Chronic renal failure

b. Chronic obstructive pulmonary disease (COPD)

c. Hepatitis C

d. Osteoarthritis

e. Type 2 DM

11. A 3-year-old child is admitted after ingesting an unknown number of chewable multiple vitamins including vitamin D. Which assessment finding, if present, would be of most concern to the nurse?

a. BP 80/50 mm Hg

b. Flank pain

c. Irritability

d. Pulse 102 beats/min

12. Calcitonin (Miacalcin)

a. is usually administered once a week.

b. is the safest effective drug for osteoporosis in men.

c. require nasal pumps be primed before each use.

d. promotes bone formation.

13. Which outcome would be of most concern to the nurse when a patient is taking a biphosphonate for Paget's disease?

a. Decrease in alkaline phosphatase (ALP)

b. Decrease in aspartate aminotransferase (AST)

c. Decrease in blood urea nitrogen (BUN)

d. Decrease in erythrocyte sedimentation rate (ESR)

14. A patient has received information regarding a new prescription for alendronate (Fosamax). Which statement would suggest understanding of the teaching?

a. "Fosamax helps my bones build up."

b. "Fosamax prevents the breakdown of bone."

c. "Fosamax only works for women."

d. "I should take Fosamax with food to prevent heartburn."

▶ 15. Which assessment finding, if identified in a patient who is receiving a biphosphonate, such as alendronate (Fosamax), should the nurse report to the prescriber immediately?
   a. Dysphagia
   b. Dysphasia
   c. Headache
   d. Muscular pain

16. Monitoring of creatinine clearance, urine output, weight, and intake and output is especially important for the nurse to monitor when a patient is receiving the biphosphonate
   a. alendronate (Fosamax).
   b. etidronate (Didronel).
   c. tiludronate (Skelid).
   d. zoledronic acid (Zometa).

17. Taking calcium supplements at the same time as a dose of a biphosphonate for osteoporosis
   a. increases bone building.
   b. interferes with absorption of the biphosphonate.
   c. potentiates the action of the biphosphonate.
   d. prevents adverse effects.

18. The nurse is instructing a 52-year-old woman regarding newly prescribed alendronate (Fosamax) for osteopenia. The prescriber also wants the patient to take supplemental calcium. Which supplement would be best?
   a. 600 mg of calcium citrate with 200 international units of vitamin D twice a day without other medications
   b. 1200 mg of calcium citrate with 400 international units of vitamin D once a day without other medications
   c. 600 mg of calcium citrate with 200 international units of vitamin D with the alendronate
   d. 1200 mg of calcium citrate with 400 international units of vitamin D with the alendronate

19. A patient who has just started taking tiludronate (Skelid) for Paget's disease calls the prescriber's office and reports that she is experiencing nausea since starting the drug. The nurse should advise the patient to
   a. stop taking the drug.
   b. take the drug with a full glass of water and call back if the nausea persists.
   c. take the drug with an antacid.
   d. take the drug with food.

▶ 20. A patient with skeletal metastasis of breast cancer who has been prescribed intravenous (IV) pamidronate (Aredia) to treat osteolytic hypercalcemia. A priority nursing assessment is
   a. DTR.
   b. hydration.
   c. nausea.
   d. pain.

▶ 21. A patient with hypercalcemia of malignancy (HCM) receives zoledronate (Zometa). Which symptom, if present, suggests that the patient may be experiencing drug-induced hypomagnesemia?
   a. Anorexia
   b. Dry, sticky mucous membranes
   c. Muscle weakness
   d. Neuromuscular irritability

22. When a patient is prescribed a biphosphonate, which nursing measure would be most effective to prevent the possible adverse effect of osteonecrosis?
   a. Emphasizing the importance of excellent oral hygiene
   b. Taking calcium supplementation with the drug
   c. Teaching the importance of weight-bearing exercise
   d. Teaching the importance of avoiding alcohol and tobacco

23. Raloxifene (Evista), a selective estrogen receptor modulator (SERM)
   a. may damage the eyes so the nurse should teach to report blurring of vision.
   b. may stimulate the occurrence of hot flushes (hot flashes).
   c. reduces the risk of hip, forearm, and vertebral fractures.
   d. should be avoided in women with a history of breast cancer.

▶ 24. Which of the following, elicited from a patient who is receiving raloxifene (Evista), would be most important for the nurse to communicate to the prescriber?
   a. Has an aunt who has been diagnosed with estrogen receptor positive breast cancer
   b. Has had a hysterectomy
   c. Is experiencing hot flashes
   d. Work requires frequent, long airplane trips

▸ 25. Which laboratory test result, if found in a woman who has just been prescribed raloxifene to prevent recurrence of breast cancer, would be of most concern to the nurse?
   a. Calcium 11.1 mg/dL
   b. Hemoglobin (Hb) 11.6 g/dL
   c. Hemoglobin A$_{1C}$ (HbA$_{1C}$) 6.8%
   d. Human chorionic gonadotropin (hCG) positive

26. To increase bone mineral density, teriparatide (Forteo) should be administered
   a. continually.
   b. intermittently.
   c. intravenously.
   d. orally.

27. Which action should the nurse perform when scheduled to administer teriparatide (Forteo) to a patient with osteoporosis?
   a. Administer in the deltoid or vastus lateralis muscle with a 1-inch needle.
   b. Administer subcutaneously in the upper arm, alternating arms daily.
   c. Date the injection pen for disposal 28 days after first use.
   d. Remove the pen from refrigeration 20 minutes before administration to allow the solution to warm.

28. Teriparatide (Forteo) administration has a risk of bone cancer. A patient receiving teriparatide complains to the nurse of bone pain. Which of the following could be symptoms of an electrolyte imbalance often seen in bone cancer and should be included in the nurse's assessment of this patient?
   a. Constipation and bloating
   b. Diaphoresis and thirst
   c. Diarrhea and abdominal cramps
   d. Weakness and fatigue

▸ 29. The nurse would withhold cinacalcet (Sensipar) and consult with the prescriber if which of the following were new findings on patient assessment?
   a. Anorexia
   b. Diarrhea
   c. Headache
   d. Numbness

30. Intravenous furosemide has been prescribed for a patient in a hypercalcemic emergency. The nurse knows that which imbalance would be least likely to occur as a result of this therapy?
   a. Hypocalcemia
   b. Hypoglycemia
   c. Hypokalemia
   d. Hyponatremia

CASE STUDIES AND PATIENT TEACHING

(Use a separate piece of paper for your responses.)

Case Study 1

A 50-year-old woman, who states that she is going through menopause, is undergoing a thyroidectomy today. The literature states that the nurse should be sure IV calcium is available postoperatively. She has just been admitted to the nursing unit from the postanesthesia care unit (PACU).

1. Knowing the anatomy of the thyroid gland, why would the nurse anticipate a potential need for IV calcium?

2. What is the average normal value for total serum calcium?

3. The patient's calcium level drops to 6.8 mg/dL. Intravenous 10% calcium gluconate 5 mL via IV (push) infusion is prescribed. The nurse's drug book recommends that the drug be infused at a rate of 0.5 to 2 mL/min. If the nurse infuses the solution at 0.6 mL/min, how long will it take to infuse the entire amount?

4. The patient is sitting in a chair when the nurse prepares to administer the calcium gluconate? Why is it important for the nurse to assist the patient back to bed before the drug is administered?

5. What should be monitored while the nurse is administering the calcium gluconate?

6. The patient's husband states that he thought calcium is in the bone. He asks how surgery on the neck can cause an imbalance in the calcium in the body. What could the nurse include in the discussion of the functions of calcium and the mechanism for calcium regulation?

Case Study 2

The orthopedic office nurse is preparing for a visit with a 56-year-old woman to review bone mineral density (BMD) test results after an ulnar and radial fracture occurred when she tripped and fell. DEXA scan results showing a BMD 2.5 SD (standard deviations) below the norm are reviewed with the patient. She is diagnosed with osteoporosis and prescribed ibandronate (Boniva) 150 mg once a month.

1. What information is essential to teach this patient regarding taking ibandronate?

2. The patient asks how it is possible to take a drug once a month to help improve bone density. What should the nurse include in the response?

3. The patient asks about taking calcium supplements. What recommendations can the nurse share?

4. Besides taking calcium supplements for osteoporosis, what other measures to promote bone density should the nurse include in teaching?

75

Drugs for Asthma

Answers can be reviewed online at http://evolve.elsevier.com/Lehne/.

OBJECTIVES

See page 28 for the Objectives.

CRITICAL THINKING AND STUDY QUESTIONS

✳ 1. Which of these outcomes would be a priority for a patient who has been diagnosed with asthma?
  a. Avoiding pollution
  b. Increasing exercise tolerance
  c. Preventing airway inflammation
  d. Stimulating release of eosinophils

2. Common triggers of asthmatic bronchospasm include (Select all that apply.)
  a. airway inflammation.
  b. cold air.
  c. environmental allergens.
  d. exercise.
  e. mast cell degranulation.
  f. pain.
  g. tobacco smoke.
  h. upper respiratory infection.

3. When caring for a patient with asthma, the nurse should be prepared to administer which of the following drugs if an uncontrolled asthmatic episode occurs?
  a. Budesonide
  b. Epinephrine
  c. Terbutaline
  d. Theophylline

4. A patient has received instructions from the nurse regarding administration of 2 puffs of a beta$_2$-agonist drug via a metered-dose inhaler (MDI). Which of the following statements, if made by the patient, would indicate the need for further teaching?
   a. "I need to inhale more slowly if the spacer whistles."
   b. "I need to count the MDI doses that I use so that I know when it is empty."
   c. "I should inhale immediately after activating the inhaler."
   d. "It is best to wait 1 full minute before I take the second puff."

▸ 5. A patient with a long history of asthma has developed peripheral muscle weakness limiting activity and exercise. It would be particularly important for the nurse to develop a plan to prevent loss of bone mass if the patient is receiving
   a. flunisolide (AeroBid) MDI.
   b. fluticasone-salmeterol (Advair) DPI.
   c. nebulized levalbuterol (Xopenex).
   d. prednisolone oral tablets.

▸ 6. A hospitalized patient is scheduled to receive budesonide (Pulmicort Turbuhaler) and salmeterol (Serevent) 2 puffs every 12 hours. She also has albuterol (Proventil) MDI 2 puffs prescribed every 4 hours as needed, which has not been administered in the last 24 hours. When preparing to administer the 0900 budesonide and salmeterol dose, the nurse notes audible wheezing, and the patient is anxious and short of breath. The patient states that she is having an asthma attack. The nurse should administer the
   a. albuterol only.
   b. albuterol, wait 5 minutes, and then administer the salmeterol and budesonide.
   c. salmeterol and reassess in 15 minutes for the need for albuterol.
   d. budesonide and salmeterol and reassess in 15 minutes for the need for albuterol.

✳ 7. The nurse is caring for several patients who receive a beta-agonist inhalation treatment for asthma. After treatments are administered, it would be a priority to reassess the patient who also has a history of
   a. heart failure (HF).
   b. deep vein thrombosis (DVT).
   c. gastroesophageal reflux (GERD).
   d. rheumatoid arthritis (RA).

8. Which of the following statements, if made by an asthmatic patient who is prescribed inhaled beclomethasone (QVAR) would indicate a need for further teaching?
   a. "This inhaler decreases the secretion of mucus in my airways."
   b. "This inhaler helps my bronchodilator work better."
   c. "This inhaler helps the hairs in my airways move the mucus upward."
   d. "This inhaler prevents swelling in my airway."

▸ 9. A 42-year-old female asthmatic patient who is prescribed budesonide (Pulmicort Turbuhaler) and formoterol (Foradil Aerolizer) 2 puffs every 12 hours is admitted for a Roux-en-Y surgical procedure for morbid obesity. Which of the following information obtained in the patient's history is most critical for the nurse to share with the surgeon?
   a. This patient experiences an asthma attack whenever exposed to tobacco smoke.
   b. The patient has degenerative joint disease (osteoarthritis) of the knees.
   c. The patient is lactose intolerant.
   d. The patient was recently changed from long-term oral methylprednisolone to inhaled beclomethasone.

▸ 10. The nurse administers an "as needed" treatment of albuterol via nebulizer when an asthmatic patient experiences severe wheezing throughout the lung fields while attempting to eat lunch. After 1 minute of treatment, the patient is resting quietly with his eyes closed. The nurse should
   a. allow the patient to rest.
   b. assess the patient's breathing.
   c. inform the dietary department that another lunch will be needed later.
   d. wake the patient and encourage him to try to finish his lunch.

▸ 11. Which of the following assessment findings in a patient who is prescribed a beta$_2$-adrenergic agonist would be a reason for the nurse to consult the prescriber?
   a. BP 140/90 mm Hg
   b. SMBG 165 mg/dL
   c. Unexplained fainting
   d. Unexplained tremor

▶ 12. A patient has been prescribed intravenous methylprednisolone and inhaled fluticasone (Flovent) during a severe asthma attack. The prescriber discontinues the intravenous drug on the eighth day. The nurse should
   a. administer the fluticasone as prescribed and continue nursing care.
   b. consult the prescriber regarding the need for an oral glucocorticoid drug.
   c. consult the prescriber regarding the need for an oral glucocorticoid drug that should have the dose tapered before the drug is discontinued.
   d. consult the prescriber regarding the need to taper the intravenous methylprednisolone before discontinuing the drug.

13. Which of the following drugs contains a component that has been associated with a risk of increased asthma severity and possibly death?
   a. Advair
   b. AeroBid
   c. Intal
   d. Pulmicort

▶ 14. If flunisolide (AeroBid) and pirbuterol (Maxair) are both ordered to be administered at 0900, how should they be administered?
   a. Flunisolide first, then pirbuterol 1 minute later, using a spacer for both drugs
   b. Flunisolide first, using a spacer, then pirbuterol 3 minutes later
   c. Pirbuterol first, then flunisolide 5 minutes later, using a spacer for both drugs
   d. Pirbuterol first, using a spacer, then flunisolide 10 minutes later

▶ 15. The nurse is caring for a patient who is prescribed zafirlukast (Accolate) for asthma and warfarin for atrial fibrillation. Because of the interaction of these two drugs, it is important for the nurse to monitor which of the following laboratory tests?
   a. BNP
   b. BUN
   c. FBG
   d. INR

16. The nurse would be most concerned about drug interactions if an asthmatic patient was prescribed both zileuton (Zyflo) and
   a. albuterol.
   b. prednisolone.
   c. terbutaline.
   d. theophylline.

▶ 17. Zafirlukast (Accolate) is scheduled to be administered at 7:00 AM (0700). Breakfast is served at 8:30 AM (0830). The nurse should
   a. administer the drug as ordered.
   b. change the timing of the drug to 8:30 AM (0830).
   c. change the timing of the drug to 10:00 AM (1000).
   d. consult the prescriber.

18. The nurse is explaining therapy with cromolyn (Intal) to an asthmatic patient. Which of the following would not need to be included in the teaching?
   a. Cromolyn must be taken on a regular basis to control inflammation.
   b. Rinse the mouth immediately after administration to remove the unpleasant taste.
   c. Timing of doses 15 minutes before activities involving exertion or exposure to known allergens may prevent bronchospasm.
   d. The drug is not effective in stopping an episode once it has begun.

✳ 19. The nurse is working triage in an emergency department. The nurse would prioritize the patient to immediate care if a patient with uncontrolled allergy-related asthma who is prescribed omalizumab (Xolair) presents complaining of
   a. fever.
   b. headache.
   c. perioral edema.
   d. severe pharyngitis.

▶ 20. Which of these findings, if identified in a patient who has been prescribed ipratropium-albuterol (Combivent), should the nurse report to the prescriber immediately?
   a. Allergy to peanuts
   b. Complaint of sore throat
   c. Consumes 4 to 6 cups of coffee per day
   d. Smokes two packs of cigarettes per day

21. Which of the following adverse effects would the patient be most likely to experience when prescribed the anticholinergic bronchodilator drug tiotropium (Spiriva)?
   a. Blurred vision
   b. Constipation
   c. Dry mouth
   d. Urinary retention

22. In teaching about administration of tiotropium (Spiriva), the nurse should include which of the following instructions?
    a. Swallow whole with a full glass of water.
    b. Do not use as a rescue inhaler.
    c. Take 15 minutes before activities involving exertion or exposure to known allergens.
    d. Use of a spacer increases the amount of drug delivered to the lungs and decreases the amount deposited in the throat.

▸ 23. The nurse is caring for an asthmatic patient who is receiving zafirlukast (Accolate) and who complains of abdominal pain. Which of the following laboratory test results should the nurse review?
    a. ALT
    b. BUN
    c. CBC
    d. ESR

24. A patient's peak expiratory flow rate has been around 70% of his personal best. Current treatment recommendations state that he should
    a. continue regularly prescribed treatment.
    b. use his rescue inhaler and continue his regularly prescribed treatment.
    c. use his rescue inhaler and consult his prescriber for possible treatment changes.
    d. seek immediate emergency medical attention.

▸ 25. A child with moderate asthma is distressed because he has just learned that he is allergic to the family dog. Which of the following interventions would most effectively address the physical and psychosocial needs of the child?
    a. Advise the family that there are no interventions that will help.
    b. Advise the family to increase the dose of the child's asthma drugs when the dog is around.
    c. Advise the family to take the dog to the local shelter.
    d. Advise the family to train the dog to stay out of bedrooms and off of furniture.

CASE STUDIES AND PATIENT TEACHING

(Use a separate piece of paper for your responses.)

Case Study 1

A 7-year-old boy, who was first diagnosed with asthma at 4 years of age, has been admitted to a medical unit from intensive care after experiencing status asthmaticus. Based on the frequency, characteristics, and severity of his symptoms, he is currently classified as having severe persistent asthma. The pediatrician has ordered oral prednisolone 10 mg every 8 hours, budesonide (Pulmicort respules) 0.2 mg and albuterol 1.25 mg via nebulizer every 6 hours as needed.

1. What is the difference between administering budesonide and albuterol via nebulizer?

2. The budesonide is available as 250 mcg/2 mL. How much budesonide should be administered via nebulizer at each dose?

3. The boy's mother tells the nurse that she does not like steroids and is concerned about her son receiving them. What does the nurse need to teach regarding the importance of steroid therapy for this child?

4. The mother has heard that steroids prevent growth. What information can the nurse provide about the effects of steroids on growth?

5. What teaching does the nurse need to provide about the inhaled steroid therapy to prevent adverse effects?

6. The nebulizer is more time consuming to use than dry-powder inhalers (DPI) and metered-dose inhalers (MDI). What are possible reasons why this route was prescribed for this child?

7. Allergy work-up identified that this child was allergic to house dust mites. What teaching should be provided regarding exposure to allergens?

8. After 2 years of standard allergy treatment, the child is still experiencing asthma attacks 2 to 3 times a week, and he is missing many days of school. The allergist has prescribed omalizumab (Xolair) 200 mg to be administered subcutaneously every 4 weeks. What is the procedure for administering this drug?

Case Study 2

An 18-year-old college freshman has had asthma since she was 5 years old. During the past year, she has had occasional asthma attacks and used an albuterol (Ventolin) inhaler 2 to 4 times a week on an as needed (PRN) basis. As she tries to make the adjustment to college life and participate in all the various activities, her attacks begin to occur more frequently, and she has had to use her albuterol inhaler once or twice a day. She comes to the student health center for management of her asthma.

1. What information would be helpful for the nurse to obtain before the student is seen by the certified registered nurse practitioner (CRNP)?

2. The CRNP prescribes cromolyn (Intal) 3 puffs, 10 minutes apart, 3 times a day and montelukast (Singulair) 10 mg by mouth once a day. She is instructed that she may use her albuterol inhaler 2 puffs, every 4 hours as needed if asthma symptoms are present. The patient questions why cromolyn has been prescribed. What should the nurse include in the explanation?

3. The patient returns to the health center for follow-up care. She is still using her albuterol inhaler several times a day and is discouraged that her asthma is still "out of control." She provides a record of when she has been in the yellow zone and today was in the red zone. The CRNP discontinues the cromolyn and montelukast and prescribes fluticasone (Flovent HA) and formoterol (Foradil) 2 puffs each every 12 hours as her regular medication regimen in addition to the PRN albuterol. The student asks the college health nurse what the difference is between the formoterol and albuterol if they are both bronchodilators. How should the nurse respond?

4. What teaching should the nurse provide about administration of the prescribed drugs?

5. The nurse knows that many college students study before examinations for long periods at a time. Colas, coffee, and over-the-counter (OTC) drugs containing caffeine are commonly used to prevent drowsiness. How should the nurse use this knowledge?

Case Study 3

A patient has been prescribed high-dose oral prednisone every other day for severe persistent asthma. Every-other-day dosing increases the risk of medication errors.

1. Why has this dosing schedule been prescribed?

2. What care should the nurse provide including prevention of adverse effects and when to notify the prescriber?

OBJECTIVES

See page 28 for the Objectives.

CRITICAL THINKING AND STUDY QUESTIONS

1. A patient exhibits allergic rhinitis symptoms every winter when the house is closed and the forced-air furnace is running. This is classified as
   a. perennial rhinitis.
   b. seasonal rhinitis.

2. Allergic rhinitis involves the release of (Select all that apply.)
   a. epinephrine.
   b. glucocorticoids.
   c. immunoglobulins.
   d. histamine.
   e. leukocytes.
   f. leukotrienes.
   g. prostaglandins.

3. The nurse teaches a patient with allergic rhinitis that antihistamines are not effective in reducing the symptom of
   a. nasal congestion.
   b. nasal itching.
   c. rhinorrhea.
   d. sneezing.

4. A patient has received instructions regarding administration of a second-generation oral antihistamine for seasonal allergic rhinitis. Which of these statements made by the patient would indicate the patient needs further teaching?
   a. "I should only use the medication when I am experiencing symptoms."
   b. "I should take the medication as prescribed throughout the season when I have allergy symptoms."
   c. "This drug can still cause sedation, so I need to be careful when driving."
   d. "This drug is not any more effective than over-the-counter antihistamines."

5. The most effective drugs for prevention and treatment of symptoms of seasonal and perennial rhinitis are
   a. first-generation oral antihistamines.
   b. intranasal corticosteroids.
   c. oral glucocorticoids.
   d. second-generation oral antihistamines.

6. The school nurse notes that a child is receiving chronic therapy with intranasal glucocorticoids for seasonal rhinitis. It is important for this nurse to monitor the child's
   a. blood sugar.
   b. hearing.
   c. height.
   d. weight.

7. An eight-year-old child was prescribed fluticasone (Flonase) 2 sprays in each nostril two weeks ago. Her mother calls the pediatric telephone advice nurse reporting that the drug has not helped. Which of the following questions should the nurse ask to identify a common cause of early treatment failures?
   a. "Does she have nasal congestion?"
   b. "How often are you admistering the sprays?"
   c. "Is she having any nasal burning after administration?"
   d. "What is the expiration date on the bottle?"

8. An advantage of intranasal cromolyn (Nasal-Crom) in allergic rhinitis is that it
   a. can be used prophylactically.
   b. has once a day dosing.
   c. is effective.
   d. is safe.

9. Which of these assessment findings, if identified in a patient who is taking an oral decongestant, should the nurse report to the prescriber immediately?
   a. Agitation
   b. Chest pain
   c. Epistaxis
   d. Sore throat

▸ 10. In which of the following situations would it be most beneficial for the nurse to administer a prescribed as needed dose of an antitussive medication?
  a. Barking cough of croup
  b. Cough that interferes with work because patient cannot carry tissues at work in which to expectorate the mucus
  c. Cough that is associated with upper respiratory infection and keeps the patient awake at night
  d. Severe episodes of coughing with sputum production that only occurs on arising

11. Two nurses are discussing the problems with commercials for prescription products aimed toward the general population. One recently saw a commercial for montelukast (Singulair). The nurses know that one reason prescribers may not readily prescribe this drug for allergic rhinitis is because it
  a. frequently causes irritation inside the nose.
  b. has many adverse effects.
  c. is limited in effectiveness as a decongestant.
  d. only treats sneezing and itching.

12. A patient is prescribed omalizumab (Xolair) for allergic rhinitis. Which of the following statements, if made by the patient, suggests a need for further teaching about this drug therapy?
  a. "I can finally go to a Labor Day picnic and not sneeze all day."
  b. "I need to continue taking this drug during the winter to control my allergy to house dust."
  c. "The doctor has prescribed this drug to control my allergy symptoms because allergies trigger my asthma."
  d. "This drug will be injected into the fat under my skin."

13. Research suggests that codeine, dextromethorphan, and diphenhydramine are not effective in suppressing coughs induced by
  a. chemical irritation.
  b. common cold.
  c. mechanical irritation.
  d. smoking.

14. Match the following drugs and their descriptors.
  _____ a. Acetylcysteine
  _____ b. Benzonatate
  _____ c. Dextromethorphan
  _____ d. Diphenhydramine
  _____ e. Guaifenesin
  _____ f. Hydrocodone

  1. Acts in CNS but lacks potential for abuse
  2. Decreases sensitivity of cough-reflex pathway
  3. Potentiates action of opiate analgesics
  4. Smells like rotten eggs
  5. Suppresses cough at doses that cause sedation
  6. Toxicity can be reversed by naloxone

15. A patient has received instructions regarding administration of benzonatate (Tessalon Perles). Which of these statements made by the patient would indicate the patient needs further teaching?
  a. "The drug should not be given to infants."
  b. "I can take the drug three times a day."
  c. "I need to be careful because the drug may make me drowsy."
  d. "I should crush the beads and mix them in a soft food such as applesauce."

16. Despite instruction by the nurse to swallow the benzonatate (Tessalon Perles) whole, the patient proceeds to chew the capsule. A priority nursing concern until the effect of this drug has diminished is
  a. aspiration.
  b. bronchospasms.
  c. respiratory depression.
  d. severe constipation.

17. Which statements are true about the common cold? (Select all that apply.)
  a. Antibiotics are not effective.
  b. Antihistamines do not help.
  c. It is best treated with multiple symptom medications.
  d. Fever usually means there is a bacterial infection.
  e. Research has not supported that vitamin C prevents colds.
  f. Zinc lozenges are not beneficial.

5. A patient with rough, scaling skin and sore tongue may be experiencing niacin deficiency. The nurse teaches that foods high in niacin include
   a. all enriched grain products, green leafy vegetables, and legumes.
   b. chicken, peanuts, and cereal bran.
   c. dairy and fortified cereal and bread.
   d. pork and enriched breads and cereals.

6. The outpatient surgery nurse is completing the history of a 62-year-old female patient admitted for carpal tunnel surgery. Medication history includes hydrochlorothiazide 25 mg once a day, calcium 400 mg 4 times a day, a senior multivitamin once a day, cholestyramine (Questran) 4 g 4 times a day, and vitamin E 1000 mg twice a day. The patient has not consumed any food, fluids, or medication since midnight. The nurse should document the findings and notify the surgeon of the medication history because the patient is at risk for
   a. excessive bleeding during surgery.
   b. hypotension during surgery.
   c. poor wound healing.
   d. vomiting during surgery.

7. The nurse would teach a patient who is a vegan the importance of supplementation with
   a. alpha-tocopherol.
   b. ascorbic acid.
   c. cyanocobalamin.
   d. folic acid.

8. The nurse would be particularly concerned if which of the following patients was self-prescribing megadoses of vitamin A for healthy skin?
   a. Adolescent female
   b. Adolescent male
   c. Elderly female
   d. Elderly male

9. The nurse should be aware that which of the following disorders puts the patient at greatest risk for bleeding and bruising because of vitamin K deficiency?
   a. Addison's disease
   b. Celiac disease
   c. Gastroesophageal reflux disease (GERD)
   d. Peptic ulcer disease (PUD)

10. A neonate who was born in an automobile in a traffic jam is admitted to the hospital 3 hours after birth. Which of the following symptoms, if it occurred, would be of most concern to the neonatal nurse relating to the delay in administering vitamin K?
    a. Bilateral edema over top of head
    b. Deep blue color of skin over sacrum
    c. Seizures 24 to 72 hours after birth
    d. Yellow color of skin

11. The nurse includes in her health promotion teaching that vitamin C supplementation has been approved for
    a. decreased bronchoconstriction of asthma.
    b. prevention of colds.
    c. promotion of wound healing.
    d. treatment of scurvy.

12. An oncology nurse is providing health teaching to a patient who is starting chemotherapy. The patient has heard that chemotherapy can cause painful "mouth ulcers." The patient would like to know if there is anything that she can do to help prevent these ulcers. The nurse's response would include trying to eat servings of which foods that are rich in the vitamin that protects mucous membrane integrity?
    a. Citrus fruits, strawberries, red peppers
    b. Deep yellow, orange, and green colored vegetables and fruits
    c. Nuts and vegetable oils
    d. Pork and enriched breads and cereals

13. The nurse is working with a patient with advanced esophageal cancer because of poor nutritional intake relating to nausea and epigastric discomfort. It is most important for the nurse to assess if the patient is self-medicating with which of the following vitamins that has been promoted as a treatment for cancer and can cause upper GI irritation?
    a. Vitamin A
    b. Vitamin B
    c. Vitamin C
    d. Vitamin E

14. Health promotion for aging adults should include the importance of adequate amounts of vitamin D because older adults often
    a. buy less fresh fruit because it is expensive.
    b. consume less dairy products.
    c. do not eat fresh vegetables because they cause gas.
    d. have difficulty chewing meat.

▸ 15. An 66-year-old female who is scheduled for a knee replacement is being seen by a pre-admission screening nurse. She has a history of cardiac valve replacement and is receiving warfarin. She was recently diagnosed with hypercholesterolemia and was prescribed cholestyramine (Questran) 4 g twice a day. Which of the following laboratory test results could be altered by the effect of this drug on vitamin K absorption and would warrant notification of the surgeon?

    a. ESR 10 mm/hr
    b. INR 5.2
    c. MCV 90 mm^3
    d. RDW 12%

▸ 16. A teacher sends a Hispanic migrant worker's child to the nurse's office because she is concerned that the child has a smooth, swollen tongue and cracks in the corners of her mouth and lips. The nurse knows that this may be a vitamin deficiency that can be caused by a diet whose main component is

    a. home-ground corn.
    b. commercial cereal.
    c. dairy products.
    d. vegetables picked at parent's work.

CASE STUDIES AND PATIENT TEACHING

(Use a separate piece of paper for your responses.)

Case Study 1

A 46-year-old male has been admitted to a medical unit after 4 days in an alcohol detoxification center. He was admitted because of complaints of extreme weakness and an unsteady gait. His wife provided a history that his alcohol intake has steadily increased since he lost his job 3 years ago. During the past 6 months, he has been living on the street and drinking 1 to 2 quarts of wine daily. He is a poor historian and does not recall being admitted to the hospital. His response when asked about his diet is, "Whatever I can get." Physical assessment reveals ataxia, edema of the lower extremities, nystagmus, dry skin with cracks in the corners of his mouth, and multiple bruises. He states that the bruises are caused by any slight pressure. He is anorexic, taking sips of fluid and eating only a few bites of his lunch. He complains that his mouth is "too sore" to eat many foods. Endoscopy reveals severe gastritis with no obvious bleeding. The patient is diagnosed with vitamin deficiency and started on an IV drip with one ampule of vitamin C and B complex per liter.

1. What symptoms led to a diagnosis of vitamin deficiency, and which vitamins are probably deficient?

2. Why is the patient less likely to be showing symptoms of fat-soluble vitamin deficiencies?

3. Blood studies include hemoglobin 8.4 g and hematocrit 25%. Which vitamins are essential in red blood cell production?

4. The patient's wife has agreed that he may come home with her after his discharge from the hospital as long as he continues to stay in an outpatient rehabilitation program and does not drink. She asks the nurse to tell her some of the foods she should prepare to be certain that he gets the necessary vitamins. What foods or food groups would you suggest to her to ensure intake of the following vitamins?

    a. A
    b. C
    c. Niacin
    d. Pyridoxine
    e. Riboflavin
    f. Thiamine
    g. Folate

5. The patient's wife asks the nurse whether it would be a good idea to go to the health-food store and buy him some high-dose vitamin pills with all vitamins included. What is the best response?

Case Study 2

The high school nurse has developed a relationship with a female student who has acne. The student states that she has been seeing a dermatologist without success. At the last appointment, the doctor stated that he would be considering isotretinoin (Accutane), a megadose form of vitamin A, as the next step in therapy.

1. What precautions and instruction should the nurse provide?

Case Study 3

There have been studies of the effects of antioxidant vitamins that have had conflicting results.

1. How are observational studies conducted?

2. What characteristics of a research study promote reliability?

3. How does a meta-analysis differ from a randomized controlled trial?

81
Drugs for Obesity

Answers can be reviewed online at http://evolve.elsevier.com/Lehne/.

OBJECTIVES

See page 28 for the Objectives.

CRITICAL THINKING AND STUDY QUESTIONS

▶ 1. A man who is 6' tall, weighs 225 lb. and has a waist circumference of 42" is classified as what risk for type 2 diabetes mellitus (DM) and cardiovascular disease?
   a. Increased
   b. High
   c. Very high
   d. Extremely high

2. The nurse is teaching health promotion to adolescent females. Developmentally, which of the following risks associated with obesity would most likely be a motivator for change to healthier eating and exercise?
   a. Cardiovascular disease
   b. Decreased fertility
   c. Diabetes mellitus
   d. Hypertension

▶ 3. What is the most important factor when the nurse is devising a weight reduction plan for a patient?
   a. Developing strategies to minimize stress
   b. Including aerobic exercise
   c. Limiting processed carbohydrates in diet
   d. Patient input in creating and revising the plan

4. Recommendations for drug therapy for obesity include to
   a. expect at least 6 lb of weight loss per week for the first 6 weeks.
   b. limit drug therapy to 6 months or less.
   c. only start drug treatment after a 6-month program of diet and exercise has failed to produce results.
   d. start regular exercise after the body mass index (BMI) is less than 40 to reduce the strain on the heart.

✳ 5. Which of the following assessments would be a priority if a patient were prescribed sibutramine (Meridia) for weight loss?
   a. Blood glucose
   b. Intake and output
   c. Other medications that the patient is taking
   d. Vital signs

✳▶ 6. A patient who is prescribed fluoxetine (Prozac) for depression admits to taking her sister's prescription drug sibutramine (Meridia) to try to lose the weight she has gained while on the antidepressant. Which of the following assessment findings, if identified by the nurse, would be of most concern?
   a. Constipation and anorexia
   b. Diaphoresis and incoordination
   c. Difficulty falling asleep and nervousness
   d. Headache and dry mouth

7. Which of the following statements, if made by a patient receiving orlistat (Xenical), would indicate a need for further teaching?
   a. "I will eat less because my appetite should decrease."
   b. "Limiting the fat in my diet will decrease unpleasant adverse effects."
   c. "This drug may help reduce my bad fat and increase my good fat."
   d. "Unpleasant gas and oily bowel movements that are difficult to control may occur."

✴ 8. Which of the following nursing concerns would be a priority when the nurse is teaching a patient who has just been prescribed toprimate for weight loss?
   a. Decisional conflict
   b. Fluid volume
   c. Safety
   d. Therapeutic regimen

9. Match the following calorie-saving foods to their descriptors.

   _____ a. aspartame (Equal)   1. Bitter aftertaste
   _____ b. saccharin (Sweet'N Low)   2. Patients with phenylketonuria (PKU) cannot use
   _____ c. sucralose (Splenda)   3. Best for cooking

10. An obese patient has been diagnosed with osteopenia. Which of the following drugs for weight loss and calorie-saving foods has the potential to potentiate this loss of bone density? (Select all that apply.)
    a. Aspartamine (Splenda)
    b. Buproprion (Wellbutrin)
    c. Fluoxetine (Prozac)
    d. Olestra (Olean)
    e. Orlistat (Xenical)
    f. Sibutramine (Meridia)
    g. Toprimate (Topimax)
    h. Zonisamide (Zonegran)

CASE STUDIES AND PATIENT TEACHING

(Use a separate piece of paper for your responses.)

Case Study 1

A 48-year-old male with a history of sleep apnea, hypertension, and type 2 diabetes weighs 385 lb and is 5' 8" tall. His waist circumference is 54". His total cholesterol is 330 mg.

1. What is this patient's BMI?

2. His physician has proposed a program of diet, exercise, and drug therapy. The patient's wife, who is 5' 5" and 165 lb and has a pear-shaped body, states that she has sought drug therapy for her weight, but her primary care provider (PCP) refused. She asks the nurse why drugs are being offered to her husband when drugs have adverse effects and he has a family history of heart disease. What could the nurse include in her explanation of guidelines for drug therapy for obesity?

3. The patient asks the nurse what is a realistic goal for weight loss, and how much does he need to cut back in eating. How should the nurse respond?

OBJECTIVES

See page 28 for the Objectives.

CRITICAL THINKING AND STUDY QUESTIONS

1. Match the following terms and descriptors.

_____ a. Antibiotic
_____ b. Antimicrobial
_____ c. Bacteriocidal
_____ d. Bacteriostatic
_____ e. Chemotherapy

1. Using chemicals against invading organisms
2. Chemical produced by one microbe that can harm another microbe
3. Drugs that slow microbe reproduction
4. Any agent that can harm microbes
5. Drugs that kill microbes

2. Which of the following are true about conjugation as a mechanism to change microbial DNA? (Select all that apply.)
   a. A single transfer of DNA can cause formerly drug-sensitive bacteria to become resistant to several antibiotics.
   b. Conjugation occurs primarily among gram-positive bacteria.
   c. Genetic material can only be transferred between members of the same species (staph to staph; strep to strep).
   d. Normal flora bacteria can transfer drug resistance to disease causing bacteria by conjugation.
   e. Conjugation results in resistance to only one drug.
   f. The resistance factor (R factor) of a donor microbe must include a DNA segment that codes for the mechanism of drug resistance and a sexual apparatus for DNA transfer.

3. Antibiotics promote drug resistance by (Select all that apply.)
   a. altering the number of nonpathogenic microbes that produce toxins against pathogenic organisms.
   b. causing spontaneous mutation of microbes.
   c. creating a situation where there is less competition for nutrients.
   d. destroying drug-sensitive normal flora.
   e. encouraging DNA transfer between microbes.

▸ 4. A patient had a specimen sent for culture and sensitivity (C&S) while in the emergency department (ED). He was admitted to a medical unit and prescribed intravenous (IV) ampicillin/sulbactam (Unasyn) 1.5 gm every 6 hours. The nurse knows the priority reason for notifying the prescriber of culture results as soon as they become available is that this
   a. antibiotic has many more adverse effects than many other antibiotics.
   b. is a broad-spectrum antibiotic, and an effective narrow-spectrum antibiotic may be effective.
   c. is an expensive antibiotic.
   d. is a narrow-spectrum antibiotic and may not be effective for the cultured organism.

▸ 5. Which of the following patients would most likely have an infection that is resistant to antibiotic therapy?
   a. A child with asthma who develops pneumonia
   b. An adult construction worker who drinks from a work site water supply and develops giardiasis
   c. An adult who developed a wound infection while in the hospital after surgery
   d. An elderly adult who got an infected paper cut

6. Describe how microbial DNA can change to result in inheritable drug resistance with the different mechanisms of antibiotic action.

235

7. Which of the following would be classified as a suprainfection?
   a. Monial vaginal infection that developed during antibiotic therapy
   b. Peritonitis that developed after surgery for a ruptured appendix
   c. Pneumonia in a patient with emphysema
   d. Varicella outbreak after injection with varicella vaccine

▶ 8. The nurse has consulted the prescriber because a patient reports an allergy to the prescribed penicillin antibiotic. The prescriber is aware of the allergy, but the patient is experiencing a life-threatening infection and no other suitable antibiotic is available. The nurse should
   a. administer the antibiotic.
   b. ask the patient if they are willing to take the antibiotic.
   c. obtain orders for treatment of a possible allergic reaction.
   d. refuse to administer the antibiotic.

9. It is most important to identify if a patient could be pregnant if she is prescribed
   a. amikacin.
   b. amoxicillin.
   c. azithromycin.
   d. cephalexin.

▶ 10. The nurse is administering a sulfonamide antibiotic to a male child of color who has not previously received this class of medication. The child was rescued after being separated from his family after a hurricane and his genetic history is unknown. Because of the possibility the child could have a glucose-6-phosphate dehydrogenase deficiency, the nurse should monitor
   a. AST and ALT.
   b. BUN and creatinine.
   c. glucose and HbA$_{1C}$.
   d. hemoglobin and hematocrit.

11. In most infections, the level of antibiotic at the site of infection needs to be
   a. at the minimum inhibitory concentration (MIC).
   b. 2 to 3 times the MIC.
   c. 4 to 8 times the MIC.
   d. 10 to 20 times the MIC.

12. A valid reason for prescribing two different antibiotics is (Select all that apply.)
   a. results of the C&S indicate multiple drugs are effective.
   b. results of C&S indicate multiple organisms sensitive to different drugs are present.
   c. severe infection in the immune compromised patient.
   d. suppressing the emergence of drug-resistant *Enterococcus faecium*.
   e. suppressing the emergence of drug-resistant *Mycobacterium tuberculosis*.
   f. the presence of foreign material.
   g. when the microbe is sensitive to both penicillin and tetracycline.

13. It is important for the nurse to teach a patient who has had surgery for placement of a prosthetic heart valve to take prescribed antibiotic therapy
   a. before dental procedures.
   b. before examination of the eyes where dilating drops are instilled.
   c. when experiencing yellowish or yellow-green nasal discharge.
   d. whenever they have a fever.

CASE STUDIES AND PATIENT TEACHING

(Use a separate piece of paper for your responses.)

Case Study 1

A 78-year-old nursing home patient with a history of hypertension, type 2 DM, and chronic obstructive pulmonary disease (COPD) is brought into the ED with a history of fever for 72 hours and moist cough. The extended care nursing report states that he was very irritable last night, and then was difficult to awaken this morning. Assessment findings include temperature 103°F (39.4°C), pulse 112 beats/min, BP 100/56 mm Hg, respirations 26 and labored, fine late inspiratory crackles (rales) throughout the lung fields, Glasgow coma scale 12. Chest x-ray demonstrates lung consolidation. Intravenous fluids are infusing. Other orders include admit, sputum (C&S), and cefotetan (Cefotan) 1 gm every 12 hours.

1. What are nursing responsibilities regarding these orders?

2. What type of antibiotic would the nurse expect to be ordered and why?

3. The IV antibiotic that was ordered is cefotetan (Cefotan) 1 gm every 12 hours. The unit nurse reviews the following (C&S) results. What action should the nurse take?

Organism: *Moraxella catarrhalis*	
Antibiotic	**Sensitivity (S = sensitive; R = resistant)**
Amikacin	R
Amoxicillin	R
Azithromycin	S
Cefepime	R
Cefotetan	R
Clarithromycin	R
Gatafloxacin	S
Levofloxacin	S
Pipericillin	R
Tobramycin	R

4. The cultured organism is sensitive to more than one drug. In this case, what other factors are considered when choosing between the effective antibiotics?

5. What assessment should be monitored by the nurse to determine clinical response to the antibiotic?

Case Study 2

A neighbor asks a student nurse why her pediatrician does not prescribe antibiotics for her young son's "ear infections" like he used to for her older children, and her doctor will not phone in prescriptions when she has a "sinus infection" anymore.

1. How can the nurse explain these changes in antibiotic prescription practices?

2. What type of chronic pediatric conditions would warrant earlier treatment of sinus and ear infections?

3. The neighbor states that she has antibiotics left over from the last infection. "I always save some in case I need it." She asks the nurse if it is okay to give this drug to her son since it was prescribed for him. How should the student nurse respond?

4. The neighbor asks what she can do to prevent resistance to antibiotics. What suggestions should the student nurse make?

5. Where can the student nurse direct people for more information on preventing antibiotic resistance?

Case Study 3

Student nurses are studying the immune system. During clinical conference, they are discussing why some patients are admitted when they have an infection and others are treated as outpatients.

1. Discuss these questions.
   a. Why is a cancer chemotherapy patient admitted for two days of IV antibiotic therapy if the drug administered is available orally?
   b. Why do patients with an abscess have to have an incision and drainage (I&D) in order to effectively eradicate the infection?
   c. How can meningitis be treated if the effective antibiotics do not cross the blood-brain barrier?
   d. A severe infection warrants use of an ototoxic drug. The patient is breast-feeding. What teaching should the nurse provide?
   e. Why is it important to know the half-life of this drug?

Case Study 4

1. What role can the nurse play in reducing infections and antibiotic resistance?

Answers can be reviewed online at http://evolve.elsevier.com/Lehne/.

OBJECTIVES

See page 28 for the Objectives.

CRITICAL THINKING AND STUDY QUESTIONS

1. Penicillins (Select all that apply.)
   a. all are able to penetrate the gram-negative cell membrane.
   b. are able to destroy many bacteria if taken as prescribed.
   c. are in the same antibiotic family as macrolides.
   d. are only active against bacteria that are undergoing growth and division.
   e. are more effective against gram-negative than gram-positive bacteria.
   f. are toxic to human tissue when prescribed in high doses.
   g. can cause diarrhea by altering the normal GI flora.
   h. must bind to special proteins on the outer surface of cytoplasmic membrane to be effective.

✳ 2. Which of the following assessments is most critical for the nurse to complete before administering a penicillin antibiotic?
   a. Allergy history
   b. BUN
   c. Temperature
   d. Wound drainage

3. A patient has read scary stories about methicillin-resistant *Staphlococcus aureus* (MRSA) in the newspapers. Which of the following statements, if made by the patient, suggest that the patient has some misconceptions about MRSA? (Select all that apply)
   a. "Because people in hospitals need a lot of antibiotics, many of the germs that survive are resistant to penicillin because they do not allow penicillin to bind to germ proteins."
   b. "I can drastically reduce my chance of catching MRSA by simple hygiene measures."
   c. "MRSA can be treated by penicillinase-resistant penicillin such as nafcillin."
   d. "Many people have MRSA in their nose and do not know it."
   e. "Most infections with MRSA come from sports equipment."
   f. "The germ that causes MRSA is commonly found on the skin."
   g. "You can always tell when skin is infected by MRSA because it turns black."

4. A mother asks why her son has been prescribed amoxicillin and calcium clavulanate (Augmentin) if amoxicillin (Amoxil) has been ineffective in the past. The nurse's response is based on the fact that the addition of calcium clavulanate
   a. aids the penicillin with attaching to microbial penicillin-binding proteins.
   b. affects a wider spectrum of bacteria.
   c. prevents penicillinase from inactivating the amoxicillin.
   d. provides additional activity to disrupt the bacterial cell wall.

5. Which of the following organisms was previously susceptible to penicillin but has developed the greatest resistance to penicillin G?
   a. Gas gangrene caused by *Clostridium perfringes*
   b. Gonorrhea caused by *Neiserria gonorrhoeae*
   c. Meningitis caused by *Streptococcus pneumoniae*
   d. Syphilis caused by *Treponema pallidum*

6. A child is prescribed amoxicillin. When asked if her son is allergic to penicillin, the child's mother states that she does not know if he has ever received any medication before except immunizations. The nurse knows that it is important to assess for an allergic response despite this history because
   a. most people who experience a penicillin allergy experience the first incident in childhood.
   b. most people who are allergic to penicillin do not know of the allergy.

c. parents often are poor historians.

d. people can have an initial exposure to penicillin present in foods.

▸ 7. A pediatric office triage nurse speaks with a mother who calls complaining that her child gets diarrhea every time he is prescribed an oral antibiotic for an ear infection. An intervention that the nurse can suggest to restore normal flora is to teach the mother to offer her son which of the following foods 30 minutes after each dose of antibiotic?

a. Cheese

b. Ice cream

c. Milk

d. Yogurt

▸ 8. The nurse is preparing to administer 8 AM (0800) medications to a patient who is to receive nafcillin (Unipen) 2 g via secondary intravenous (IV) infusion. The drug is dissolved in 100 mL of normal saline solution. The drug handbook states the drug should be infused over 30 to 90 minutes. Just before the nurse hangs the nafcillin, the nurse is informed the patient is to be placed on a cart to go off the unit for a critical test in 30 to 45 minutes. The patient is expected to be off the floor for 30 minutes. The nurse should

a. hold the drug infusion until the patient returns from the test.

b. infuse the drug in 30 minutes before placing the patient on the cart.

c. infuse the drug in 45 minutes while loading the patient on the cart.

d. set the infusion to run over 90 minutes.

9. When the nurse is assisting with skin testing for penicillin allergy with the minor determinant mixture (MDM),

a. the nurse instructs the patient how to assess for a local reaction during the following week.

b. the nurse knows that the test carries little risk of a systemic reaction.

c. respiratory support and epinephrine should be available.

d. the test involves injection of a small amount of penicillin under the skin.

10. The nurse would be concerned about the increased possibility of an allergic reaction when administering which of the following antibiotics if the patient's allergy record includes penicillin allergy? (Select all that apply.)

a. Ampicillin/sulbactam (Unasyn)

b. Azithromycin (Zithromax)

c. Carbenicillin (Geocillin)

d. Cefadroxil (Duricef)

e. Clindamycin (Cleocin)

f. Erythromycin (EES)

g. Gatafloxacin (Tequin)

h. Imipenem and cilastatin (Primaxin)

i. Piperacillin/tazobactam (Zosyn)

j. Tobramycin (Nebcin)

k. Vancomycin (Vancocin)

11. A patient is prescribed IV ticarcillin (Ticar) every 4 hours and amikacin (Amikin) every 8 hours. In order for the patient to receive maximum benefit from both of these antibiotics, the nurse should administer the drugs

a. amikacin first, then ticarcillin.

b. at the same time at a Y-site.

c. in the same solution.

d. in a separate IV line.

▸ 12. Ampicillin 1 g/sulbactam 0.5 g (Unasyn) is supplied in 50 mL of solution to be infused over 15 minutes. The nurse should program the IV pump to deliver how many milliliters per hour?

13. The drug of choice for MRSA is

a. dicloxacillin.

b. nafcillin.

c. oxacillin.

d. vancomycin.

▸ 14. Which of these findings, if identified in a patient who is receiving ticarcillin (Ticar), should the nurse report to the prescriber immediately?

a. Capillary refill 2 seconds

b. Respirations 16 per minute

c. Temperature 101° F

d. Weight gain of 2 lb in 24 hours

▸ 15. The nurse reviews current laboratory test results before administering ticarcillin (Ticar). Which of the following laboratory results warrants consultation with the prescriber?

a. BNP 65 picograms/dL

b. BUN 22 mg/dL

c. Hgb 8 g/dL

d. WBC 15,000 mm³

16. A patient has just been prescribed carbenicillin (Geocillin) 500 mg 4 times a day. Which of the following timing of administration would be most therapeutic?
    a. 2 AM – 8 AM – 2 PM – 8 PM
    b. 4 AM – 10 AM – 4 PM – 10 PM
    c. 9 AM – 1 PM – 5 PM – 9 PM
    d. 12 Midnight – 6 AM – 12 Noon – 6 AM

17. The nurse would be concerned about toxicity if a patient receiving penicillin had which of the following laboratory results?
    a. ALT 52 international units/L
    b. BUN 20 mg/dL
    c. Creatinine 2.2 mg/dL
    d. Potassium 3.3 mEq/L

CASE STUDIES AND PATIENT TEACHING

(Use a separate piece of paper for your responses.)

Case Study 1

An 8-year-old is diagnosed with streptococcal pharyngitis. She is prescribed amoxicillin 250 mg 3 times a day for 10 days.

1. What important information should the nurse obtain before the penicillin is administered?

2. What information about the possible side effects and adverse reactions of penicillin does the nurse need to provide to the patient's mother?

3. Describe the types of allergic reactions that might develop with the administration of penicillin and the interventions that should be included in nursing care to prevent complications from an allergic reaction.

4. The patient's mother asks how and when amoxicillin should be given. How should the nurse respond?

5. Why is it critical that the nurse teach the patient's mother not to stop the medication even if the child's throat stops hurting in 4 to 5 days?

6. What outcomes would indicate that the antimicrobial effects were successful?

Case Study 2

The nurse is working in a public health clinic. A 15-year-old with no known allergies is diagnosed with syphilis and prescribed 1 dose of 2 million units of procaine penicillin G 2 intramuscularly (IM).

1. Developmentally, why is this drug a good choice for this patient?

2. The patient asks why she cannot get this medication in a pill. How should the nurse respond?

3. Describe the technique the nurse should use to administer this IM injection, including precautions to prevent administration complications.

4. The patient has denied allergy to penicillin. Why does the nurse need to be cautious about possible allergy?

5. What actions/policies should the clinic have in place to prevent death from an anaphylactic reaction?

84
Drugs That Weaken the Bacterial Cell Wall II: Cephalosporins, Carbapenems, Vancomycin, Aztreonam, Teicoplanin, and Fosfomycin

Answers can be reviewed online at http://evolve.elsevier.com/Lehne/.

OBJECTIVES

See page 28 for the Objectives.

CRITICAL THINKING AND STUDY QUESTIONS

1. Characteristics of cephalosporins are most like
   a. aminoglycosides.
   b. macrolides.
   c. penicillins.
   d. sulfonamides.
   e. tetracyclines.

2. Which of the following statements about cephalosporins is false?
   a. First-generation cephalosporins are effective for non-MRSA staphylococcal infections of the skin.
   b. Second-generation cephalosporins are more resistant to destruction by beta-lactamase enzymes.
   c. Third-generation cephalosporins are considerably more effective in treating gram-negative infections.
   d. Fourth-generation cephalosporins are the only class that has good penetration of the CSF.

▶ 3. Which of the following should be reported to the prescriber of cefotaximine?
   a. Albumin 3.4 g/dL
   b. ALT 58 international units/L
   c. eGFR 48 mL/min
   d. INR 1

4. Nursing interventions when administering cephalosporins include
   a. always administering on an empty stomach.
   b. assessment for severe allergy to carbapenems due to cross-allergy.
   c. instructing the patient to immediately report pain or warmth at IV site.
   d. oral suspensions to be kept at room temperature.

5. A patient is admitted to the hospital. She is alone and dazed and unable to provide an accurate past medical history. She is prescribed cefotetan 1 g q 12 hr IV for urosepsis. The patient's daughter arrives and provides her PMH. Which of the following should be reported to prescriber immediately?
   a. Cholecyctitis
   b. Type 2 DM
   c. Gastroesophogeal reflux disease
   d. von Willibrand disease

▶ 6. A patient who is receiving ceftazidime (Fortaz) has three loose brown bowel movements in 24 hours. The nurse should
   a. administer the drug and continue nursing care.
   b. continue to administer the drug and notify the prescriber of the change in bowel movements.
   c. discontinue administering the drug and notify the prescriber.
   d. page the prescriber STAT.

▶ 7. A patient with hospital-acquired pneumonia has just been prescribed cefotaxime (Claforan) and probenecid (Benemid). The patient has no history or evidence of gout. The nurse should
   a. administer both medications as ordered.
   b. administer the cefotaxime as ordered and ask the patient if they were taking probenecid at home.
   c. administer the cefotaxime, but contact the prescriber before administering the probenecid.
   d. contact the prescriber before administering either of the medications.

✳ 8. An alert and oriented patient with a history of penicillin allergy is prescribed cephalexin (Keftab). The initial action by the nurse should be to
   a. administer the cephalexin.
   b. administer the cephalexin and carefully assess for allergic reaction.
   c. assess the type of reaction that the patient had to the penicillin.
   d. notify the prescriber of the allergy and ask for a different antibiotic order.

▶ 9. The nurse is reviewing new laboratory results, including creatinine clearance results of 82 mL/min for a 74-year-old male patient receiving cefotetan (Cefotan) 2 g every 12 hours. The nurse should
   a. administer the medication.
   b. withhold the medication and notify the prescriber of the laboratory results.

 10. Cefoperazone (Cefobid) has been prescribed at discharge for a patient with pelvic inflammatory disease. Due to the possibility of a disulfiram-like reaction, during discharge teaching it is important for the nurse to teach the patient to avoid
   a. alcohol.
   b. antacids.
   c. aspirin.
   d. ibuprofen.

▶ 11. The nurse is preparing to administer an IV minibag of ceftriaxone in 50 mL of 5% dextrose to an infant. The infant has an IV of lactated Ringer's solution infusing at 35 mL/hour. The nurse should
   a. start a second IV for concurrent administration of the minibag and IV fluids.
   b. run the minibag as a piggyback at a Y site.
   c. consult with the prescriber.
   d. stop the running IV, infuse the minibag, then restart the running IV.

▶ 12. Which of the following laboratory results, if present, would be a reason to withhold administering cefotetan (Cefotan) to an adult male and to notify the prescriber?
   a. ALT 254 international units/L
   b. BUN 34 mg/dL
   c. Creatinine 3.5 mg/dL
   d. FBS 380 mg/dL

 13. Cefditoren (Spectracef) is prescribed on discharge for a patient diagnosed with bronchitis caused by *Moraxella catarrhalis,* type 2 DM, GERD, and end-stage renal failure. Why is this antibiotic a good choice for this patient?
   a. Its absorption is not affected by antacids.
   b. Cefditoren is effective for beta-lactamase producing *M. catarrhalis*.
   c. Cefditoren is inexpensive.
   d. Cefditoren has once-a-day dosing.

▶ 14. Ceftriaxone (Rocephin) 1 gram intramuscular is ordered for a 130-lb woman. The drug is reconstituted to a solution of 250 mg/mL. The nurse should administer
   a. 1 mL each in the right and left vastus lateralis and deltoid muscles.
   b. 2 mL each in the right and left ventrogluteal muscles.
   c. 2 mL each in the right and left deltoid muscle.
   d. 4 mL in the right or left gluteus maximus muscle.

 15. The carbapenem antibiotic imipenem (Primaxin) is a combination of the antibiotic and cilastatin. The purpose of the additive cilastatin is to
   a. decrease adverse effects of nausea and vomiting.
   b. improve absorption in the GI tract.
   c. prevent destruction of the antibiotic by beta-lactamase.
   d. prevent inactivation by a kidney enzyme.

▶ 16. The doctor has prescribed meropenem (Merrem) 250 mg every 8 hours for a 14-lb child who has been diagnosed with bacterial meningitis. The recommended safe pediatric dose of meropenem (Merrem) for meningitis is 40 mg/kg every 8 hours. Is this a safe dose?

 17. The nurse is preparing to administer an intermittent infusion of ertapenem (Invanz). This drug cannot be administered concurrently with which of the following intravenous (IV) solutions? (Select all that apply.)
   a. 5% dextrose in water
   b. 0.9% sodium chloride (normal saline)
   c. 0.45% sodium chloride
   d. 0.45% sodium chloride/5% dextrose solution
   e. 0.225% sodium chloride/5% dextrose solution
   f. Lactated Ringer's solution

▸ 18. Vancomycin is being administered by mouth for pseudomembranous colitis caused by *Clostridium difficile*. The nurse receives laboratory results on the patient that include creatinine 2.2 mg/dL. The nurse should
   a. administer the medication.
   b. hold the medication and notify the prescriber.

CASE STUDIES AND PATIENT TEACHING

(Use a separate piece of paper for your responses.)

Case Study 1

A 45-year-old, gravida 4, para 4, obese female admitted to the nursing unit with the diagnosis of cholelithiasis and cholecystitis. She complains of abdominal pain. She has a fever of 101°F and a white count of 12,000 mm³. A nasogastric tube is placed, an IV is started, and 1 g of cefazolin (Ancef) is ordered every 6 hours. Pain management is provided by IV meperidine (Demerol). Her cholecystectomy will be scheduled when her temperature returns to normal, probably in 2 to 3 days.

1. The nurse should assess the patient for which possible adverse reactions to the antibiotic?

2. What are the steps the nurse must take when administering a slow bolus intravenous infusion (IV push) of the antibiotic?

3. How can the possibility of thrombophlebitis be minimized?

4. Why would a broader spectrum antibiotic not be prescribed for this patient?

5. What should the nurse do if the nurse discovers the patient has had an anaphylactic reaction to penicillin?

Case Study 2

The nurse is caring for a patient who is prescribed IV cefoperazone (Cefobid) 2 g every 12 hours and Amikacin (Amikin) 300 mg 3 times a day after surgery for a ruptured appendix.

1. What assessments and laboratory results should be monitored while this patient is on this drug therapy?

2. What precautions does the nurse need to take when administering these two antibiotics through the same IV site?

3. The nurse notes that the patient's INR is 3.5. What should the nurse do?

4. Three days postoperatively, the patient has progressed to a soft diet and develops severe watery diarrhea. What are possible causes of the diarrhea?

5. What are possible electrolyte imbalances that could occur and what are their symptoms?

Case Study 3

A patient is prescribed vancomycin (Vancocin) 1 g every 12 hours scheduled at 0900 (9 AM) and 2100 (9 PM). The pharmacy provides a solution of 1 g in 200 mL.

1. Why is it critical to use an IV pump when administering this drug rather than hanging this drug by gravity?

2. If the drug is administered at 0900, at what time should blood be drawn to assess peak levels of the drug?

3. The drug will reach its therapeutic level after how many doses of the drug?

4. Describe red man syndrome and the nursing measures that can be taken to prevent this reaction?

5. Does experiencing red man syndrome create a contraindication for further administration of vancomycin?

6. Describe how the nurse will assess for the possible adverse effects of
   a. ototoxicity.
   b. immune-mediated thrombocytopenia.

Case Study 4

A child was treated with amoxicillin for otitis media. The child became more listless and developed a high fever. The parents are directed to seek care at the emergency department of the local hospital. The child is diagnosed with bacterial meningitis and prescribed IV cefotaxime.

1. The child's father asks why his child is being given a cephalosporin if amoxicillin did not work. The father is allergic to penicillin and has been told of the similarity and cross allergy between penicillins and cephalosporins. He wants to know why they are they not giving his child something stronger. How should the nurse respond?

85

Bacteriostatic Inhibitors of Protein Synthesis: Tetracyclines, Macrolides, and Others

Answers can be reviewed online at http://evolve.elsevier.com/Lehne/.

OBJECTIVES

See page 28 for the Objectives.

CRITICAL THINKING AND STUDY QUESTIONS

1. Tetracycline (Select all that apply.)
   a. absorption of long-acting agents is decreased by food.
   b. easily crosses mammalian cell membranes.
   c. is active against the bacilli that cause anthrax.
   d. is a narrow-spectrum antibiotic.
   e. kill bacteria.
   f. low doses prevent destruction of gingival connective tissue.
   g. reduces symptoms of rheumatoid arthritis.
   h. resistance to the drug is increasing.

2. The nurse teaches a patient who has been prescribed oral tetracycline (Sumycin) that the medication should not be taken with which of the following over-the-counter medications? (Select all that apply.)

   a. Ascorbic acid
   b. Centrum silver
   c. Ferrous sulfate
   d. Folic acid
   e. TUMs

▶ 3. A patient who was admitted with severe abdominal pain has been diagnosed with *H. pylori* associated peptic ulcer. Tetracycline 500 mg, metronidazole 250 mg, and bismuth subsalicylate 525 mg have been prescribed 4 times a day. The nurse notes that the patient's 24-hour fluid intake has been approximately 2500 mL and urine output has been 600 to 800 mL for each of the past 2 days. The nurse should
   a. administer the medications and continue nursing care.
   b. administer the medications and report the changes.
   c. withhold the medication and continue nursing care.
   d. withhold the medication and notify the prescriber of the changes.

▶ 4. Tetracycline can cause esophageal ulceration. What can the nurse teach to minimize the risk of this adverse effect?
   a. Stay upright for at least 30 minutes after taking the medication.
   b. Take the medication at bedtime.
   c. Take the medication with an antacid.
   d. Take the medication with milk.

▶ 5. A patient is prescribed a tetracycline antibiotic. Which of the following patient data are reasons that the medication should be withheld by the nurse and the prescriber consulted?
   a. Allergic to penicillin
   b. 12-year-old child
   c. Pregnancy status unknown
   d. Theophylline for asthma is also prescribed

6. The nurse should assess for adverse effects of lightheadedness and dizziness when a patient is receiving
   a. demeclocycline.
   b. doxycycline.
   c. minocycline.
   d. oxytetracycline.

✳ 7. The nurse prepares to administer prescribed demeclocycline (Declomycin) to a patient whose chart and assessment findings do not suggest the presence of infection, acne, peptic ulcer, periodontal disease, or rheumatoid arthritis. A priority nursing issue for this patient is
   a. fluid balance.
   b. pain.
   c. safety.
   d. tissue perfusion.

8. A patient with a penicillin allergy is prescribed erythromycin ethylsuccinate 250 mg every 6 hours for pneumonia caused by *Haemophilus influenzae*. The medication administration record (MAR) has the medication scheduled at 0600, 1200, 1800, and 2400. On the second day of therapy, the patient complains that he does not like taking the drug because it causes heartburn. An appropriate intervention by the nurse would be to
   a. administer the drug with food.
   b. change the timing of the drug to 0800, 1200, 1730, and 2400 so that most doses are administered with meals.

   c. explain that administering the drug with food or antacids will prevent absorption of the drug.
   d. withhold the drug and notify the prescriber.

▶ 9. Which of these findings would be most significant for the nurse if a patient was receiving erythromycin estolate?
   a. Cheesy vaginal discharge and vaginal itching
   b. Dark urine and abdominal pain
   c. Dyspepsia and flatulence
   d. Headache and insomnia

10. Enteric-coated erythromycin base should be administered (Select all that apply.)
   a. on an empty stomach.
   b. whole, not chewed.
   c. with a full glass of water.
   d. with food.

▶ 11. Erythromycin oral suspension 200 mg 4 times a day has been prescribed for a child. The pharmacy provided erythromycin 250 mg/5 mL. How much erythromycin should the nurse teach the parent to administer per dose?

12. Because of the risk of prolonged QT interval and torsades de pointes, the nurse would consult the prescriber before administering erythromycin to a patient who has experienced
   a. frequent headaches.
   b. nausea.
   c. unexplained fainting.
   d. wheezing.

13. Careful review of all of the drugs that a patient is prescribed is important when a patient is prescribed erythromycin because erythromycin
   a. action is prevented by clindamycin.
   b. becomes ineffective because metabolism is increased by nondihydropine CCCB.
   c. can increase levels of warfarin and cause bleeding.
   d. prevents the absorption of -azole antifungals.

14. The nurse teaches that to be well absorbed, which of the following forms of clarithromycin (Biaxin) must be administered with food?
    a. Standard tablets
    b. Extended-release tablets
    c. Granules

15. What teaching can the nurse provide regarding administration of antibiotics that helps decrease the development of resistance?
    a. Always take antibiotics with food.
    b. Only take antibiotics when symptoms are present.
    c. Go to the doctor and ask for antibiotics as soon as you think you have an infection.
    d. When prescribed, take the full course as directed even if symptoms are gone.

▶ 16. It is important for the nurse to monitor which of the following laboratory tests when a patient is prescribed erythromycin and warfarin?
    a. BUN
    b. CK-MM
    c. INR
    d. RBC

▶ 17. The MAR has azithromycin (Zithromax) listed to be administered at 0800. Breakfast arrives on the nursing unit around 0800, lunch at 1230 and supper at 1730. The patient does not receive any antacids. The nurse should
    a. administer the drug at 0730, within the acceptable time frame.
    b. administer the drug at 0800 and hold the patient's breakfast until 0900.
    c. consult the prescriber.
    d. reschedule the drug for 1030.

✳ 18. Which of the following assessment findings would be of most concern if a patient is receiving troleandomycin (Tao)?
    a. Acne-like rash
    b. Dark urine and nausea
    c. Productive cough
    d. Urine output of 500 mL/8 hours

19. A diabetic patient is receiving clindamycin (Cleocin) for gas gangrene. Which of the following is most suggestive of the development of antibiotic-associated membranous colitis (AAPMC) caused by *Clostridium difficile*?
    a. Dyspepsia and flatulence
    b. Five watery stools a day

    c. Hypoactive bowel sounds
    d. Nausea and vomiting

20. The nurse would consult the prescriber regarding administration of linezolid (Zyvox) if the nurse discovered the patient has a history of
    a. asthma.
    b. celiac disease.
    c. gout.
    d. phenylketonuria.

▶ 21. The nurse would consult the prescriber of linezolid (Zyvox) if the patient did not have a baseline of which of the following laboratory tests?
    a. Arterial blood gases
    b. Cardiac enzymes
    c. CBC and differential
    d. Liver function tests

22. A patient with a history of hypertension controlled by an angiotensin-converting enzyme inhibitor is prescribed linezolid (Zyvox) for a vancomycin-resistant enterococcal (VRE) infection. The patient should be instructed to avoid eating which of the following foods while on this antibiotic?
    a. Aged cheese
    b. Milk
    c. Red meat
    d. Seafood

23. The nurse should include in teaching to a patient who has been receiving linezolid (Zyvox) to immediately report which of the following symptoms of a *rare* adverse effect that has been associated with prolonged therapy?
    a. Dizziness when changing positions
    b. Headache
    c. Numbness or tingling in any extremity
    d. Vomiting

✳ 24. A patient was receiving telithromycin (Ketek) for CAP caused by *Chlamydia pneumoniae*. The patient developed nausea, vomiting, dark urine, and fatigue. The prescriber discontinued the drug after evaluating ALT levels at 287 international units/L. A priority teaching for this patient is
    a. if you take this drug, you should take it with food to minimize adverse effects on the GI tract.
    b. if you take this drug, you need to drink 80 to 100 ounces of fluids each day.

c. if you take this drug, you should look at your stool and contact the prescriber if it turns black or bloody.

d. you can never take this drug again.

25. It is important for the nurse to notify the prescriber if a patient is prescribed which of the following cholesterol lowering drugs and telithromycin (Ketek)? (Select all that apply.)
    a. Atorvastatin (Lipitor)
    b. Fluvastatin (Lescol)
    c. Lovastatin (Mevacor)
    d. Pravastatin (Pravachol)
    e. Simvastatin (Zocor)

✱ 26. Which of these laboratory tests, if identified in a patient who is receiving dalfopristin/quinupristin (Synercid), should the nurse report to the prescriber immediately?
    a. ALT 250 international units/L
    b. BUN 20 mg/dL
    c. CK-MM 50 units/mL
    d. FBS 250 mg/dL

▶ 27. The nurse is caring for a patient whose peak chloramphenicol level is 28 mcg/mL. Which of the following assessment findings is most important to report to the prescriber relating to administration of this drug?
    a. BP 135/80
    b. Facial flushing with activity
    c. Pallor
    d. Vomiting

28. A major advantage of tigecycline (Tygacil) in treating VRE is
    a. it does not change the metabolism of any drugs including warfarin.
    b. less development of antibiotic resistance.
    c. oral administration.
    d. it is safe for use in pregnancy and with children.

29. When used to treat colonized MRSA, mupirocin (Bacroban) is administered
    a. intranasally.
    b. intravenously.
    c. orally.
    d. topically.

CASE STUDIES AND PATIENT TEACHING

(Use a separate piece of paper for your responses.)

Case Study 1

A 30-year-old office worker reports to the healthcare facility with a fever of 101°F and a nonproductive cough that has lasted 10 days. Her medical history reveals that she is an asthmatic, takes theophylline (Theo-Dur), and is allergic to penicillin. On physical exam, her respiratory rate is 24 and nonlabored, and bilateral basilar crackles (rales) are heard. The patient is given a prescription for erythromycin 250 mg 4 times a day for 10 days to treat what is suspected to be mycoplasma pneumonia. She is advised to take Tylenol 325 mg q4hr for fever, to increase her fluids to 6 to 8 glasses of water per day, and to stay home from work for 2 to 3 days.

1. What serious adverse effect is this patient at risk for based on drug interactions, and what symptoms would suggest this syndrome?

2. What should the nurse do regarding the possibility of this syndrome?

Case Study 2

A 15-year-old male patient is readmitted after being discharged following an appendectomy with shaking chills, fever of 103°F, and purulent drainage from the incision site. Culture and sensitivity results of the wound drainage reveal Enterococcus faecium *that is resistant to vancomycin. Dalfopristin/quinupristin (Synercid) 500 mg intravenous every 12 hours is prescribed.*

1. What laboratory tests and symptoms should the nurse monitor to assess for hepatotoxicity?

2. What nursing assessments and interventions should the nurse include in the plan of care relating to the significant risk of infusion-related thrombophlebitis?

3. Dalfopristin/quinupristin (Synercid) inhibits CYP3A4 hepatic drug-metabolizing enzyme. What are the ramifications for nursing care?

Answers can be reviewed online at http://evolve.elsevier.com/Lehne/.

OBJECTIVES

See page 28 for the Objectives.

CRITICAL THINKING AND STUDY QUESTIONS

1. Major adverse effects of aminoglycoside antibiotics include damage to (Select all that apply.)
   a. cochlea (hearing).
   b. heart (pumping).
   c. kidneys (tubular necrosis).
   d. lungs (fluid accumulation).
   e. stomach (ulcers).
   f. vestibular apparatus (balance).

2. Aminoglycosides (Select all that apply.)
   a. are administered intravenously (IV) to treat meningitis.
   b. are all equally susceptible to inactivation by enzymes.
   c. are narrow-spectrum antibiotics.
   d. are never administered orally.
   e. are primarily used to treat serious infections with aerobic gram-negative bacilli.
   f. can be toxic to the kidneys and nervous system.
   g. cannot kill bacteria when serum levels drop below the minimal bactericidal concentration.
   h. effectiveness correlates to serum concentration levels.

3. Facultative bacteria survive in
   a. the absence of oxygen.
   b. both the absence and presence of oxygen.
   c. the presence of oxygen.

4. Neomycin topical drops have been prescribed for a patient with external otitis. Which of the following assessment findings would be a reason for the nurse to consult with the prescriber?
   a. Foul odor from the external canal
   b. Pain when straightening the pinna to instill the drops
   c. Tasting the drops after they are instilled
   d. Temperature 100.4°F (38°C)

5. A patient, who is prescribed tobramycin (Nebcin), complains of a headache. The nurse should
   a. assess the onset, characteristics, and associated symptoms of the headache.
   b. medicate with acetaminophen and reassess in 1 hour.
   c. withhold the tobramycin and notify the prescriber when making rounds.
   d. withhold the tobramycin and notify the prescriber STAT.

6. The nurse is assessing a patient who is scheduled to receive a dose of gentamicin (Garamycin). In the last 12 hours, fluid intake has been 900 mL, urine output has been 300 mL, and the patient's bladder is not distended. The nurse should
   a. administer the drug.
   b. administer the drug and notify the prescriber of the output.
   c. instruct the patient that he needs to drink a full glass of water each time the medication is administered.
   d. withhold the drug and notify the prescriber of the output.

7. The nurse is taking a history from the wife of a patient who was admitted in a septic state and prescribed an aminoglycoside antibiotic. Which of the following questions is most important to ask the wife about her husband's history?
   a. "Has he ever had any surgery performed?"
   b. "Has he been told to follow any specific diet?"
   c. "Has he received a flu vaccine this year?"
   d. "What medications is he currently taking?"

8. The nurse is assessing for adverse effects of IV tobramycin. Which of the following changes would be most significant?
   a. Dilute urine
   b. Headache
   c. Limp, weak muscles
   d. Ringing in the ears

248

9. The nurse is aware that the risk of ototoxicity is increased if a hypertensive patient is also receiving
   a. bumetanide.
   b. ethacrynic acid.
   c. furosemide.
   d. hydrochlorothiazide.

10. A patient is prescribed IV ticarcillin (Ticar) every 4 hours and amikacin (Amikin) every 8 hours. In order for the patient to receive maximum benefit from both of these antibiotics, the nurse should administer the drugs
    a. amikacin first, then ticarcillin.
    b. at the same time at a Y-site.
    c. in the same solution.
    d. in a separate IV line.

11. Match the interaction of drugs with aminoglycosides.

    _____ a. Amphotericin B
    _____ b. Aspirin
    _____ c. Cephalosporin
    _____ d. Cyclosporine
    _____ e. Ethacrynic acid
    _____ f. NSAID
    _____ g. Penicillin
    _____ h. Pancuronium
    _____ i. Polymyxin
    _____ j. Tubocurarine
    _____ k. Vancomycin

    1. Aid aminoglycoside getting into cell
    2. Inactivate aminoglycosides when in the same solution
    3. Directly increase risk of damage to the inner ear
    4. Indirectly increase risk of damage to the inner ear
    5. Increase risk of kidney damage
    6. Risk of respiratory arrest

▸ 12. The nurse would be most concerned about the possibility of toxicity when a patient is prescribed the same daily dose of an aminoglycoside divided into which of the following regimens?
    a. Once a day
    b. Every 8 hours
    c. Every 12 hours

13. When aminoglycosides are prescribed IV as a once daily dose, it is important to monitor the
    a. trough levels 1 hour after completing the infusion.
    b. peak levels 15-30 minutes after completing the infusion and trough levels 30 minutes before the next dose.
    c. peak levels 1 hour after completing the infusion and trough levels 30 minutes before the next dose.
    d. trough levels up to 1 hour before the next dose.

14. The most important reason why amikacin (Amikin) should only be used in cases where other aminoglycosides are known to be resistant is
    a. it must be dosed more frequently.
    b. its sensitivity to aminoglycoside-inactivating enzymes.
    c. to delay emergence of organisms' resistance to amikacin.
    d. toxicity.

▸ 15. The nurse is caring for a patient who is receiving gentamicin twice a day. Peak and trough levels were drawn after the fourth dose. Results were peak 3 mcg/mL and trough 0.6 mcg/mL. The nurse should
    a. administer an additional dose.
    b. continue nursing care.
    c. consult with the prescriber.
    d. withhold future doses until the prescriber can be consulted.

✳ 16. Which of these laboratory tests would be most important for the nurse to assess when a patient is receiving an aminoglycoside?
    a. Creatinine
    b. Fasting glucose
    c. Hemoglobin and hematocrit
    d. INR

▸ 17. A patient received a neuromuscular blocking agent during surgery. In the recovery room, the prescriber orders gentamicin 40 mg IV stat. What is the most appropriate nursing action?
    a. Administer the drug as quickly as possible.
    b. Assess the patient's vital signs.
    c. Clarify the order.
    d. Refuse to administer the drug.

CASE STUDIES AND PATIENT TEACHING

(Use a separate piece of paper for your responses.)

Case Study 1

A 72-year-old man with a history of diabetes mellitus (DM) treated with metformin and rheumatoid arthritis treated for many years by nonsteroid anti-inflammatory drugs had a prostatectomy 14 days earlier. He is readmitted to a medical-surgical unit for a surgical site infection. Assessment findings include BP 100/70 mm Hg, pulse 98 beats/min, respirations 24 breaths per minute, and temperature 104° F (40°C). He is difficult to arouse and his skin is hot and dry. Escherichia coli cultured from the wound drainage is sensitive to amikacin (Amikin). The nursing drug handbook lists the recommended IV dose as a loading dose of 7.5 mg/kg followed by 15 mg/kg/day in 2 to 3 divided doses every 8 to 12 hours for 7 to 10 days. This patient weighs 65 kg and has been prescribed a loading dose of 250 mg of amikacin followed by 175 mg every 8 hours.

1. Calculate the recommended dose of amikacin for this patient.

2. What are possible reasons for the prescribed dose not being equivalent to the recommended dose?

3. The drug is to be administered at 0600 (6 AM), 1400 (2 PM), and 2200 (10 PM). Peak and trough levels of the amikacin are ordered. When will the nurse schedule the collection of the blood sample for this testing?

4. Why are serum trough levels more significant than serum peak levels?

5. The trough level of the amikacin (Amikin) is 15 mcg/mL. What should the nurse do?

Case Study 2

A 40-year-old male patient is recovering in the trauma unit from a major accident. He is on a ventilator and has a central line for IVs and antibiotics, a Swan-Ganz catheter to measure cardiac status, an arterial line to measure continuous blood pressures, a small-bore feeding tube, 2 chest tubes, and a Foley catheter. After 3 days, he develops gram-negative septicemia and pneumonia and is started on gentamicin sulfate (Garamycin) and ampicillin (Unasyn) IV.

1. Describe the assessments the nurse should perform to detect nephrotoxicity and neurotoxicity.

2. How does nephrotoxicity increase the risk of developing ototoxicity?

3. Which toxicity is most likely to be permanent?

4. How can the nurse prevent drug interactions?

5. What type of urine collection bag should the nurse use with this patient?

6. What changes in the dosages of medications would be necessary if the patient were 80 years old instead of 40?

Case Study 3

A mother needs to instill antibiotic ear drops in her child's ear.

1. Describe the teaching the nurse would provide.

Answers can be reviewed online at http://evolve.elsevier.com/Lehne/.

OBJECTIVES

See page 28 for the Objectives.

CRITICAL THINKING AND STUDY QUESTIONS

1. Sulfonamides (Select all that apply.)
   a. are chemically related to glipizide, glyburide, furosemide, and hydrochlorothiazide.
   b. are narrow-spectrum antibiotics.
   c. are no longer active against many microbes for which they initially were effective.
   d. are usually administered intramuscularly or intravenously.
   e. are widely used because of low toxicity.
   f. can cause folic acid deficiency in the patient.
   g. cross the placenta.
   h. do not cause toxicity when applied topically.
   i. inhibit microbial synthesis of folic acid.
   j. were the first systemic antibiotics developed.

2. The primary reason why the nurse teaches a patient who is prescribed sulfamethoxazole to take this medication with a full glass of water is to
   a. decrease the risk of esophageal irritation.
   b. minimize crystal formation.
   c. prevent nausea.
   d. stimulate frequent voiding.

▶ 3. A patient who has liver impairment has been prescribed a sulfamethoxazole. The nurse should assess for which of the following symptoms that would be a result of increased acetylation of the drug?
   a. Clay-colored stool
   b. Pallor
   c. Rash
   d. Urine output of 100 mL in 4 hours

▶ 4. Sulfonamides can cause the adverse effect of kernicterus. This presents as
   a. damage to the brain in neonates from products of Hgb breakdown.
   b. damage to the kidney tubules by crystals in the urine.
   c. inability of the bone marrow to produce blood cells.
   d. unusual sensitivity to sunlight.

▶ 5. A patient who takes glyburide for type 2 diabetes mellitus (DM) is prescribed sulfamethoxazole-trimethoprim (Septra). Because of possible drug interactions, the nurse should assess for
   a. bleeding and bruising.
   b. diaphoresis and tachycardia.
   c. hot, dry skin, and thirst.
   d. paresthesias and abdominal cramps.

▶ 6. The patient has been receiving mafendine (Sulfamylon) application to a second-degree burn for over 2 weeks. Which of the following laboratory results would be a reason for withholding mafendine application and consulting the prescriber?
   a. pH 7.32, HCO_3 18 mEq/L, pCO_2 36 mm Hg
   b. pH 7.35, HCO_3 22 mEq/L, pCO_2 37 mm Hg
   c. pH 7.41, HCO_3 24 mEq/L, pCO_2 40 mm Hg
   d. pH 7.45, HCO_3 21 mEq/L, pCO_2 47 mm Hg

▶ 7. The nurse is preparing to apply topical mafendine (Sulfamylon) to second-degree burns on the anterior of a 7-year-old patient's arms, upper legs, and trunk. To gain compliance with this therapy, it would be important for the nurse to
   a. employ aseptic technique.
   b. explain the importance of therapy.
   c. prevent pain.
   d. shield so the patient cannot see the wounds.

▶ 8. The nurse is administering trimethoprim to a patient who has a history of alcohol use disorder. Because folate deficiency is associated with alcohol use disorder, the nurse should assess for symptoms of possible adverse effects of trimethoprim including
   a. nausea and vomiting.
   b. rash and malaise.
   c. pallor and sore throat.
   d. photosensitivity and drug fever.

9. Trimethoprim (Proloprim) is classified as pregnancy category C. This means
   a. animal studies have shown a risk for fetal problems, but human studies have not shown any problems.
   b. controlled studies have shown no risk to the developing fetus.
   c. do not use this drug in pregnancy.
   d. risks are possible, but potential benefits may justify the risk.
   e. there is definite evidence of risk to the developing fetus.

10. Benefits of trimethoprim-sulfamethoxazole (TMP/SMZ) over the components used alone include
    a. lack of interactions with drugs that have a narrow therapeutic range.
    b. fewer adverse effects.
    c. less resistance has developed.
    d. lower incidence of toxicity.

11. A physician who is on call for another physician gives a verbal order for sulfamethoxazole-trimethoprim (Septra) for a patient. The nurse would consult the prescriber about this order if the patient had a history of
    a. chronic obstructive lung disease.
    b. diabetes mellitus.
    c. hypertension.
    d. megoblastic anemia.

▸ 12. An allergy to which of the following diabetic medications would be a reason for the nurse to contact the prescriber if a patient is prescribed trimethoprim plus sulfamethoxazole for Pneumocystis pneumonia (PCP)?
    a. Glimepiride (Amaryl)
    b. Rosiglitazone (Avandia)
    c. Metformin (Glucophage)
    d. Acarbose (Precose)

▸ 13. The recommended dose of sulfamethoxazole-trimethoprim (Septra) for children is $150\,mg/m^2$ BSA of trimethoprim and $750\,mg/m^2$ BSA of sulfamethoxazole daily in three doses, not to exceed 320 mg of trimethoprim and 1600 mg of sulfamethoxazole per day. What is the recommended dose for a child who is 96 cm tall and weighs 18 kg?

CASE STUDIES AND PATIENT TEACHING

(Use a separate piece of paper for your responses.)

Case Study 1

A 30-year-old IV drug addict who is HIV positive has been treated with AZT for more than 1 year. She presents to the clinic with a low-grade fever, nonproductive cough, and shortness of breath. A chest x-ray shows diffuse infiltrates. A diagnosis of pneumocystis pneumonia *(PCP) caused by* Pneumocystis jiroveci *is made.*

1. The patient becomes tearful. She states that she knows about getting pneumonia from *Pneumocycstis carnii*. Now she has something new and she is sure that she is going to die. How should the nurse respond?

2. The patient is started on trimethoprim-sulfamethoxazole (TMP/SMZ). Why is TMP/SMZ a good choice for this patient?

3. Why is it important to wait for the results of hCG levels before this patient starts taking TMP/SMZ?

4. What adverse effects should the nurse teach the patient to report, should they occur?

5. What can the nurse teach to decrease the incidence and severity of these possible adverse effects to TMP/SMZ?
   a. Photosensitivity
   b. Stevens-Johnson syndrome
   c. Renal damage

6. What forms of sulfonamide drugs have less risk of Stevens-Johnson syndrome?

Case Study 2

The nurse has volunteered to do a health mission trip to provide healthcare to Rwandan refugees in Uganda. A clinic has been set up and doctors and nurse practitioners are diagnosing cases and providing donated samples of medications. The RN is providing teaching via an interpreter. Sulfonamides are being provided to patients with urinary tract infections.

1. What adverse effect would these patients be at greater risk for than the general population?

2. What type of sulfonamides would be more likely to cause hemolytic anemia?

3. The nurse should assess for what symptoms that suggest possible development of hemolytic anemia?

4. An HIV-positive mother comes to the clinic with a 2-week-old infant who appears toxic. The only antibiotic the team has in a liquid form is a sulfonamide. Why is this dangerous to give to this infant?

88

Drug Therapy of Urinary Tract Infections

Answers can be reviewed online at http://evolve.elsevier.com/Lehne/.

OBJECTIVES

See page 28 for the Objectives.

CRITICAL THINKING AND STUDY QUESTIONS

1. An example of a complicated urinary tract infection (UTI) is a UTI
   a. acquired in the hospital.
   b. caused by an enlarged prostate.
   c. caused by multiple organisms.
   d. of the kidney pelvis.

2. A female patient has been prescribed ciprofloxacin (Cipro) 250 mg by mouth twice a day for 7 days. The patient asks why she has to take the antibiotic for so long. Her friend had a UTI and only had to take her antibiotic for 3 days. The nurse knows that a possible explanation for the need for the longer therapy includes
   a. fewer adverse effects.
   b. less potential for antibiotic resistance.
   c. lower cost.
   d. upper urinary tract involvement.

✳ 3. A prescriber's orders for a new admission include urine culture and sensitivity and ciprofloxacin 400 mg intravenously (IV) every 12 hours. A priority nursing responsibility is to
   a. calculate the drip rate for the IV infusion.
   b. flush the IV cap.
   c. mix the antibiotic in the correct IV solution.
   d. obtain the urine culture specimen before administering the antibiotic.

4. Nitrofurantoin, methenamine, nalidixic acid, and cinoxacin.
   a. are first-line agents for prostatitis.
   b. are not absorbed from the GI tract.
   c. concentrate in the urine much greater than in the blood.
   d. have few adverse effects.

✳ 5. Which of these assessment findings, if identified in a patient who is receiving nitrofurantoin (Macrodantin), should the nurse report to the prescriber immediately?
   a. Brown-colored urine
   b. Paresthesia
   c. Nausea
   d. Headache

6. A patient is receiving 50 mg of nitrofurantoin (Macrodantin) at bedtime for prophylaxis of recurrent cystitis. This means the patient
   a. is taking very high doses of the drug because she cannot get rid of the infection.
   b. is taking low doses of the drug to prevent reinfection.
   c. is taking low doses to prevent relapse.
   d. has a UTI caused by a resistant microorganism.

▶ 7. The nurse is reviewing the other over-the-counter products taken by a patient who has been prescribed methenamine (Mandelamine). Which of these home treatments might reduce the urinary antiseptic action of methenamine?
   a. A vegetarian diet that includes a large amount of tomatoes, strawberries, and oranges
   b. Drinking 10 glasses of water each day for general health
   c. Ibuprofen taken twice a day for joint pain
   d. Megadoses of vitamin C (ascorbic acid) to prevent colds

8. A patient has been prescribed nalidixic acid (NegGram) for recurrent UTIs. The nurse should teach the patient to (Select all that apply.)
   a. report musculoskeletal pain.
   b. report unusual bruising.
   c. stop taking the drug if you note changes in your vision.
   d. stop taking the drug if urinary discomfort does not resolve in 48 hours.
   e. take the medication with milk.
   f. use sunscreen.

▶ 9. Which of the following laboratory test results is most important to review before the nurse administers cinoxacin (Cinobac)?
   a. ALT
   b. bilirubin
   c. creatinine
   d. sodium

CASE STUDIES AND PATIENT TEACHING

(Use a separate piece of paper for your responses.)

Case Study 1

A 75-year-old man with known benign prostatic hypertrophy (BPH) has had numerous episodes of cystitis.

1. If the patient develops flank pain, chills, fever, or other signs of infection higher in the urinary tract suggesting pyelonephritis, what actions should be taken?

2. The patient has been successfully treated with TMP/SMZ and has been prescribed nitrofurantoin (Macrodantin) to prevent recurrence of UTIs until he can be evaluated for surgery for his enlarged prostate. The nurse should teach the patient to be alert for what possible adverse effects from Macrodantin?

3. What nursing assessments and teaching can the nurse employ to prevent complications from nitrofurantoin (Macrodantin) therapy?

4. The patient calls to tell the office nurse that his urine has changed to a brown color. What should the nurse tell him?

5. Why is it important to monitor creatinine levels in this patient?

Case Study 2

A female student is seen at the college health center. She constantly feels that she needs to urinate, but does not want to because it hurts, and the urge to urinate persists after she voids. She denies fever and flank pain and has not looked at her urine.

1. What additional questions should the nurse ask the patient to assist the practitioner with diagnosing?

2. Why is it important to determine how frequently the patient has had UTIs in the past?

3. The college health nurse knows that most UTIs treated with sulfonamides are due to *Escherichia coli* infection. Why are females more prone to get this infection?

4. What instruction should the nurse provide the student to prevent future infections?

89

Antimycobacterial Agents: Drugs for Tuberculosis, Leprosy, and *Mycobacterium avium* Complex Infection

Answers can be reviewed online at http://evolve.elsevier.com/Lehne/.

OBJECTIVES

See page 28 for the Objectives.

CRITICAL THINKING AND STUDY QUESTIONS

1. Select all that apply to tuberculosis (TB).
   a. Drug treatment is best if medications can be taken daily at home.
   b. Infected, but symptom-free individuals cannot infect other people.
   c. Infected individuals have a risk of developing active TB without additional exposure to the bacteria even if the infection has been dormant for many years.
   d. Infection is best treated in the hospital.
   e. TB is an infection limited to the lungs.
   f. TB is more prevalent in jail and homeless populations than the general population.
   g. Primary infection usually is evident on chest x-ray.
   h. Resistance to drugs is increasing.
   i. Treatment of active infection should always include at least two drugs.

▶ 2. Describe nursing actions that can decrease the emergence of resistance of *Mycobacterium tuberculosis* to drug therapy?

3. A patient who has been diagnosed with active TB has been prescribed isoniazid, rifampin, ethambutol, and pyrazinamide. The patient asks the nurse why he has to take so many drugs. The basis of the nurse's response should include that this multiple drug therapy (Select all that apply.)
   a. confers immunity to *M. tuberculosis*.
   b. decreases adverse effects.
   c. decreases the risk of relapse.
   d. does not increase the risk of suprainfection.
   e. eliminates actively dividing and resting tuberculosis mycobacteria.
   f. prevents the mycobacteria from developing resistance to a drug.

4. A patient asks the nurse why he has to continue to take medication after completion of the initial induction phase if his sputum is "clean." The nurse explains that
   a. dormant bacteria are still present inside cells and can become active at a later time.
   b. sputum cultures are not sensitive enough to ensure that the active bacteria are eliminated.
   c. sputum cultures are not specific for mycobacterium.
   d. this therapy is in case the person comes into contact with the person who originally infected him.

5. An HIV-infected patient who is receiving drug therapy including delavirdine (Rescriptor) and saquinavir (Fortovase) is diagnosed with an active TB infection. Because of the drug interaction that decreases the effect of these drugs for HIV infection, this patient should not be prescribed
   a. ethambutol.
   b. isoniazid.
   c. pyrazinamide.
   d. rifampin.

6. A college nursing student with no medical problems, no symptoms of disease, and no risk factors for contracting TB is being screened for TB before starting a clinical nursing course. He has a 20 mm area of erythema surrounding an 11 mm area of induration 48 hours after receiving a PPD tuberculin test. Chest x-ray and sputum culture are negative. The nurse would expect prophylactic treatment to involve
   a. multiple drug therapy.
   b. watchful waiting.
   c. isoniazid.
   d. rifampin.

✳ ▸ 7. The nurse is receiving isoniazid therapy for latent TB. It would be most important to contact the prescriber if the nurse experiences
   a. headache.
   b. dry mouth.
   c. right upper quadrant (RUQ) pain.
   d. heartburn.

▸ 8. The public health nurse would withhold administration of TB drug therapy with rifampin and pyrazinamide and contact the prescriber if the patient's laboratory testing results include
   a. AST 75 international units/L.
   b. bilirubin, total 3 mg/dL.
   c. BUN 22 mg/dL.
   d. creatinine 1 mg/dL.

9. The nurse should be particularly vigilant with monitoring intake and output and creatinine levels when a patient is receiving which of the following anti-tubercular drugs? (Select all that apply.)
   a. Amikacin
   b. Cycloserine
   c. Ethambutol
   d. Ethionamide
   e. Gatifloxacin
   f. Kanamycin
   g. Isoniazid
   h. Pyrazinamide

   i. Rifampin
   j. Streptomycin

10. A patient with a history of peripheral vascular disease, type 2 diabetes mellitus, and latent TB is prescribed isoniazid and pyridoxine. The purpose of the pyridoxine is to
    a. improve arterial blood flow.
    b. prevent hypoglycemia.
    c. prevent peripheral neuropathy.
    d. treat resting mycobacteria within cells.

11. The interaction of isoniazid and phenytoin is especially important because
    a. isoniazid levels can become subtherapeutic.
    b. phenytoin has a narrow therapeutic range.
    c. phenytoin levels can become subtherapeutic.
    d. the risk of hepatotoxicity increases.

▸ 12. A paranoid schizophrenic patient who has been involuntarily committed to a psychiatric institution has been diagnosed with latent TB and is refusing drug therapy with isoniazid. An appropriate nursing response would be to
    a. consult the prescriber and psychiatrist regarding possible intramuscular administration of isoniazid.
    b. explain the importance of drug therapy.
    c. withhold the drug and isolate the patient until he agrees to take the drug.
    d. withhold the drug, the patient cannot infect others.

13. The nurse knows that rifampin may not reach therapeutic levels if it is administered orally
    a. on an empty stomach.
    b. with food.
    c. with other drugs that are metabolized by the hepatic cytochrome P450 enzymes.
    d. with protease inhibitors and non-nucleoside reverse transcriptase inhibitors (NNRTIs) for HIV infection.

▸ 14. A patient takes prophylactic warfarin because of a history of atrial fibrillation, which can cause the release of clots that become emboli. The patient has recently been diagnosed with TB and prescribed antimicrobial drugs, including rifampin. Because of the interaction between warfarin and rifampin, it is important for the nurse to assess the patient for
    a. abdominal pain.
    b. bleeding.
    c. change in mental status.
    d. oliguria.

15. A patient has received instructions regarding TB therapy with rifampin. Which of these statements made by the patient would indicate the patient needs further teaching?
    a. "I should contact my prescriber if I experience significantly decreased urine output."
    b. "I should contact my prescriber if I experience reddish colored urine."
    c. "I should contact my prescriber if I experience right upper quadrant pain."
    d. "I should contact my prescriber if I experience yellowish color to my skin or eyes."

▶ 16. The nurse is preparing to administer rifampin 420 mg intravenously. The solution was prepared by dissolving 600 mg of powdered rifampin in 10 mL of sterile water. Six milliliters of the prepared solution was added to a 500 mL intravenous (IV) bag of 5% dextrose. The infusion is to run over 3 hours. What is the hourly rate of infusion that the nurse should program into the IV infusion pump?

17. Several second-line agents for TB have the potential to damage the eighth cranial nerve. The nurse would assess for this damage by noting changes in (Select all that apply.)
    a. balance.
    b. extraocular movements.
    c. facial movements.
    d. hearing.
    e. sense of smell.
    f. swallowing.
    g. vision.

18. Benefits of the new antitubercular drug R207910 include that it (Select all that apply.)
    a. concentrates in lung tissue.
    b. does not interact with drugs for HIV.
    c. has no known incidence of resistance.
    d. requires once-a-month dosing.
    e. is safe for long term use.

19. Multidrug therapy for Hansen's disease (leprosy) is considered
    a. curative.
    b. prophylactic.
    c. unnecessary.

20. Current recommendation for administration of rifampin for Hansen's disease (leprosy) is once a
    a. day.
    b. week.
    c. month.
    d. year.

21. The nurse teaches a patient with G-6-PD deficiency who is receiving dapsone for leprosy the importance of having blood specimens drawn because the patient is at increased risk for
    a. destruction of red blood cells.
    b. fluid retention.
    c. infection.
    d. liver damage.

✳ 22. Which of these assessment findings, if identified in a patient who is receiving clofazimine, should the nurse report to the prescriber immediately?
    a. Darkening of the skin
    b. Diarrhea, nausea, and vomiting
    c. Hyperactive bowel sounds in right upper quadrant (RUQ) and absent bowel sounds in the left lower quadrant (LLQ)
    d. Red tinged sputum and urine

CASE STUDIES AND PATIENT TEACHING

(Use a separate piece of paper for your responses.)

Case Study 1

A 36-year-old, single mother and social worker is prescribed rifampin, isoniazid, ethambutol, and pyrazinamide after being diagnosed with active TB.

1. Why is therapy for active infection always initiated with at least two drugs?

2. What information should the nurse provide to ensure that these medications are taken exactly as prescribed?

3. What obstacles might this patient face regarding compliance with drug therapy?

4. What will be necessary to determine the effectiveness of drug therapy?

5. The public health nurse is consulted regarding the need to identify all of the people who share facilities with the patient to screen them for TB and prophylactically treat the individual without active infection with isoniazid. Why is it essential to treat TB contacts prophylactically for TB?

6. When evaluating the contacts associated with an active TB patient, what considerations are made to determine whether they are candidates for isoniazid prophylactic therapy?

7. What is the drug of choice as the primary agent for treatment and prophylaxis of TB, and why is this true?

8. Two months into therapy, the nurse is reviewing laboratory results for this patient, which includes ALT 65 international units/L, AST 80 units/L, total bilirubin 0.3 mg/dL, creatinine 0.8 mg/dL, and uric acid 12 mg/dL. What questions should the nurse ask this patient?

Case Study 2

A homeless 45-year-old male comes to the emergency department with weight loss, lethargy, a low-grade fever, and a productive cough streaked with blood. His chest x-ray indicates a suspicious area in the middle right lobe. He is hospitalized, and sputum cultures are ordered. The sputum cultures reveal **M. tuberculosis.** *His active TB is to be treated with a combination of drugs based on the sputum culture drug sensitivity. The patient is started on isoniazid, ethambutol, and pyrazinamide in the initial phase of therapy.*

1. What organ function is the nurse most concerned about when a patient is taking this combination of drugs? What symptoms would suggest this adverse effect?

2. What are the benefits of directly observed therapy (DOT) for this patient?

3. What interventions could the public nurse implement to improve compliance with drug therapy with this patient?

4. If this patient was found to be HIV positive, what drug-drug interactions may occur between the TB drug regimen and his HIV drug therapy?

5. The nurse is evaluating the patient when he comes in for DOT. The patient reports vision changes in which he feels like he is looking through a tunnel. What could possibly be causing this visual change? What should the nurse do?

6. The nurse is writing a letter to her legislator because of proposed cuts to funding for healthcare that would affect patients with TB. What could the nurse include in the letter to justify the expense of the government providing assistance for people who cannot afford to pay for therapy for TB?

OBJECTIVES

See page 28 for the Objectives.

CRITICAL THINKING AND STUDY QUESTIONS

1. Ciprofloxacin is highly active against the microbe that commonly causes (Select all that apply.)
   a. anthrax when used as postexposure prophylaxis.
   b. gastroenteritis from eating raw eggs.
   c. gas gangrene.
   d. methicillin-resistant *Staphylococcus aureus* (MRSA).
   e. pseudomembranous enterocolitis.
   f. tetanus.
   g. uncomplicated urinary tract infection (UTI).

▶ 2. The nurse is preparing to administer IV ciprofloxacin to a patient with septic arthritis after arthroscopic surgery. The nurse would ask the unit clerk to notify him/her when the results from which of the following tests becomes available?
   a. culture and sensitivity (C & S)
   b. MRI
   c. urinalysis
   d. X-ray

3. The nurse assesses a 6-year-old child who is receiving ciprofloxacin (Cipro) for a complicated UTI. What problem is a consequence of a common adverse effect of the drug?
   a. Difficulty walking
   b. Fluid deficit
   c. Seizures
   d. Tooth discoloration

▶ 4. Which of the following would warrant further investigation if the nurse is caring for a 6-month-old breastfed infant who is prescribed ciprofloxacin for pyelonephritis?
   a. Mother supplements breastfeeding with rice cereal
   b. Stool after every feeding
   c. Stool mushy and seedy
   d. Suckling interrupted by crying

5. A consulting urologist orders ciprofloxacin 250 mg twice a day for a 72-year-old woman with a UTI. The patient is also receiving ferrous sulfate 300 mg for anemia and calcium carbonate 400 mg 4 times a day for osteopenia. The nurse should
   a. administer the ciprofloxacin 1 hour before the other medications.
   b. administer the ciprofloxacin 2 hours after the other medications.
   c. consult with the prescriber for directions.
   d. hold the ferrous sulfate and calcium during ciprofloxacin therapy.

6. The nurse is administering ciprofloxacin (Cipro) to a patient who receives theophylline for asthma. Because of potential drug interactions the nurse should monitor theophylline levels and assess for
   a. constipation.
   b. drowsiness.
   c. tachycardia.
   d. weakness.

✳ 7. Because of common adverse effects of ciprofloxacin in the elderly, a nursing priority is
   a. altered sensory perceptions.
   b. fluid volume deficit.
   c. impaired urinary elimination.
   d. ineffective gas exchange.

8. The nurse teaches a patient who has been prescribed ciprofloxacin because of possible exposure to anthrax spores to take the medication as prescribed for a period of
   a. 10 to 14 days.
   b. 30 days.
   c. 60 days.
   d. 6 months.

＊ 9. It is less of a priority than for other fluoroquinolones for the nurse to teach strict sun protection measures to a patient who is prescribed
   a. ciprofloxacin (Cipro).
   b. lomefloxacin (Maxaquin).
   c. ofloxacin (Floxin).
   d. sparfloxacin (Zagam).

10. A common symptom of suprainfection that can occur with extended ciprofloxacin therapy is
   a. circumoral cyanosis.
   b. high fever.
   c. pin-point maculopapular rash.
   d. white patches in the mouth.

11. The primary reason why sparfloxacin (Zagam) is used for community acquired pneumonia is because
   a. it is effective against all common respiratory tract pathogens.
   b. of convenience of dosing.
   c. food does not affect absorption.
   d. possible adverse effects are insignificant.

▶ 12. When a patient is prescribed a fluoroquinolone that is known to cause prolongation of the QT interval on ECG, the nurse should monitor the electrolytes for which of the following results that are most likely to increase the risk of this adverse effect?
   a. Chloride less than 98 mEq/L
   b. Magnesium less than 1.3 mEq/L
   c. Potassium less than 3.5 mEq/L
   d. Sodium less than 135 mEq/L

13. Gemifloxacin (Factive) is generally not a preferred agent because it
   a. causes more adverse effects.
   b. costs more than other fluoroquinolones.
   c. is less effective.
   d. is only available in intravenous (IV) formula.

14. Metronidazole (Flagyl) is an antibacterial agent that
   a. is effective against aerobic and anaerobic bacteria.
   b. is limited by rapidly developing resistance by microbes.
   c. is used as prophylaxis for gastrointestinal (GI) surgery.
   d. penetrates the central nervous system (CNS).
   e. should not be used if a patient ingests alcohol.

▶ 15. The nurse is preparing to administer daptomycin (Cubicin). The nurse should withhold the medication and contact the prescriber if
   a. the patient is diagnosed with MRSA of the skin.
   b. the patient's INR is 1.8.
   c. the patient reports sudden severe muscle pain.
   d. peak and trough plasma levels have not been ordered.

▶ 16. A nursing measure to prevent the most common adverse effect of daptomycin (Cubicin) is to
   a. assist the patient with frequent ambulation around the nursing unit.
   b. dim the lights in the room.
   c. elevate the IV site.
   d. limit noise in the halls during the night.

▶ 17. Which of the following isoenzymes of CPK would be most helpful when monitoring for the most common serious adverse effect if a patient is prescribed daptomycin (Cubicin) and simvastatin (Zocor)?
   a. CPK
   b. CPK BB
   c. CPK MB
   d. CPK MM

▶ 18. The nurse is preparing to administer daptomycin (Cubicin). The patient has an IV infusion of 5% dextrose in 0.45% sodium chloride infusing at a rate of 125 mL/hr. What action should the nurse take?

19. The prescriber has asked the nurse to provide teaching for a 34-year-old female patient who has requested a prescription for rifaximin (Xifaxan) before a mission trip to Central America. Teaching should include not administering the drug if the patient experiences (Select all that apply.)
    a. amenorrhea.
    b. bloody stool.
    c. fever.
    d. flatulence.
    e. nausea.

CASE STUDIES AND PATIENT TEACHING

(Use a separate piece of paper for your responses.)

Case Study 1

A 68-year-old female, returns to her prescriber after taking 10 days of ampicillin for her upper respiratory infection. She continues with a low-grade fever and does not seem to have improved. She has a productive cough and thick secretions. Her x-ray does not indicate pneumonia. The patient has a past history of atrial fibrillation, for which she takes an anticoagulant. She is given ciprofloxacin 250 mg, orally, 2 times a day for 7 more days. The nurse in the's office wants to be sure she understands this medication.

1. What in the patient's history may contribute to potential drug-drug interactions?

2. What foods should the patient avoid when taking oral ciprofloxacin?

3. The patient calls the prescriber's office in two days to report that she is much better. She asks whether she can stop taking the medication since it is so expensive and she is improving so much. How should the nurse respond?

4. What new problem might the patient develop while taking this antibiotic?

Case Study 2

A 15-year-old Amish boy is admitted to the nursing unit after emergency surgery for a ruptured appendix. He is prescribed IV metronidazole (Flagyl) 500 mg in 100 mL D_5W every 6 hours and ampicillin/sulbactam (Unasyn) 1.5 g (in 50 mL NSS) every 8 hours. Both are to run at a rate of 100 mL per hour.

1. The drug handbook states that the therapeutic dose of metronidazole is 7.5 mg/kg every 6 hours. The child is 5'6" and weighs 145 lb. Is the dose safe and effective?

2. Metronidazole is scheduled at 0000-0600-1200-1800 at a rate of 100 mL/hr. Ampicillin/sulbactam is scheduled at 0600-1400-2200. Which would the nurse administer first at 0600, when would the nurse start each drug?

3. What procedures need to be followed when administering these drugs?

4. The nurse finds the pharmacy prepared a minibag of metronidazole in the refrigerator. The nurse should
    a. administer the drug.
    b. discard the solution and get a new bag from the pharmacy.
    c. examine the solution and administer it if no visible particles are present in the solution.
    d. determine how long the bag has been refrigerated and infuse if it has been less than 30 minutes.

5. Because the Amish family delayed seeking treatment for their child's abdominal pain and GI bacteria were expelled into the peritoneum, the nurse would monitor for what symptoms that suggest the bacteria have invaded the retroperitoneal region?

Answers can be reviewed online at http://evolve.elsevier.com/Lehne/.

OBJECTIVES

See page 28 for the Objectives.

CRITICAL THINKING AND STUDY QUESTIONS

1. Amphotericin B (Select all that apply.)
   a. can bind to cholesterol in human cell membranes causing toxicity.
   b. damages the kidneys.
   c. doses must be decreased if initial creatinine clearance is less than 40 mL/min.
   d. is rarely associated with fungal resistance.
   e. has broad-spectrum bactericidal activity.
   f. is used for system fungal infections.
   g. readily penetrates the central nervous system (CNS).
   h. remains in human tissue more than a year after treatment is discontinued.

2. At what point is the patient most likely to experience fever, chills, rigors, nausea, and headache when receiving amphotericin B?
   a. Immediately after the infusion begins
   b. 20 to 30 minutes after the infusion begins
   c. 1 to 3 hours after the infusion begins
   d. 3 to 6 hours after the infusion begins

▶ 3. A patient receiving amphotericin B experiences sudden episodes of shaking chills after receiving a dose of amphotericin B. Which of the following drugs, which are ordered as needed for this patient, should the nurse administer at this time?
   a. Acetaminophen
   b. Dantrolene (Dantrium)
   c. Diphenhydramine (Benadryl)
   d. Lorazepam (Ativan)

▶ 4. The nurse is reviewing laboratory tests before preparing to administer the first dose of amphotericin B. The patient's creatinine level is 3 mg/dL. The nurse should
   a. administer the medication.
   b. administer the medication and assess intake and output.
   c. withhold the medication and assess skin color.
   d. withhold the medication and page the prescriber STAT.

▶ 5. Because amphotericin causes fungal death by increasing leakage of intracellular cations, it is important for the nurse to assess the patient for
   a. abdominal cramps and peaked T waves on ECG.
   b. positive Chvostek's and Trousseau's signs.
   c. thirst and flushed skin.
   d. weakness and abdominal distention.

▶ 6. Which of the following laboratory results of an adult male patient suggest bone marrow suppression caused by amphotericin B?
   a. Hemoglobin 10 g/dL; hematocrit 30%; MCV 110 mcg^3; MCH 28 pg/cell
   b. Hemoglobin 10 g/dL; hematocrit 30%; MCV 67 mcg^3; MCH 30 pg/cell
   c. Hemoglobin 10 g/dL; hematocrit 30%; MCV 89 mcg^3; MCH 28 pg/cell
   d. Hemoglobin 10 g/dL; hematocrit 30%; MCV 105 mcg^3; MCH 20 pg/cell

7. A patient with a systemic fungal infection is prescribed amphotericin B and flucytosine. The nurse expects the drug interaction of
   a. decreased risk of amphotericin toxicity.
   b. increased risk of renal damage.
   c. increased risk of rigors.
   d. potentiation of amphotericin effect.

8. Itraconazole is
   a. always administered intravenously (IV).
   b. capable of inhibiting hepatic metabolizing enzymes.
   c. effective against more fungi than amphotericin.
   d. nephrotoxic.

9. To achieve maximum absorption of itraconazole (Sporanox) capsules, the nurse administers the drug with
   a. apple juice.
   b. milk.
   c. Pepsi-cola.
   d. water.

▶ 10. The nurse is reviewing test results for a patient who is prescribed itraconazole (Sporanox). Which of the following results would warrant immediate consultation with the prescriber?
   a. AST 35 international units/L
   b. BNP 745 pg/mL
   c. Echocardiogram—ejection fraction 75%
   d. Potassium 3.8 mEq/L

▶ 11. The nurse is administering itraconazole (Sporanox) to a patient who has a history of hypertension treated with hydrochlorothiazide and hypercholesterolemia treated with simvastatin (Zocor). Because of the effect of itraconazole on hepatic isoenzyme CYP3A4, the nurse should monitor the patient for symptoms of
   a. bleeding.
   b. hypoglycemia.
   c. hypotension.
   d. muscle pain.

12. Which of the following drugs may prevent absorption of itraconazole (Sporanox) no matter when they are administered?
   a. Cyclosporin (Sandimmune)
   b. Digoxin (Lanoxin)
   c. Esomeprazole (Nexium)
   d. Ranitidine (Zantac)

▶ 13. Which of these patient findings would suggest a serious adverse effect in a patient who is receiving the azole antifungal drug fluconazole (Diflucan)?
   a. Abdominal pain and diarrhea
   b. Fever and rash
   c. Headache
   d. Nausea and vomiting

14. The nurse is most concerned about alterations in metabolism of several of the antifungal drugs that are metabolized by the P-450 cytochrome system if a patient's diet includes
   a. grapefruit.
   b. green leafy vegetables.
   c. milk.
   d. red meat.

▶ 15. The nurse reviews the laboratory results of a female patient who is prescribed voriconazole (Vfend) 200 mg by mouth. Which of the following laboratory results warrants withholding the drug and immediately notifying the prescriber?
   a. AST 37 international units/L
   b. FBG 222 mg/dL
   c. Hb 11.8 g/dL
   d. hCG 72 international units/mL

▶ 16. A patient who has been receiving ketoconazole for 5 days experiences nausea and vomiting. The initial response of the nurse should be to
   a. administer the medication with food.
   b. assess the skin, abdomen, urine, and stool.
   c. consult the prescriber.
   d. withhold the medication.

▶ 17. When administering drugs that are potentially nephrotoxic, the nurse should consult the prescriber before administering which over-the-counter (OTC) drugs?
   a. Antacids
   b. Acetaminophen
   c. NSAIDs
   d. Laxatives

▶ 18. A patient is prescribed posaconazole (Noxafil) for thrush (oral candidiasis) that occurred after treatment of pneumonia with IV antibiotics. It would be most important to promptly inform the prescriber if drug reconciliation reveals that the patient takes which of the following drugs for his cluster headaches
   a. aspirin, acetaminophen, caffeine (Excedrin Migraine).
   b. dihydroergotamine (Migranal).
   c. ibuprofen (Motrin IB).
   d. sumatriptan (Imitrex).

19. What can the nurse teach a patient who is prescribed flucytosine (Ancobon) to prevent nausea and vomiting?
   a. Take the medication over a 15-minute interval.
   b. Take the medication with a cola beverage.
   c. Take the medication with food.
   d. Take the medication with milk.

▸ 20. The nurse is preparing to administer anidu-lafungin (Eraxis) 100 mg IV push to a patient with esophageal candidiasis. The drug is diluted to a concentration of 0.5 mg/mL. The drug book states that infusions should not exceed 1.1 mg/min. The hospital pharmacy directions are to administer at a rate of 1 mg/min. How many milliliters will the nurse administer every 10 seconds?

21. The nurse reviews the CBC of a patient who is prescribed flucytosine (Ancobon) and notes neutropenia. This patient is especially at risk for
a. fatigue.
b. fluid volume deficit.
c. impaired skin integrity.
d. infection.

▸ 22. The nurse would be concerned that a patient who is receiving caspofungin is experiencing a histamine reaction if the patient reports
a. bloated.
b. feeling flushed.
c. headache.
d. nausea.

23. Match the following fungal infections to their site of occurrence.

_____ a. Tinea capitis   1. Body
_____ b. Tinea corporis   2. Foot
_____ c. Tinea cruris   3. Groin
_____ d. Tinea pedis   4. Scalp

24. A common cause of recurrence of tinea corporis is

25. The medication administration record lists a clotrimazole troche to be administered at 0900. The nurse administers this medication by
a. applying it to the skin.
b. dissolving it in 8 ounces of water.
c. instructing the patient to chew it.
d. instructing the patient to let it dissolve in the mouth.

▸ 26. A postoperative patient who had knee replacement surgery is prescribed Lovenox (low-molecular-weight heparin) to prevent clot formation related to immobility. The patient develops candidiasis under the breasts and in the groin. The prescriber orders miconazole cream. The nurse should
a. administer both the Lovenox and miconazole and monitor INR.
b. administer the Lovenox, but consult the prescriber regarding the miconazole.
c. administer the miconazole but consult the prescriber regarding the Lovenox.
d. withhold both the Lovenox and miconazole and consult the prescriber.

27. What is a potential problem of patients' self-prescribing OTC miconazole for vaginal discharge?
a. Local irritation
b. Systemic toxicity
c. The cause may not be a yeast infection.
d. The treatment is usually not effective.

CASE STUDIES AND PATIENT TEACHING

(Use a separate piece of paper for your responses.)

Case Study 1

A 25-year-old female was recently diagnosed with acute myelogenous leukemia (AML). She is admitted for the induction phase of chemotherapy. Her platelet count is low, and she has vaginal candidiasis. OTC topical treatments for vaginal candidiasis are available.

1. What problems might this produce?

2. The treatment of choice for this patient's fungal infection is clotrimazole. It is essential that extreme care be taken in providing nursing care to this patient because she is at high risk for additional infections that could now be lethal. The nurse must consider many areas when treatment includes combining the treatment for fungus with the numerous other physical problems a patient with AML faces. What possible adverse effects of intravaginal clotrimazole tablets should the nurse instruct this patient to report?

3. The patient asks why she must use the vaginal tablets when she already has an IV for chemotherapy administration. What should the nurse tell her?

4. The patient's fungal infection has advanced because of her severely immunocompromised state. She now has systemic mycoses requiring amphotericin B for treatment. All of her medications must be carefully evaluated to determine whether they are toxic. What system is almost always damaged in some way by amphotericin B and can increase the risk of toxicity of other drugs?

5. What intervention can the nurse employ to reduce the risk of kidney damage by amphotericin B?

6. Why is it important for the prescriber to first order a 1-mg test dose of amphotericin B (Fungizone) before starting full therapy?

7. The drug book recommends after a successful test dose that the first dose of amphotericin B should be 0.25 mg/kg of drug. The patient weighs 110 lb. The prescriber has ordered 12 mg. Is this a safe dose?

8. The amphotericin B vial is supplied as a powder. This 50 mg of powder must be reconstituted using 10 mL of sterile water that does not contain a bacteriostatic agent to a concentration of 5 mg/mL. This solution is further diluted in sterile water to provide a concentration of 0.1 mg/mL for infusion. Why must the drug be mixed this way?

9. How much solution will the nurse administer if the drug is diluted to 0.1 mg/mL, and the prescribed dose is 12 mg?

10. What nursing measures should the nurse take when infusing amphotericin to prevent infusion-related adverse effects?

Case Study 2

1. What can the nurse teach to decrease the incidence and complications of opportunistic infections in
   a. the general population?
   b. debilitated patients?
   c. immunocompromised patients?

Case Study 3

A 42-year-old truck driver has been prescribed voriconazole (Vfend) for esophageal candidiasis secondary to immune deficiency caused by HIV.

1. What teaching does the nurse need to provide this patient regarding drug therapy?

2. Why is this patient more at risk for hepatotoxicity and drug interactions than the average person?

Answers can be reviewed online at http://evolve.elsevier.com/Lehne/.

OBJECTIVES

See page 28 for the Objectives.

CRITICAL THINKING AND STUDY QUESTIONS

1. A significant challenge to scientists who are trying to develop antiviral drugs is developing a drug that
   a. can be administered orally.
   b. does not harm human tissue.
   c. is broad spectrum.
   d. is not metabolized by the liver.

2. When researching antiviral drugs and vaccines, epidemiologically, it is a priority for the researchers to identify if the drug decreases
   a. active viral shedding.
   b. duration of illness.
   c. frequency of symptomatic episodes.
   d. symptoms.

3. A college student who has been diagnosed with her first genital herpes infection is discussing the disorder and prescribed topical acyclovir treatment with the college health center nurse. Which of the following statements, if made by the patient, would suggest that the patient needs teaching about this disorder and drug therapy?
   a. "I can get a different infection in the sores if I am not careful about cleaning after having a bowel movement."
   b. "I should use gloves when applying the ointment, immediately dispose of them, then wash my hands because I can spread the infection to other parts of my body."
   c. "If I apply the ointment as prescribed, it will decrease the chance that I spread the infection but the sores won't heal faster."
   d. "Using the ointment as soon as I feel the first signs of a new outbreak may prevent the outbreak."

▸ 4. What should the nurse teach a patient who is currently in a long-term committed monogamous relationship and who has been prescribed continuous oral acyclovir therapy for recurrent genital herpes regarding condom use?
   a. Condoms prevent the spread of infection, even during active outbreaks.
   b. Use a condom if any symptoms of outbreak are present.
   c. Use a condom with every sexual contact except if outbreak-free, and conception is desired.
   d. Your partner is already infected so condom use does not matter.

✳ 5. Which of the following actions by the nurse would be a priority for preventing the most common complications of intravenous (IV) acyclovir (Zovirax) therapy?
   a. Assessing the IV site before infusing the drug
   b. Ensuring a fluid intake of 2500 to 3000 mL/24 hr
   c. Reporting vomiting to the prescriber
   d. Teaching perineal hygiene

✳ 6. The nurse is preparing to administer intravenous acyclovir. It would be a priority for the nurse to provide nursing interventions for which of the following assessment findings?
   a. BP 160/85
   b. Creatinine 0.9 mg/dL
   c. Dry, sticky mucous membranes
   d. Eight-hour urine output 750 mL

▸ 7. It would be a priority to report which of the following laboratory results to the prescriber if a patient is prescribed valacyclovir (Valtrex)?
   a. CD4 $100/mm^3$
   b. Hgb (Hb) 11 g/dL
   c. Platelets $220,000/mm^3$
   d. WBC $12,800/mm^3$

8. The nurse is preparing to administer oral famciclovir (Famvir) 500 mg prescribed orally once a day to a patient admitted with exacerbated chronic obstructive pulmonary disease (COPD) who has developed shingles. The nurse reviews laboratory test results that include eGFR 35 mL/min. The nurse should
   a. administer the drug as ordered.
   b. consult the prescriber STAT regarding timing of doses.
   c. consult the prescriber STAT regarding the need for more laboratory tests.
   d. withhold the drug and consult the prescriber during her next hospital rounds.

▶ 9. The nurse would withhold ganciclovir and notify the prescriber if patient laboratory test results include
   a. BUN 20 mg/dL.
   b. hCG positive.
   c. neutrophils 2000/mm³.
   d. platelets 75,000/mm³.

▶ 10. The nurse is discussing planned care with the certified nursing assistant who is assigned to a patient who is receiving oral ganciclovir for CMV retinitis. Which of the following precautions would the nurse include in instructions regarding care?
   a. Do not provide any food 1 hour before or 2 hours after drug administration.
   b. Elevate all 4 side rails.
   c. Turn and reposition the patient every 2 hours.
   d. Use an electric razor to shave the patient.

▶ 11. Which of the following steps is most important for the nurse to follow when administering valganciclovir?
   a. Administer with the patient in an upright position.
   b. Assess vital signs before administering the drug.
   c. Dissolve the drug completely in 8 ounces of water or juice.
   d. Wear gloves when handling the tablet.

▶ 12. When administering adefovir (Hepsera), which of the following assessments would suggest that therapy could be toxic?
   a. Decreased sperm count
   b. Nausea

c. Oliguria
d. Yellow-colored sclera

▶ 13. Laboratory results for a patient who is prescribed foscarnet (Foscavir) include FBS 90 mg/dL, AST 87 units/L, potassium 3.6 mEq/L, calcium 8.4 mg/dL, and magnesium 2 mEq/L. The nurse should assess for
   a. cool, clammy skin.
   b. headache.
   c. muscle spasms.
   d. thirst.

14. When explaining prescribed pegylated interferon (peginterferon), the nurse should include that, compared with conventional interferon, this drug
   a. can be administered orally.
   b. prevents relapse when discontinued.
   c. produces less adverse effects.
   d. produces more consistent therapeutic blood levels.

15. It is important for the nurse to assess for suicidal ideation if a patient is prescribed
   a. interferon alfa.
   b. lamivudine.
   c. ribavirin.
   d. valacyclovir.

16. When administering ribavirin and interferon alfa for hepatitis C, loss of detectable serum HCV RNA for at least what period of time after cessation of treatment would indicate that therapy has achieved the desired effect?
   a. 6 weeks
   b. 6 months
   c. 1 year
   d. 5 years

17. When teaching a patient self-administration of subcutaneous interferon alfa, the nurse should stress the importance of
   a. applying pressure to the site after injection to prevent hematoma formation.
   b. aspirating to check for blood before injecting.
   c. changing the needle after drawing the solution into the syringe.
   d. sterile technique.

18. The nurse teaches sexually active patients who are prescribed ribavirin of the need to use two reliable forms of contraception during treatment and for at least what period of time after treatment ends?
    a. 1 month
    b. 3 months
    c. 6 months
    d. 12 months

▸ 19. Which of these assessment findings, if identified in a patient who is receiving lamivudine (Epivir HBV), adefovir (Hepsera), or entecavir (Baraclude) for hepatitis B, should the nurse report to the prescriber immediately?
    a. Deep rapid breathing
    b. Fever
    c. Poor appetite
    d. Nausea

▸ 20. A patient is prescribed adefovir (Hepsera) 10 mg by mouth once a day. Results of her recent laboratory tests include CrCl 62 mL/min. The nurse should
    a. administer the medication as prescribed.
    b. consult the prescriber regarding the need for dose reduction.
    c. withhold the medication and contact the prescriber immediately.

21. The nurse is reviewing the chart of a patient prescribed telbivudine (Tyzeka). The nurse would consult the prescriber if which of the following was noted?
    a. ALT 287 to 350 international units/L over the past year
    b. Evidence of active HBV replication
    c. HBV, acute episode, recently diagnosis
    d. Patient 17 years old

▸ 22. The nurse would be concerned about administering live flu vaccine to which of the following patients?
    a. 7-year-old male with a seizure disorder
    b. 12-year-old female receiving aspirin for its cardioprotective effects
    c. 28-year-old male with type 1 diabetes
    d. 38-year-old female with multiple sclerosis

23. When preparing to administer a dose of LAIV (FluMist) for a 5-year-old child, who has never received a flu vaccine in the past, the office nurse notes a dose sitting on the counter. The seal is intact, and the expiration date is okay. On questioning, no other nurse remembers getting the dose out, and no other nurse needs the drug. The nurse should
    a. administer 1 spray in each nostril.
    b. administer 1 spray in each nostril and remind the parents that a second dose will be needed in about 7 to 10 weeks.
    c. discard the dose and thaw a new dose, administering 1 spray in each nostril.
    d. discard the dose and thaw a new dose, administering 1 spray in each nostril, and remind the parents that a second dose will be needed in about 7 to 10 weeks.

▸ 24. A priority of nursing teaching to a patient prescribed amantadine (Symmetrel) for influenza prophylaxis is
    a. elimination.
    b. fluid volume.
    c. nutrition.
    d. safety.

25. The nurse is aware that the most significant factor in determining the effectiveness of oseltamivir (Tamiflu) in treating influenza is
    a. administration with food.
    b. influenza A is the causative organism.
    c. starting therapy as soon as symptoms occur.
    d. vaccination for influenza has already been administered.

▸ 26. Which of the following new assessment findings would be most significant if noted in an infant who is receiving inhaled ribavirin for RSV?
    a. Coarse rhonchi (gurgles) in upper airways
    b. Pulse 120 beats/min
    c. Respirations 30 breaths per minute
    d. Wheezing throughout lung fields

CASE STUDIES AND PATIENT TEACHING

(Use a separate piece of paper for your responses.)

Case Study 1

A 25-year-old married female graduate student comes to the college health center clinic complaining of painful sores in her genital region. She has a round ulcerated area on the labia minora and also on the cervix. She informs the nurse that she plans to get pregnant in the near future. She states she had these "sores" 3 months ago, but thought they were caused by the irritation of swimming every day. The CRNP diagnoses herpes simplex genitalis and prescribes oral acyclovir. The patient states that she hates to take pills and has heard that this drug is available in a cream.

1. What information can the nurse provide as to why oral acyclovir was ordered instead of the topical acyclovir?

2. The patient asks whether this medication will cure the herpes. How should the nurse respond?

3. What information should the nurse provide regarding transmission of genital herpes?

4. How should the nurse respond to the woman's concerns about how this infection will affect her becoming pregnant?

Case Study 2

An elderly patient who has a history of smoking, diabetes mellitus (DM), hypertension, and COPD has come to the flu shot clinic at the public health department to receive a flu vaccine.

1. What questions should the nurse ask the patient before administering the vaccine?

2. If the patient complains of coughing and runny nose, should the vaccination be withheld?

3. The patient is complaining to the nurse about needing to get a flu shot every year. She hates the shot and has heard that people can still get the flu after receiving the shot. She asks why they cannot just come up with a pill that is effective to treat the infection. What could the nurse include in her explanation?

4. The patient asks why she cannot get the nasal spray that her grandson received yesterday. What is a possible explanation for why this drug is limited to people aged 5 to 49 years?

5. What teaching should the nurse provide regarding close contact with her grandson?

Case Study 3

The public health nurse receives a call from a school nurse questioning whether a child who received intranasal LAIV (FluMist) should be in school. The nurse is concerned because the child's teacher is pregnant.

1. How should the nurse respond?

2. What intervention would be most important for the school nurse to emphasize when discussing with the teacher prevention of becoming infected with influenza from active cases or live vaccine?

Answers can be reviewed online at http://evolve.elsevier.com/Lehne/.

OBJECTIVES

See page 28 for the Objectives.

CRITICAL THINKING AND STUDY QUESTIONS

1. Which of the following regarding human immunodeficiency virus (HIV) infection is true? (Select all that apply.)
   a. A patient can have HIV without having detectable levels of the virus in the blood.
   b. A CD4 T-cell count below 200 cells/mL is needed for diagnosis.
   c. Infection increases the risk of other infections.
   d. HIV is synonymous with AIDs.
   e. Kaposi's sarcoma is a risk factor for HIV infection.
   f. HIV kills helper T lymphocytes.
   g. HIV kills CD4 T cells within 2 hours of infection.
   h. The virus needs a host cell in order to reproduce.
   i. The virus does not replicate during the latent phase of infection.
   j. The virus can reside in microglial cells in the central nervous system (CNS).

2. Match the following drugs and mechanisms of action.

   _____ a. CCR5 antagonists
   _____ b. Fusion inhibitor
   _____ c. Integrase inhibitor
   _____ d. Protease inhibitor
   _____ e. Reverse transcriptase

   1. Block viral entry into cells
   2. Hampers enzymes required for HIV replication

3. The nurse is teaching a patient about the need for multiple-drug therapy for HIV. Which of the following statements, if made by the patient, would indicate a need for further teaching?
   a. "If I don't take all of the drugs as prescribed, the virus is more likely to become resistant to drugs."
   b. "The higher the number of viruses in my body, the greater the chance one will become resistant."
   c. "The virus recognizes the antibiotic and is able to change to prevent being destroyed."
   d. "When the HIV is changing RNA into DNA within the host cell, genetic changes can occur spontaneously."

✳ 4. The nurse is caring for an AIDS patient admitted with *P. jiroveci* pneumonia. The patient's HAART includes zidovudine (Retrovir). It would be a priority to report which of the following assessment findings to the prescriber?
   a. Deep rapid breathing
   b. Rales (crackles) in lower lobes
   c. Temperature 101.6°F
   d. Warm, moist skin

▸ 5. Which nursing intervention can decrease the risk of lactic acidosis in a patient who is prescribed zidovudine (Retrovir)?
   a. Encouraging coughing and deep breathing
   b. Maintaining adequate hydration
   c. Monitor blood glucose
   d. Preventing skin breakdown

6. The prescriber has informed a patient who has been prescribed a nucleoside/nucleotide reverse transcriptase inhibitor (NRTI) of the risk of hepatic steatosis. The patient asks the nurse "What is hepatic steatosis?" The nurse should explain that this is a possible severe adverse effect involving
   a. fatty degeneration of the liver.
   b. increased secretions of glands.
   c. infection of the liver.
   d. stools that are foamy and float.

7. The nurse is preparing to administer 60 mg of intravenous zidovudine to a patient who weighs 135 lb. Before administering this dose, the nurse would ensure that it was diluted in at least
   a. 2 mL of bacteriostatic water.
   b. 5 mL of sterile water.
   c. 15 mL of 5% dextrose for injection.
   d. 50 mL of normal saline.

✳ 8. An HIV-positive patient is prescribed trimethoprim/sulfamethoxazole for a urinary tract infection (UTI). A priority nursing action is to monitor which of the following laboratory tests? (Select all that apply.)
   a. AST and ALT
   b. BUN and creatinine
   c. CBC and differential
   d. Electrolytes
   e. Lipids
   f. PT and INR

9. A patient has received instructions regarding administration of didanosine (Videx EC). Which of these statements made by the patient would indicate the patient understood the directions?
   a. "I can open this capsule and sprinkle the contents on applesauce."
   b. "I need to notify the prescriber if I cannot swallow this capsule whole."
   c. "I should keep the medicine in my bathroom medicine cabinet so I remember to take it every morning."
   d. "I should take this drug with meals."

▶ 10. Which of these nursing assessment findings would be most significant if a patient was receiving didanosine?
   a. Diarrhea
   b. Foot tingling
   c. Itching
   d. Vomiting

▶ 11. A patient receiving highly active antiretroviral therapy (HAART) develops a sore throat and cough. The nurse should consult the prescriber immediately if the HAART includes which of the following drugs?
   a. Abacavir (Ziagen)
   b. Didanosine (Videx)
   c. Stavudine (Zerit)
   d. Zidovudine (Retrovir)

12. Nursing interventions and teaching relating to the most common adverse effects of efavirenz (Sustiva) should focus on
   a. circulation.
   b. nutrition.
   c. safety.
   d. skin integrity.

▶ 13. When a patient who is receiving nevirapine (Viramune) or delavirdine (Rescriptor) complains of muscle and joint pain, it would be important for the nurse to assess if the patient is also experiencing
   a. dizziness.
   b. nausea.
   c. paresthesias.
   d. rash.

14. It would be a priority for the nurse to inform the prescriber that an HIV-positive patient has admitted to engaging in unprotected sex if the patient's HAART includes
   a. efavirenz (Sustiva).
   b. emtricitabine (Emtriva).
   c. indinavir (Crixivan).
   d. zidovudine (Retrovir).

▶ 15. An HIV-positive patient who has recently been prescribed a HAART, including the NNRTI efavirenz, calls the prescriber's office and reports experiencing drowsiness and dizziness. An appropriate recommendation by the telephone triage nurse is for the patient to
   a. discontinue all drugs and make an appointment to be seen as soon as possible.
   b. discontinue taking the drug, but continue the other drugs in the regimen.
   c. take the drug at bedtime.
   d. take the drug with food.

16. Weight-bearing exercise and adequate calcium intake are most important if HAART includes a
   a. fusion inhibitor.
   b. nucleoside/nucleotide reverse transcriptase inhibitor (NRTI).
   c. non-nucleoside reverse transcriptase inhibitor (NNRTI).
   d. protease inhibitor (PI).

17. The nurse would be most concerned that the patient may not adhere to HAART therapy with which of the following classes of antiviral drugs if the patient verbalized that body image is an important priority?
   a. Fusion inhibitor
   b. Nucleoside/nucleotide reverse transcriptase inhibitor (NRTI)
   c. Non-nucleoside reverse transcriptase inhibitor (NNRTI)
   d. Protease inhibitor (PI)

18. The nurse is aware that the HIV-seropositive community often shares the belief that garlic supplementation decreases HIV reproduction and boosts the immune system. This belief can be particularly dangerous if the patient is prescribed
    a. indinavir.
    b. lopinavir.
    c. nelfinavir.
    d. saquinavir.

19. Patients who are prescribed protease inhibitors (PI) should be instructed to not self-prescribe the herbal product St. John's wort because this product can increase the
    a. metabolism and excretion of the PI.
    b. MAO inhibitor effects of the St. John's wort.
    c. likelihood of suicidal ideation.
    d. likelihood of toxicity from the PI.

▸ 20. Use of which of the following substances, if noted in the history of a patient who is prescribed the PI, amprenavir (Agenerase), would be of most concern to the nurse?
    a. Alcohol
    b. Cocaine
    c. Heroin
    d. Tobacco

▸ 21. Which of the following, if identified in the history of a patient who has been taking atazanavir (Reyataz), would be most important for the nurse to report to the prescriber immediately?
    a. Diabetes treated with a sulfonylurea
    b. Erectile dysfunction treated with sildenafil
    c. Gastroesophageal reflux disease (GERD) treated with a proton pump inhibitor
    d. Hyperlipidemia treated with a statin

22. The nurse has just provided instructions regarding administration of enfuvirtide (Fuzeon). Which of these statements made by the patient would indicate the need for further teaching?
    a. "I need to refrigerate the dissolved powder for up to 24 hours if I do not use it immediately after mixing."
    b. "I should discontinue using the drug if it causes a rash or itching at the injection site."
    c. "I should inject the drug into the fat beneath the skin of my belly or thigh."
    d. "I should inspect the solution for discoloration, bubbles, and undissolved particles before drawing it up into the syringe."

▸ 23. Which of these assessment findings, if identified in a patient who is receiving enfuvirtide (Fuzeon), should the nurse report to the prescriber immediately? (Select all that apply.)
    a. Chills
    b. Dizziness
    c. Headache
    d. Pain at injection site
    e. Positive pregnancy test
    f. Sudden muscle weakness in the legs

24. The recommended dose of enfuvirtide (Fuzeon) for an 8-year-old child who weighs 44 lb is
    a. 20 mg.
    b. 40 mg.
    c. 45 mg.
    d. 90 mg.

✳ 25. A HIV+ patient who is receiving HAART, including maraviroc (Selzentry), reports to the nurse that he has vomited and is experiencing severe abdominal pain. Assessment reveals a generalized pruritic rash. The priority nursing action is to
    a. obtain an order for diphenhydramine (Benadryl) for the itching.
    b. withhold all prescribed drugs and contact the prescriber.
    c. withhold all food and fluids until the source of the abdominal pain is identified.
    d. withhold the maraviroc (Selzentry) drug and contact the prescriber.

26. What is the most important role of the nurse when treatment failure occurs?
    a. Identifying individual factors that may have contributed to treatment failure
    b. Identifying the patient's immune status
    c. Supporting the patient emotionally
    d. Teaching the new drug regimen

27. Principles of treating HIV-seropositive pregnant women include (Select all that apply.)
    a. administering the drugs to the neonate.
    b. benefits of treatment normally outweigh risks.
    c. considering C-section for delivery.
    d. HAART should not be used during pregnancy.
    e. the drugs are not teratogenic.
    f. the drug regimen should only include one drug at a time.

28. When emptying a urinal from an HIV-seropositive patient, the nurse splashes urine on intact skin. The nurse should
    a. go to the emergency department (ED) at the end of the shift for blood work.
    b. immediately go to the ED for initiation of postexposure prophylaxis (PEP).
    c. make an appointment with his/her primary care provider on the next off day to discuss if postexposure prophylaxis (PEP) is appropriate.
    d. report the incident immediately to a supervisor.

29. Which of the following assessment findings would best indicate that HAART is currently effective?
    a. CD4 T count 600 cells/mm³
    b. Neutrophils 2750/mm³
    c. Plasma HIV RNA 30, virions/mL
    d. WBC 5000/mm³

CASE STUDIES AND PATIENT TEACHING

(Use a separate piece of paper for your responses.)

Case Study 1

A 30-year-old female has been HIV seropositive for 4 years. She had been prescribed HAART therapy, including zidovudine (Retrovir), indinavir (Crixivan), and lamivudine (Epivir), but until now she has never taken any antiviral agent.

1. What are reasons for an HIV-seropositive patient, who does not feel ill, being prescribed drug therapy?

2. The patient asks if there are any reasons for not taking HAART when she still feels well. How should the nurse respond?

3. The patient asks the nurse why she feels better now than she did when she was first diagnosed. How can the nurse explain the presence of symptoms during the initial phase and lack of symptoms during the middle phase?

4. The patient asks why she needs so many drugs. She would rather take a large dose of one drug than multiple doses of different drugs. How should the nurse respond?

5. When consulting with the prescriber, what might the nurse discuss that might increase the chance that this patient will adhere to drug therapy?

6. The patient agrees to start taking the prescribed drugs. The original HAART included zidovudine (Retrovir), indinavir (Crixivan), and lamivudine (Epivir). The prescriber changes the HAART to zidovudine, saquinavir (Invirase), and lamivudine to improve the likelihood of adherence. The patient asks the nurse why the prescriber wants her to take saquinavir instead of indinavir. How can the nurse explain this change?

7. What symptoms of adverse effects of these NRTIs should the nurse teach the patient to report to the prescriber?
    a. Zidovudine (Retrovir)
    b. Lamivudine (Epivir)

8. What interventions can the nurse teach to prevent adverse effects from the protease inhibitor saquinavir (Invirase)?

9. The patient is sexually active. What teaching should the nurse provide to this patient regarding the possibility of pregnancy?

Case Study 2

A 38-year-old male who has been HIV seropositive for 12 years comes to the ED complaining of anorexia, nausea, chest and abdominal pain. He is currently prescribed a HAART of lopinavir, lamivudine, and stavudine.

1. What factors relating to this drug therapy would support a triage nurse's decision to have this patient evaluated immediately?

2. During assessment the ED nurse notes a pale and anxious patient who weighs 147 lb and is 5 feet 10 inches tall. Temperature is 103.2°F, BP 90/65 mm Hg, pulse 118 beats/min, respirations 27 breaths per minute and labored. Crackles are noted throughout the lung fields with bronchial breath sounds in the upper lobes. The nurse notes a cough productive of purulent sputum and multiple enlarged lymph nodes. Chest x-ray, laboratory, and sputum specimens are obtained. Laboratory results include troponin I 0.01 ng/mL; troponin T 0.1 ng/mL; CPK 68 units/mL; CK MB 0.2%; WBC 750/mm³, neutrophil count 500/mL; CD4 T 180 cells/mL; hemoglobin 7.5 gm/dL; hematocrit 22.7%; AST 65 Units/L; BUN 27 mg/dL; and creatinine 1.4 mg/dL. What nursing concerns must the unit nurse address after receiving this report when planning for transfer of this patient to the nursing unit?

3. The patient is diagnosed with *P. jiroveci* pneumonia and dehydration and is prescribed antibiotic therapy with pentamidine (Pentam) and intravenous fluids. What precautions must the nurse take when administering this antibiotic?

4. The patient develops rapport with the nurse and expresses his fears. He has heard from friends that there is a new injected drug that "works wonders." The nurse facilitates the patient in verbalizing his concerns and thoughts with his prescriber. What reason might the prescriber have for not prescribing enfuvirtide (Fuzeon) at this time for this patient?

Case Study 3

A 35-year-old male has been HIV seropositive for 12 years. His HAART includes zidovudine. When being interviewed by the nurse during a routine clinic appointment, he complains of declining vision, headaches, and daily temperature elevations. Physical examination findings include multiple enlarged lymph nodes and several white retinal patches.

1. What complications of HIV are likely to be occurring?

2. The patient is diagnosed with CMV retinitis. The treatment of choice for CMV retinitis caused by cytomegalovirus (CMV) is ganciclovir. What concern does the nurse have about the addition of ganciclovir to a drug regimen including zidovudine?

3. The prescriber wants to begin with intravenous therapy. What strategies can the nurse employ when administering intravenous ganciclovir to reduce the risk of and identify possible damage to the patient's renal system?

4. The patient tells the nurse that he has no job or insurance at present. What would the nurse be concerned about?

Case Study 4

1. What are important contributions that the nurse can make toward improving outcomes for patients infected with HIV?

94

Drug Therapy of Sexually Transmitted Diseases

Answers can be reviewed online at http://evolve.elsevier.com/Lehne/.

OBJECTIVES

See page 28 for the Objectives.

CRITICAL THINKING AND STUDY QUESTIONS

1. The nurse obtains the most accurate information about nursing care of sexually transmitted diseases/infections (STDs/STIs) from the
   a. Centers for Disease Control and Prevention.
   b. drug manufacturers.
   c. Food and Drug Administration.
   d. textbooks.

2. Annual screening for *Chlamydia trachomatis* is recommended for all sexually active women under the age of
   a. 20 years.
   b. 25 years.
   c. 30 years.
   d. 35 years.

3. Doxycycline would not be prescribed for a female patient for whom pregnancy status is unknown because it
   a. can damage fetal bones.
   b. causes nausea.
   c. is hepatotoxic.
   d. is not effective 25% of the time.

4. A patient asks why she has been prescribed doxycycline 100 mg twice a day for a chlamydia infection when a friend was prescribed a single dose of azithromycin. What factors must be considered when a prescriber is selecting an antibiotic for a patient?

5. A 7-pound neonate develops *Chlamydia trachomatis* pneumonia following intrapartal exposure. The recommended safe dose of erythromycin succinate for neonates is 50 mg/kg/day divided into 4 doses. The nurse calculates that the safe single dose for this patient is approximately
   a. 20 mg.
   b. 40 mg.
   c. 160 mg.
   d. 350 mg.

6. A friend tells the nurse that a sexual partner has informed her that he has gonorrhea. She has a refillable prescription of ciprofloxacin (Cipro) for recurrent cystitis. She tells the nurse she knows that she has used this drug in the past for gonorrhea. The most important reason why the nurse should discourage using this ciprofloxacin is
   a. the nurse's friend is likely to develop an allergic reaction to floxacin (Cipro).
   b. the law requires reporting of gonorrhea infections.
   c. this drug is no longer effective against *Neisseria gonorrhoeae.*
   d. the dose is too low to treat gonorrhea.

7. Which of these assessment findings would be most significant if a patient was receiving intramuscular (IM) ceftriaxone 1 g once a day 12 hours for disseminated gonococcal infection?
   a. Fever
   b. Joint pain
   c. Petechial rash
   d. Stiff neck

8. The throat culture of a 6-year-old boy is positive for *Neisseria gonorrhoeae.* A nursing priority in this situation is
   a. assessing for eye exudate.
   b. correctly calculating the dose of ceftriaxone to be administered.
   c. ensuring the safety of the child.
   d. removing the child from his home.

9. A patient is admitted to the hospital with a diagnosis of pelvic inflammatory disease (PID). She asks the nurse why her prescriber has recommended hospitalization and intravenous (IV) antibiotics instead of oral antibiotic therapy at home. The basis of the nurse's response is
   a. inadequately treated PID is more likely to cause scarring of the uterine (fallopian) tubes.
   b. PID is very contagious, and she needs to be in isolation.
   c. the recommended antibiotic for PID is only available by IV route.
   d. women who have PID have a higher incidence of cervical cancer.

10. A 32-year-old woman develops septic arthritis. When obtaining a history, it is important to evaluate for previous infection with
    a. *Chlamydia trachomatis.*
    b. *Neisseria gonorrhoeae.*
    c. *Treponema pallidum.*
    d. *Trichomonas vaginalis.*

✻ 11. The nursery nurse is caring for a neonate whose mother has an active infection with *Chlamydia trachomatis.* A priority nursing outcome for the neonate relating to possible chlamydia infection would be that the neonate will
    a. be free of conjunctival discharge.
    b. blink in response to direct light shined in the eyes.
    c. breast-feed for 10 to 15 minutes at least every 3 hours without becoming dyspneic.
    d. gain 2 ounces a week for the first 4 weeks after birth.

▸ 12. The current treatment recommendation for a pregnant patient who is allergic to penicillin and diagnosed with syphilis is
    a. azithromycin.
    b. ceftriaxone.
    c. doxycycline.
    d. penicillin-allergy desensitization and penicillin.

13. The recommended treatment for acute epididymitis is different depending on the age of the patient because usually
    a. older men have developed a resistance to the antibiotic used for younger men.
    b. the method and organism of infection is different.

    c. younger men have better kidney functioning.
    d. younger men are less likely to be adherent to multidose therapy.

▸ 14. The nurse teaches that the primary cause of recurrent STIs caused by the same organism is failure to
    a. prescribe the correct antibiotic.
    b. seek treatment early in the disease.
    c. take the medication as prescribed.
    d. treat the sexual partner.

15. A 35-year-old woman comes to her gynecologist's office with the complaint of a yellow-green vaginal discharge. She is diagnosed with trichomoniasis and prescribed metronidazole (Flagyl). It is important for the nurse to teach the patient the importance of not consuming
    a. alcohol.
    b. antacids.
    c. grapefruit juice.
    d. milk.

16. Clindamycin cream (Clindesse) requires only one dose of vaginal cream to treat bacterial vaginosis because
    a. bacterial vaginosis is not a serious infection.
    b. clindamycin has a half-life of several days.
    c. the cream adheres to the vaginal mucosa for several days.
    d. the medication immediately kills the infecting microbes.

17. A major goal of therapy with famciclovir (Famvir) for genital herpes is
    a. analgesia.
    b. to decrease length of active episodes.
    c. eradication of the virus.
    d. prevention suprainfections during outbreaks.

18. A patient has received instructions regarding administration of podofilox (Condylox) for genital warts. Which of these statements made by the patient would indicate the patient needs further teaching?
    a. "After I finish using this drug I will no longer be contagious."
    b. "I must apply this drug 2 times a day for 3 days in a row."
    c. "It will take a long while before this medication has removed the wart."
    d. "This therapy may be uncomfortable."

CASE STUDIES AND PATIENT TEACHING

(Use a separate piece of paper for your responses.)

Case Study 1

A sexually active, single, 19-year-old woman presents to the emergency department with a 2-week history of dull bilateral abdominal pain, low back pain, and mucopurulent vaginal discharge with increased pain today. She denies fever, nausea, vomiting, diarrhea, and urinary symptoms. She reports irregular periods since age 13. Her last menstrual period was 2 months ago. She does not use any measure of birth control. She was treated at the health department 3 months ago for a "female infection" and states she took the medication when she remembered and did not return for a follow-up examination. She has had two sexual partners in the past 6 months, one of whom was also treated for an infection 3 months ago at the health department. She is unsure whether he was adherent to his treatment plan or whether he is symptomatic at this time. She has no known medication allergies and takes no medication on a regular basis.

Her vital signs are as follows: BP 110/72 mm Hg, pulse 88 beats/min, respirations 20 breaths/minute, and temperature 99.4°F. The physician orders a CBC, sedimentation rate, RPR, serum pregnancy, and a catheterized urinalysis. He performs abdominal and pelvic examinations and obtains cervical cultures for gonorrhea and chlamydia and specimens for saline and KOH wet preps. The physical exam reveals a soft abdomen, right and left lower quadrant tenderness without rebound, and normal bowel sounds. The pelvic exam reveals mucopurulent vaginal discharge and mild right and left adnexal tenderness with bimanual exam. The laboratory results reveal Hgb 11.1, WBC 7.0, and negative results for urinalysis and pregnancy tests.

After review of the medical and social history, physical exam, and laboratory results (excluding the cultures), the physician makes a diagnosis of PID. Orders include administering ceftriaxone 250 mg IM now and prescriptions for doxycycline 100 mg twice a day for 10 days and Tylenol #3 1 tablet every 3 to 4 hours as needed for pain. The patient is told that she will be notified regarding the results of the cultures.

1. Why is it important to determine whether the patient is pregnant before administering doxycycline or tetracycline?

2. The patient is to be observed for 30 minutes following administration of the cephalosporin injection and then discharged home. She is given instructions for bed rest for 2 days with a reexamination in 24 to 48 hours if the signs and/or symptoms increase or persist. What teaching regarding the prescribed medication and follow-up care should the nurse provide to this patient?

3. Why is it important for the patient to avoid all forms of alcohol?

4. The patient is instructed to inform her sexual partners of the need for examination. The patient's phone number and address are verified for notification purposes. She is also advised that the culture results will be reported to the health department if they are positive, and the health department will then follow-up with her. The patient states that she does not understand why she has to inform her sexual partners of her infection and why she has to take all of the medication if she is feeling better in a couple of days. What information and instructions can the nurse provide to the patient to help her understand the importance of adherence to her treatment plan?

5. After completing the teaching, the patient's verbalizations reflect that she still does not recognize the significance of her infection or importance of adhering to therapy. How might this alter the plan of care for this patient?

Answers can be reviewed online at http://evolve.elsevier.com/Lehne/.

OBJECTIVES

See page 28 for the Objectives.

CRITICAL THINKING AND STUDY QUESTIONS

1. Antiseptics are
   a. commonly used to treat superficial infections.
   b. effective when used properly to cleanse a new wound.
   c. more potent than disinfectants.
   d. only applied to nonliving tissue.

2. Which of the following is an example of sterilization?
   a. Autoclaving surgical instruments
   b. Gowning before entering a room where a patient is in protective isolation
   c. Personal respiratory equipment for tuberculosis (TB)
   d. Standard precautions

▶ 3. Why is it important for nurses to understand the time course of action of an antiseptic?

✳ 4. Which of the following is least significant in preventing a surgical incision-site infection?
   a. Preoperative scrubbing of surgical site with an antiseptic
   b. Preoperative scrubbing of scrub nurses' hands
   c. Rigorous disinfection of operating room and fixtures before surgery
   d. Sterilization of surgical instruments

5. To ensure effectiveness of ethyl alcohol (ethanol) as an antiseptic, the nurse should
   a. apply the alcohol directly to open wounds after medicating the patient for pain.
   b. not use alcohol in combination with chlorhexidine.
   c. use an alcohol with a concentration greater than 75%.
   d. use a gel that prolongs evaporation of the alcohol.

▶ 6. The most important reason for not wiping a subcutaneous heparin injection site with an isopropyl alcohol pad immediately after injecting the medication is to avoid
   a. bruising.
   b. neutralizing the heparin.
   c. poor absorption of the heparin.
   d. significant pain.

7. Alcohol hand sanitizers are not effective against which of the following organisms because it produces spores?
   a. *Clostridium difficile*
   b. Methicillin-resistant *Staphylococcus aureus* (MRSA)
   c. Rhinovirus
   d. Vancomycin-resistant enterococci (VRE)

8. When the nurse is preparing to cleanse a wound, which preparation would be most appropriate and effective?
   a. Glutaraldehyde (Cidex)
   b. Iodine solution
   c. Iodine tincture
   d. Povidone-iodine (Betadine)

9. The nurse knows that sodium hypochlorate (household bleach) when being used as a wound irrigant needs to be diluted with water in a ratio of 1 part bleach to
   a. 1 part water.
   b. 5 parts water.
   c. 10 parts water.
   d. 20 parts water.

10. Hexachlorophene (PHisoHex) is no longer recommended as a preoperative scrub because it
    a. can be absorbed through intact skin.
    b. can depress the central nervous system (CNS) causing stupor and death.
    c. does not stop bacteria from replicating.
    d. frequently damages the liver.

11. The benefit of applying hydrogen peroxide to a wound is
    a. killing of bacteria.
    b. killing of spores.
    c. killing of viruses.
    d. loosening of debris from the wound.

12. The surgical scrub that is fast-acting, antibacterial, and remains active on the skin after rinsing is
    a. benzalkonium chloride (BAC).
    b. chlorhexidine (Hibiclens).
    c. hexachlorophene (PHisoHex).
    d. povidone-iodine (Betadine).

13. The operating room nurse is preparing to apply benzalkonium chloride (BAC) as a surgical scrub. Before applying the solution, it is important for the nurse to
    a. rinse the skin with water and alcohol.
    b. shave the area.
    c. wash the skin with soap.
    d. warm the solution.

14. It is acceptable to use an alcohol-based handrub to cleanse the hands instead of soap and water (Select all that apply.)
    a. after eating.
    b. after removing gloves.
    c. after taking linens into a patient's room.
    d. after contact with an unknown powder present on a patient.
    e. before patient contact.
    f. before taking a pulse.
    g. after using the restroom.
    h. when the hands have been exposed to wound drainage.
    i. after setting up a patient for lunch who is in isolation for TB.

15. The nurse should scrub the hands and forearms with an antimicrobial soap for surgical scrub asepsis for
    a. 1 to 2 minutes.
    b. 4 to 6 minutes.
    c. 8 to 10 minutes.
    d. 10 to 15 minutes.

16. The nurse professor is orienting student nurses to the intensive care unit. Hygiene instructions should include
    a. alcohol handrub should be used when the hands are visibly dirty.
    b. all forms of jewelry are forbidden.
    c. do not wear artificial nails.
    d. trim natural nails to no more 1/2 inch beyond the fingertip.

17. Centers for Disease Control and Prevention (CDC) classification for wearing gloves when contact with unintact skin is anticipated is
    a. recommended.
    b. required.
    c. strongly recommended.
    d. suggested.

CASE STUDIES AND PATIENT TEACHING

(Use a separate piece of paper for your responses.)

Case Study 1

The delivery room nurse needs to prepare used instruments for disinfection with glutaraldehyde (Cidex) before being sent for sterilization.

1. What steps should the nurse take before soaking the instruments?

2. How long do the instruments need to soak?

3. What precautions does the nurse need to take when disinfecting with glutaraldehyde (Cidex)?

4. Describe the hand-washing technique the nurse would use after completing this disinfection process.

Answers can be reviewed online at http://evolve.elsevier.com/Lehne/.

OBJECTIVES

See page 28 for the Objectives.

CRITICAL THINKING AND STUDY QUESTIONS

1. Helminthiasis (Select all that apply.)
   a. affects more people than any other infectious disorder.
   b. always produces symptoms.
   c. can go away without any treatment.
   d. can involve the liver and blood vessels.
   e. in some situations, teaching principles espoused by Florence Nightingale can be the most important nursing intervention.
   f. treatment with drugs is most important in situations where the patient is at high risk for reinfection.

2. A patient has just started treatment with mebendazole (Vermox) for hookworm infestation. The nurse assesses for the most common complication of hookworm infestation, which may be
   a. feculent vomiting.
   b. pale conjunctiva.
   c. perianal itching.
   d. rectal prolapse.

3. A patient who has been treated with mebendazole (Vermox) for trichinosis is now prescribed prednisone. The purpose of this medication is to
   a. kill larvae that have migrated.
   b. prevent calcification of dead larvae in skeletal muscle.
   c. prevent migration of larvae.
   d. reduce inflammation during larval migration.

4. Nursing examination of a missionary who was admitted after becoming ill in Haiti reveals severe scrotal and peripheral edema. What other assessment finding, if present, suggests possible nematode infestation?
   a. Limited range of motion of joints
   b. Multiple bruises
   c. Swollen lymph nodes
   d. Weak hand grasps

5. A patient, who works for the World Health Organization (WHO) and whose job duties include worldwide travel, complains of recent noticeable decreased visual acuity. Because of the possibility of contracting onchocerciasis from fly bites, the nurse should assess for recent travel to which of the following areas in the patient's history? (Select all that apply.)
   a. Argentina
   b. Australia
   c. Canada
   d. China
   e. Columbia
   f. Congo
   g. Guatemala
   h. Kenya
   i. Madagascar
   j. Mexico
   k. Mozambique
   l. Japan
   m. Peru
   n. Rwanda
   o. Venezuela

6. To prevent complications from therapy with praziquantel (Biltricide) prescribed for tapeworms, the nurse teaches the patient to
   a. avoid hazardous activity.
   b. chew the tablet completely before swallowing.
   c. monitor daily urine output.
   d. take the medication on an empty stomach.

▶ 7. The nurse is administering albendazole (Albenza) to an elderly patient who has been diagnosed with the larval form of the pork tapeworm. Which of the following laboratory results would warrant consultation with the prescriber regarding administration of the medication?
   a. AST 175 international units/L
   b. BUN 25 mg/dL
   c. Creatinine 1.4 mg/dL
   d. Potassium 3.4 mg/dL

✳ 8. A resident has just prescribed diethylcarbamazine (Hetrazan) for an infection with *Wuchereria bancrofti*. Which of the following symptoms, occurring after the start of administration of the drug, would be of most concern to the nurse?
   a. Dizziness
   b. Headache
   c. Nausea
   d. Personality change

CASE STUDIES AND PATIENT TEACHING

(Use a separate piece of paper for your responses.)

Case Study 1

The mother of a 2½-year-old, who attends day care, notices that her child has been restless, is not sleeping well, has been scratching her perineal area, and wetting the bed. The mother calls her pediatric office and is told by the nurse to put a loop of transparent tape in the child's anal area in the early morning before the child awakens. The nurse further instructs the mother to remove the tape later in the morning, put it in a plastic bag, and bring it to the office. On examination of the tape sample, the pediatric nurse practitioner (PNP) diagnoses enterobiasis pinworms.

1. What is the probable mode of transmission of the parasite in this case?

2. The PNP prescribes mebendazole (Vermox) for the entire family. What did the prescriber need to determine before prescribing the drug for the entire family?

3. How could the pinworm infestation have been transmitted from the child to other family members?

4. What teaching can the nurse provide these family members to prevent future infestation and spread of pinworms?

5. The entire family is adherent to the prescribed therapy. Why is there little problem with adherence with this therapy?

6. The mother is embarrassed and does not want to notify the day care of her child's infection. How should the nurse respond?

Case Study 2

A nurse is caring for victims exposed to contaminated floodwaters who have been brought into a makeshift clinic in a temporary shelter.

1. The nurse knows that which segments of the population would be more at risk for helminthiasis?

2. Several children are experiencing vomiting and massive diarrhea. The nurse should be assessing for what symptoms of these possible fluid and electrolyte imbalances?
   a. Water
   b. Potassium
   c. Magnesium
   d. Sodium

3. Some patients are diagnosed with threadworm infestation. The only medication available for these patients is thiabendazole donated by a drug company. What actions should the nurse take to prevent complications of possible adverse effects of this drug?

4. What can the nurse do in this situation to prevent spread of these infections?

97

Antiprotozoal Drugs I: Antimalarial Agents

Answers can be reviewed online at http://evolve.elsevier.com/Lehne/.

OBJECTIVES

See page 28 for the Objectives.

CRITICAL THINKING AND STUDY QUESTIONS

1. Malaria (Select all that apply.)
   a. deaths are most likely in children under the age of 5 years.
   b. cases in North America are usually contracted elsewhere.
   c. eradication has not been successful because the transmitting insect and the parasite have become resistant to the drugs.
   d. is most prevalent in the Sahara desert areas of Africa.
   e. is transmitted by the Anopheles fly.
   f. kills more people than any other infection except tuberculosis.
   g. vaccination has been effective for many years, but many African people are afraid of vaccinations.

＊ 2. The most important action by the nurse to prevent transmission of malaria is
   a. administering drugs at the correct time.
   b. placing the patient in strict isolation.
   c. universal precautions.
   d. using a mask with all patient contact.

3. The repeating episodes of fever, chills, and profuse sweating that are characteristic of malaria are due to
   a. infection at the site of the mosquito bite.
   b. ingestion of blood by the mosquito.
   c. red blood cell (RBC) rupture.
   d. toxicity of the suppressant drugs.

＊ 4. Prompt treatment of suspected cases of malaria is most urgent if the patient experiences
   a. chills.
   b. dark urine.
   c. high fever.
   d. sweating.

▶ 5. To prevent a serious complication, the most significant priority in the nursing care of a patient who has malaria caused by *Plasmodium falciparum* is
   a. assessing for crackles and respiratory distress.
   b. assessing vital signs every 4 hours.
   c. glucometer checks every 2 hours.
   d. monitoring for elevations in liver function studies.

6. Primaquine is not used for relapse prevention of infection with malaria caused by *P. falciparum* because
   a. it is a drug that is only used prophylactically to prevent infection of erythrocytes.
   b. *P. falciparum* is resistant to primaquine.
   c. the infection is mild, and relapses will decrease and disappear over time without treatment.
   d. there are no dormant forms of the organism in the liver to be eradicated.

7. A patient asks why prophylactic chloroquine (Aralen) is taken only once a week. The basis of the nurse's response is
   a. absorption is very slow after oral administration.
   b. deposition in tissue is slowly released into the blood.
   c. it is administered IM as a depot preparation.
   d. it remains fat soluble and cannot be excreted by the kidneys.

▶ 8. It is extremely important to monitor urine color during treatment with primaquine if laboratory results for an adult female include
   a. G6PD 7.8 units/g of Hb.
   b. Hemoglobin 14 g/dL.
   c. Hematocrit 40%.
   d. RBC $4.9 \times 10^6/\mu L$.

✳ 9. A patient with diabetes treated with metformin is prescribed quinine for malaria. It is most important for the nurse to assess for
  a. excessive urination.
  b. hot and dry skin.
  c. palpitations and hunger.
  d. visual disturbances.

10. Quinine is categorized as category X. This means that the nurse should
  a. administer the drug to a pregnant woman if prescribed because there are no known risks to the human fetus.
  b. administer the drug to a pregnant woman if the risk of not treating with the drug is greater than any risk to the fetus.
  c. administer the drug to a pregnant woman and carefully assess for any adverse effects.
  d. not administer the drug until the pregnancy status of the woman has been determined.

▸ 11. Which of the following changes, if noted in a patient receiving mefloquine (Lariam), is a reason for the nurse to withhold the drug and contact the prescriber?
  a. Headache
  b. Heartburn
  c. Lack of interest in things normally found to be pleasurable
  d. Nausea

▸ 12. Because of adverse effects, the nurse knows that developmentally which of the following American patients would be least likely to adhere to atovaquone/proguanil (Malarone) therapy?
  a. A 15-year-old girl
  b. A 35-year-old male
  c. A 55-year-old male
  d. A 75-year-old female

13. A prescriber in the United States tells the nurse that he needs artesunate to treat a patient with severe malaria. This drug can be obtained by contacting the
  a. Centers for Disease Control and Prevention (CDC).
  b. Food and Drug Administration (FDA).
  c. World Health Organization (WHO).

▸ 14. Tetracycline is prescribed for a female patient who has chloroquinolone-resistant malaria. Which of the following laboratory test results would warrant withholding the drug and contacting the prescriber?
  a. ALT 60 international units/L
  b. Creatinine 1 mg/dL
  c. hCG 75 milli-international units/mL
  d. RBC 4.2×10^6/mcL

15. Clindamycin 20 mg/kg is the recommended dose for a child with malaria. Which of the following is an acceptable dose schedule for a child who weighs 55 pounds?
  a. 100 mg four times a day
  b. 150 mg three times a day
  c. 200 mg twice a day
  d. 500 mg once a day

CASE STUDIES AND PATIENT TEACHING

(Use a separate piece of paper for your responses.)

Case Study 1

A 45-year-old male has just returned from Africa after 4 years of service with the World Health Organization (WHO). During that time, he had been taking chloroquine (Aralen) prophylactically to prevent malaria in case he was bitten by an infected Anopheles mosquito.

1. What does this treatment actually accomplish?

2. What other measures should he have been taught to decrease the risk of malarial infection?

3. Before his African service was completed, the man quit taking the chloroquine because he was experiencing nausea and vomiting. Soon after, he started experiencing episodes of high fever followed by chills, then diaphoresis occurring every 2 days. He was diagnosed with vivax malaria and was unable to perform his work due to the frequency and intensity of symptoms. The patient is prescribed a 3-day treatment of chloroquine for his acute attack of malaria. What teaching could the nurse provide to decrease adverse effects and to prevent serious effects?

4. The patient tells the nurse that he knows that missionaries took intravenous (IV) quinine in the past. He asks why he wasn't prescribed that drug. What information can the nurse share about the decrease in use of quinine?

5. He was advised that he should return home for treatment with primaquine to prevent relapse. Why was this patient not treated in Africa where he could continue his work?

6. When the patient completes his acute treatment, he asks why he cannot continue taking the chloroquine to prevent recurrence of the malaria symptoms. What is the basis of the nurse's response to this question?

98
Antiprotozoal Drugs II: Miscellaneous Agents

Answers can be reviewed online at http://evolve.elsevier.com/Lehne/.

OBJECTIVES

See page 28 for the Objectives.

CRITICAL THINKING AND STUDY QUESTIONS

✳ 1. A farmer is hospitalized after developing cryptosporidosis during high-dose prednisone for exacerbated chronic obstructive pulmonary disease (COPD). A nursing priority for this patient is
   a. activity intolerance.
   b. fatigue.
   c. fluid volume deficit.
   d. imbalanced nutrition.

▸ 2. Which of the following symptoms, if present in a patient who is receiving iodoquinol (Yodoxin) for amebiasis, would be of most concern to the nurse?
   a. Anal itching
   b. Blurred vision
   c. Facial pustules
   d. Palpable thyroid

3. A patient asks why he has to take a second drug, iodoquinol (Yodoxin), after he finishes a course of metronidazole (Flagyl) for amebiasis. The best explanation for administration of the iodoquinol is
   a. metronidazole does not adequately kill the amebae in the large intestine.
   b. iodoquinol is absorbed better than metronidazole.
   c. liver abscesses caused by the amebae are not affected by metronidazole.
   d. metronidazole is metabolized by the CYP3A4 hepatic enzyme.

▸ 4. The nurse teaches a patient who is prescribed metronidazole (Flagyl) that it is very important to report which possible adverse effect of the drug to the prescriber?
   a. Darkening of the urine
   b. Metallic taste
   c. Mouth ulcers
   d. Paresthesias

5. An emergency department (ED) nurse is providing discharge teaching to a breast-feeding mother who is prescribed metronidazole (Flagyl) for giardiasis after a camping trip where she drank water from a stream. It is important for the nurse to teach this patient to feed her baby formula and pump her breasts and discard the breast milk throughout the time the medication is being taken plus an additional
   a. 1 day.
   b. 3 days.
   c. 1 week.
   d. 2 weeks.

▶ 6. A patient who has been prescribed metronidazole (Flagyl) asks why he should not drink any product that contains alcohol. The nurse's response is based on alcohol combined with metronidazole can cause
   a. bradycardia.
   b. dangerous CNS depression.
   c. hypertension.
   d. psychotic symptoms.

7. Tinidazole (Tindamax) differs from metronidazole (Flagyl) in that tinidazole
   a. does not interact with alcohol.
   b. has a longer half-life.
   c. is contraindicated in the last trimester of pregnancy.
   d. is less expensive.

▶ 8. The nurse notes yellowish discoloration of the sclera of an immunocompetent 7-year-old girl who is receiving nitazoxanide (Alinia) for giardiasis. The nurse should
   a. administer the medication and continue nursing care.
   b. review the most recent BUN and creatinine.
   c. withhold the medication and review laboratory tests.
   d. withhold the medication and contact the prescriber.

9. Which of the following, if noted in the urine of a patient who is receiving suramin sodium (Germanin) for early East African sleeping sickness, should the nurse report immediately to the prescriber?
   a. Multiple casts
   b. pH 5.7
   c. Protein 2 mg/dL
   d. Specific gravity 1.015

▶ 10. The drug handbook states that melarsoprol (Arsobal) has Herxheimer-type reactions as a frequent adverse effect. The nurse observes for this immune reaction which presents as
   a. a maculopapular rash.
   b. flu-like symptoms.
   c. lesions on the oral and conjunctival mucosa.
   d. tingling around the mouth and throat.

11. Which of the following laboratory tests results would warrant withholding eflornithine (Uridyl) prescribed for late stage African sleeping sickness and consulting the prescriber?
   a. ALT 338 international units/L
   b. BNP 260 picograms/mL
   c. BUN 32 mg/dL
   d. CPK 80 ng/mL

12. A patient is admitted with American trypanosomiasis (Chagas' disease). It would be most important to inform the prescriber of the patient's history of which of the following if nifurtimox (Lampit) is prescribed
   a. asthma.
   b. bowel obstruction.
   c. type 2 diabetes mellitus.
   d. G6PD deficiency.

CASE STUDIES AND PATIENT TEACHING

(Use a separate piece of paper for your responses.)

Case Study 1

The nurse works in a busy family practice. A 17-year-old female presents to the office with complaints of stabbing right upper quadrant (RUQ) pain, anorexia, chills, and diarrhea for 10 days.

1. What subjective information would be helpful to collect before the primary care practitioner (PCP) sees the patient?

The patient was on a camping trip in the White mountains of New Hampshire a few weeks ago. She experienced nausea and fatigue toward the end of trip and has gotten worse since coming home. She denies alcohol and tobacco use and sexual activity and is currently experiencing a menstrual period. She has lost 4 pounds in the last 2 weeks. Assessment findings include T 102.7°F, pulse 98 BPM; BP 100/64 mm Hg; dry mucous membranes, abdominal guarding, weakness.

The PCP orders a CBC and differential, electrolytes, and a CT scan of the abdomen. The PCP diagnoses amebiasis. Because the patient states that she will have difficulty being compliant with three times a day dosing with metronidazole, the PCP prescribes tinadazole (Tindamax) 2 g once a day for 3 days.

2. During teaching regarding adverse effects of this drug, the nurse should explain the importance of contacting the prescriber if what symptoms occur?

3. Based on the patient's exposure to the organism, symptoms, and developmental considerations, what other teaching should the nurse provide?

4. One duty is to review laboratory tests and notify the PCPs of results. The nurse is reviewing laboratory results for the patient with amebiasis. Abnormal results include WBC 12,800/mm³, sodium 137 mEq/L, potassium 3.6 mEq/L, and multiple small abscesses in the liver on CT scan. Which test result is most important to promptly review with the PCP and why?

5. The PCP asks the nurse to have the patient come in immediately. After explaining the laboratory test results, the patient agrees to be faithful for a course of metronidazole followed by iodoquinolol. What teaching should the nurse provide?

Case Study 2

A 26-year-old patient with hemophilia is 5 feet 7 inches tall and weighs 140 pounds. Because of his hemophilia, he has received numerous transfusions since his first accident at 2 years of age when he cut his head falling down the steps. Three years ago, he was diagnosed as HIV-positive and has been on azidothymidine (AZT) since then. He was hospitalized three days ago when he complained of a cough, dyspnea, and chest discomfort. The nurse notes that he is very pale and shows some cyanosis around his nail beds. He has been diagnosed with pneumocystis pneumonia (PCP).

1. Drug orders include intravenous (IV) pentamidine isethionate (Pentam 300) 220 mg once a day for 14 days. The recommended dose is 4 mg/kg/day. Is the prescribed dose safe and therapeutic?

2. The pentamidine must be dissolved in sterile water just before use. The vial is diluted to 100 mg/mL. How much pentamidine should be withdrawn from the vial to equal a dose of 220 mg?

3. The IV pentamidine is diluted to a total of 250 mL of 5% dextrose in water. What rate should be programmed into the infusion pump if the solution is to be administered over 60 minutes?

4. What nursing measures should be implemented to prevent complications of adverse effects of IV pentamidine?

5. The patient has received pentamidine before as an aerosol inhalation. He wants to know why he must have his medication through an IV instead of the inhaler. He says he is afraid that he will bleed if something happens to the IV. How should the nurse respond?

Case Study 3

A school nurse who works in rural farming area has noted an extremely high incidence of absences due to severe diarrhea in children who live within a one-mile radius of each other.

1. What could possibly be causing these illnesses and what can the nurse do to prevent these illnesses?

Case Study 4

A patient who has a history of diabetes, seizure disorder, atrial fibrillation, and bipolar disorder is prescribed metronidazole (Flagyl). The patient's home medication regimen lists metformin (Glucophage) 500 mg twice a day, phenytoin (Dilantin) 100 mg three times a day, warfarin (Coumadin) 2.5 mg once a day on Monday and Thursday and 2 mg once a day on the rest of the days, and lithium carbonate (Eskalith) 300 mg three times a day.

1. What are the possible effects on drug levels of the interaction of each of these drugs with metronidazole (Flagyl)?

2. The nurse should assess for which symptoms of these drug reactions?

3. What are interventions the nurse should employ if symptoms occur?

99
Ectoparasiticides

Answers can be reviewed online at http://evolve.elsevier.com/Lehne/.

OBJECTIVES

See page 28 for the Objectives.

CRITICAL THINKING AND STUDY QUESTIONS

1. Match the following terms and descriptors. (You may use options more than once.)

_____ a. Pediculosis
_____ b. Scabies

1. Animals never infested
2. Common site of adult infestation is webs of fingers
3. Intense itching
4. Lice infestation
5. Mite infestation
6. Transmission possible via contact with objects
7. Treatment and how contracted differs by site
8. Visible lines where burrows

2. The nurse has taught a mother how to apply permethrin (Elimite) 5% cream to treat her 7-year-old son who has visible scabies burrows on his buttocks. Which of these statements made by the mother would indicate she understood the directions?
   a. "I should not apply the cream to his face or scalp."
   b. "The cream should be applied to the skin from head to the soles of the feet being careful to avoid eyes and mucous membranes."
   c. "The cream should be washed off after 10 minutes with warm water."
   d. "The cream should not be washed off."

3. Which of the following could be associated with a severe reaction when malathion (Ovide) has been prescribed for head lice?
   a. Absorption of the lotion through scratches on the scalp
   b. Administration concurrently with drugs that inhibit the P-450 hepatic cytochrome system
   c. Failure to use the fine-toothed comb to remove nits after application
   d. Smoking while applying the lotion

4. Which of the following treatments for scabies normally involves repeated applications?
   a. Crotamiton (Eurax)
   b. Ivermectin (Stromectol)
   c. Lindane (Kwell)
   d. Permethrin (Nix)

CASE STUDIES AND PATIENT TEACHING

(Use a separate piece of paper for your responses.)

Case Study 1

A teacher consults the school nurse about a second-grade girl in her class. The child is one of three siblings attending the elementary school. The child has very long blond hair, and over the past week, the child has been constantly scratching her head. She has scratched her head so much that her hair is tangled and almost impossible to brush, and her scalp is bleeding. The school nurse notes small white spots on her hair shaft close to the scalp. Examination under the microscope reveals nits. The nurse contacts the girl's mother to report these nits (eggs), telling her it is probably Pediculus humanus capitis *(head lice).*

1. How should the school nurse handle the possibility that other children in the school may be infested?

2. The girl's mother is quite upset about the lice. She wants to know how her child could have gotten "these bugs" and how to tell whether others in the family have them. How should the nurse respond?

3. The mother was told by a friend to cut all of Joan's hair to get rid of the lice. What are reasons why the nurse would not want the mother to do this to the child?

4. The mother contacts the pediatrician who orders permethrin (Nix) shampoo. What should the office nurse include in the explanation for using this product?

5. What is the purpose of the fine-toothed comb in head lice treatment?

6. The child's mother tells the nurse that when she had head lice as a child, her prescriber had her mother apply lindane (Kwell) shampoo. She wants to know why that is not used anymore. What would the nurse tell her?

100
Basic Principles of Cancer Chemotherapy

Answers can be reviewed online at http://evolve.elsevier.com/Lehne/.

OBJECTIVES

See page 28 for the Objectives.

CRITICAL THINKING AND STUDY QUESTIONS

1. The best description of cancer cell reproduction is
   a. abnormal.
   b. rapid.
   c. slow.
   d. unregulated.

2. A patient is admitted for surgical removal of a cancerous tumor of the colon. He is concerned about the prospect of living with a colostomy and asks the nurse why the prescriber cannot just give him some drugs to kill the cancer. The basis of the nurse's response is that solid tumors (Select all that apply.)
   a. are disseminated.
   b. have fewer cells that are actively dividing.
   c. have fewer cells in the G_0 phase.
   d. have poor blood supply at the core.
   e. have normal DNA.

3. A spouse of a cancer patient asks why some tumors become resistant to chemotherapy. Which of the following would not be included in the explanation?
   a. A transport molecule may be stimulated to pump drugs out of the cancer cell.
   b. Cancer cells in the G_0 phase have time to repair drug-induced damage before it does serious harm.

c. Chemotherapy drugs alter the cancer cell DNA, making the cell resistant.

d. Drug-resistant mutant cells have more nourishment because of the death of drug-sensitive cells.

4. The mother of a child with leukemia is concerned about her son's fear and discomfort during chemotherapy. She asks the nurse why he cannot receive one large dose of a single powerful drug instead of multiple doses of different drugs. After teaching, which statement if made by the mother, suggests that that this mother needs further explanation?

a. "Different drugs kill cancer cells in different ways."

b. "It is especially important for my son to receive multiple doses because one of the drugs that my son is getting only kills cancer cells at a particular point of cell reproduction."

c. "If multiple drugs are used, the cancer is less likely to develop resistance to all of them."

d. "My son will not experience adverse effects if he receives multiple drugs administered at different times."

5. The nurse would expect that when more than one anticancer chemotherapeutic agent is used together, the drugs

a. adverse effects primarily affect different organs.

b. are less effective than if used alone.

c. can be mixed in the same intravenous solution.

d. have the same mechanism of action.

6. A patient with brain cancer asks the nurse why they are putting the drug into her back instead of a vein. The basis of the nurse's response should be that this route

a. allows higher doses of chemotherapy to be used.

b. allows the drug to get to the tumor cells.

c. prevents many adverse effects.

d. prevents drug-resistant mutation of the cancer cells.

▶ 7. The nurse is caring for a 62-year-old female who developed pancreatitis during chemotherapy after mastectomy. Most recent laboratory results include RBC 2.8 10^6/mcL, WBC 4100/mm^3, neutrophils 18,000/mm^3, and platelets 147,000/mm^3. An expected nursing diagnosis, based on these laboratory results, would be

a. activity intolerance.

b. decreased cardiac output.

c. impaired gas exchange.

d. ineffective cerebral tissue perfusion.

▶ 8. The nurse is caring for a chemotherapy patient with neutropenic precautions. The nurse washes her hands and dons gown, mask, and gloves in the anteroom before entering the actual patient room. The patient refuses care by the nurse until the nurse washes her hands at the sink in the room and puts on new gloves. The nurse should

a. explain that she is more likely to transmit an infection if she takes off her current gloves while in the room.

b. explain that she washed her hands just outside the door before entering the room.

c. rewash her hands in the room and put on new gloves.

d. rewash her hands, put on new gown, gloves, and mask inside the room.

9. When teaching a cancer patient who is receiving chemotherapy, which of the following foods would be least likely to cause an infection if the patient develops neutropenia?

a. Commercially canned fruit

b. Fresh vegetables from the patient's garden

c. Rare meat

d. Yogurt

10. The nurse is administering subcutaneous insulin to a chemotherapy patient who is experiencing bone marrow suppression. Which of the following techniques would be best for the nurse to use to prevent an adverse effect from the bone marrow suppression?

a. Administer the insulin via an existing IV port.

b. Apply pressure to the injection site for a few minutes after injection.

c. Delay the administration of insulin until after the patient has eaten his meal.

d. Wipe the injection site with Betadine after injection.

11. A patient receiving chemotherapy develops hyperuricemia. A nursing priority addresses the effect of the urate crystals on the
    a. blood.
    b. joints.
    c. kidneys.
    d. liver.

▸ 12. When administering a known vesicant chemotherapeutic agent, it is most important for the nurse to know
    a. if the patient has been premedicated with an antiemetic.
    b. if an antidote is available should extravasation occur.
    c. the mechanism of action of the drug.
    d. whether gloves are needed during administration.

CASE STUDIES AND PATIENT TEACHING

(Use a separate piece of paper for your responses.)

Case Study 1

A 28-year-old female is admitted to the oncology unit with a diagnosis of suspected Hodgkin's disease. The diagnosis is confirmed after a biopsy. The patient is started on treatment, which consists of external radiation treatments and chemotherapy. The patient asks the nurse, "How does cancer spread?"

1. What information can the nurse provide about the characteristics of cancer cells that promote growth and metastasis?

2. The patient asks why a person is more likely to get cancer if they have a family history of cancer. How are genetics linked to cancer?

3. The nurse is discussing strategies to minimize the adverse effects of chemotherapy, including mouth ulcer (stomatitis). The patient asks why these drugs cause mouth ulcers if they are given intravenously. How should the nurse respond?

4. What interventions can the nurse suggest to minimize the effects of chemotherapy on the patient's GI tract?

Case Study 2

A nurse has just lost a sister to breast cancer. Before her sister's death, her sister challenged her to use her knowledge and energy to prevent cancer suffering and death. The nurse networks with fellow nurses to identify what they can do to work toward fulfilling her sister's wishes.

1. What actions could the nurse take?

Case Study 3

The oncology nurse is participating in a cancer support meeting for patients who are receiving chemotherapy and their families.

1. What teaching can she provide regard minimizing harm and discomfort from these effects of the chemotherapy?
    a. Bone marrow suppression
    b. Reproductive toxicity
    c. Hyperuricemia

Case Study 4

Discuss with classmates interventions that address the following nursing problems that a patient receiving chemotherapy may experience.

1. a. Activity intolerance and/or fatigue
    b. Disturbed body image
    c. Fluid volume deficit
    d. Imbalanced nutrition: less than body requirement
    e. Risk for infection

Answers can be reviewed online at http://evolve.elsevier.com/Lehne/.

OBJECTIVES

See page 28 for the Objectives.

CRITICAL THINKING AND STUDY QUESTIONS

▸ 1. An important teaching relating to a common adverse effect of cytotoxic drugs would be
   a. change positions slowly to prevent dizziness or fainting.
   b. night driving may not be safe.
   c. the importance of weight-bearing exercise.
   d. use an electric razor to prevent cutting yourself.

2. A cancer patient asks the nurse why so many drugs that are used to treat cancer cause infections. Which of the following should not be included in the nurse's response?
   a. Blood cells that protect from infection rapidly reproduce so they are easily affected by these drugs.
   b. Most drugs that kill cancer cells actually prevent them from reproducing.
   c. There are drugs available to help boost the body's production of infection-preventing and infection-fighting white blood cells.
   d. When a person has cancer, their blood cells are always invaded by the cancer so the drugs are killing cancerous blood cells.

3. To ensure that phase-specific anticancer drugs are present when cancer cells will be harmed by the drug, these drugs are administered
   a. combined with other drugs.
   b. in large doses spaced at least 3 weeks apart.
   c. with prolonged infusion or at short intervals.
   d. when cancer cells are not resting.

4. Cell-cycle–phase nonspecific drugs may not kill cells in G_0 phase because the
   a. cell has time to repair damage.
   b. cell is not cancerous if it is in G_0 phase.
   c. cell is not reproducing.
   d. cell's DNA is not harmed.

5. The nurse is teaching a patient who has been prescribed oral cyclophosphamide (Cytoxan). Which of the following statements, if made by the patient, suggests a need for further teaching?
   a. "I need to notify my doctor if I develop a fever greater than 100.4°F."
   b. "I need to take a drug to prevent nausea at least two hours before I take this drug."
   c. "I should drink at least 12 glasses of fluids every day, especially water."
   d. "It is important for me to take this drug on an empty stomach with a full glass of water."

▸ 6. The nurse prepares to obtain a sample for which of the following tests before administering ifosfamide (Ifex)?
   a. Capillary blood for SMBG
   b. Sputum for C&S
   c. Stool for hematest
   d. Urine for urinalysis

7. Which of the following is an appropriate nursing outcome for a patient who is prescribed prednisone for an adverse effect of Carmustine (BiCNU, Gliadel)?
   a. Ambulates to bathroom without shortness of breath
   b. BP 100/60 to 116/80
   c. Changes position without experiencing dizziness
   d. Performs ADL without experiencing joint pain

▸ 8. The nurse should withhold chemotherapy with cisplatin (Platinol-AQ) and consult with the oncologist if a patient reports which of the following symptoms since the last infusion?
   a. Nausea
   b. Paresthesias
   c. Sensitivity to cold
   d. Tinnitus

▶ 9. Because of the danger of fetal malformation when receiving methotrexate, the nurse teaches a 38-year-old female the importance of using two reliable forms of birth control during
   a. therapy.
   b. therapy and through at least 1 month after therapy.
   c. therapy and through at least 3 months after therapy.
   d. therapy and through at least 6 months after therapy.

▶ 10. A priority nursing concern relating to a peripheral sensory neuropathy complication of oxaliplatin (Eloxatin) is
   a. clumsiness.
   b. difficulty swallowing.
   c. difficulty writing.
   d. intolerance to cold.

▶ 11. The nurse is reviewing the laboratory tests of a female patient who is scheduled to receive methotrexate. Which of the following results, especially if a change from a previous result, would be most important to report to the attending oncologist?
   a. ALT 55 international units /L
   b. Creatinine clearance 45 mL/min
   c. Hemoglobin 10.8 g/dL
   d. Sodium 134 mEq/L

✳ 12. A patient with throat cancer is receiving massive doses of methotrexate. Which of the following actions is of the greatest priority?
   a. Administering the prescribed ondansetron (Zofran) 30 minutes before the start of the methotrexate infusion
   b. Administering the leucovorin (folinic acid, citrovorum factor) as prescribed
   c. Infusing the methotrexate over exactly the prescribed time interval
   d. Monitoring for electrolyte imbalances because of the high risk of diarrhea or vomiting

13. Which of the following statements, if made by a patient who has been receiving teaching regarding prevention of adverse effects of methotrexate therapy, suggests understanding of the teaching?
   a. "Drinking cranberry juice will help protect my kidneys from damage by methotrexate."
   b. "I should increase my fluid intake to 30 ounces each day."

   c. "If I get a cough, I should report it to my doctor."
   d. "It is important to avoid grapefruit juice when taking this drug."

▶ 14. Based on body surface area recommendations, the dose of pemetrexed (Alimta) should be $600 \, mg/m^2$ every 3 weeks. Which of the following doses of this drug would be within the therapeutic recommendations for a patient who is 5' 5" tall and weighs 135 lb?
   a. 1 g
   b. 850 mg
   c. 915 mg
   d. 925 mg

15. The nurse teaches a patient that dexamethasone is prescribed when a patient is being treated with pemetrexed (Alimta) in an attempt to prevent
   a. anemia.
   b. infection.
   c. nausea.
   d. rash.

✳ 16. The oncology nurse is administering pemetrexed (Alimta) in 100 mL of 0.9% sodium chloride (NSS). While administering the drug, the nurse notes swelling at the intravenous catheter insertion site. The area is cool and pale. The priority nursing action is to
   a. administer an antidote to prevent tissue necrosis.
   b. apply heat.
   c. apply cold.
   d. stop infusing the drug.

▶ 17. Which of the following symptoms of adverse effects of cytarabine (ara-C) would be of most concern to the nurse?
   a. Anorexia, nausea, and bruising
   b. Headache, fever, and vomiting
   c. Mouth ulcers, inflamed conjunctiva, and nausea
   d. Nausea, vomiting, and fever

18. The nurse should consult with the prescriber before administering which of the following chemotherapeutic agents if the patient reports diarrhea or mouth ulcers?
   a. Cladribine (Leustatin)
   b. Fludarabine (Fludara)
   c. Fluorouracil (Adrucil)
   d. Gemcitabine (Gemzar)

19. The nurse knows that palm and sole tingling, burning, redness, swelling, and blistering are possible adverse effects of some
    a. alkylating agents.
    b. antimetabolites.
    c. miotic inhibitors.
    d. platinum compounds.

20. The nurse assesses for which of the following symptoms of the most common effects of mercaptopurine (Purinethol) toxicity?
    a. Bleeding
    b. Constipation
    c. Diarrhea
    d. Hair loss

21. A patient is receiving doxorubicin. The nurse should emphasize the importance of reporting symptoms of the most critical adverse effects including
    a. alopecia.
    b. hyperpigmentation of extremities.
    c. mouth ulcers.
    d. shortness of breath.

22. The nurse is preparing to administer doxorubicin to a 44-year-old male with non-Hodgkin's lymphoma. The nurse would be most concerned if the patient admitted to not being adherent to taking his prescribed
    a. bupropion (Wellbutrin).
    b. enalapril (Vasotec).
    c. ibuprofen (Motrin).
    d. lorazepam (Ativan).

▶ 23. A patient who is receiving an infusion of liposomal doxorubicin (Doxil) reports back pain and chest tightness within minutes of the start of the infusion. The nurse stops the infusion. The symptoms abate, and the patient's vital signs are within normal limits, but the patient voids bright red urine. The nurse should
    a. administer an antidote.
    b. consult with the prescriber STAT.
    c. hold the drug until the next scheduled dose.
    d. restart the infusion at a slower rate and monitor for return of symptoms.

✳ 24. Which of the following information, if revealed by a patient who is scheduled to start chemotherapy with epirubicin (Ellence) for breast cancer, would be a priority for the nurse to report to the prescriber before administering the drug?
    a. Axillary nodes positive for cancerous cells
    b. Desire to have children after therapy is completed
    c. History of asthma
    d. Recent episodes of hypoglycemia

25. The nurse should warn patients that they may experience a blue-green discoloration of their urine and the whites of their eyes if they receive which of the following antitumor antibiotics?
    a. Epirubicin (Ellence)
    b. Idarubicin (Idamycin)
    c. Liposomal daunorubicin (DaunoXome)
    d. Mitoxantrone (Novantrone)

▶ 26. The nurse is preparing to administer bleomycin (Blenoxane) to a patient with testicular cancer. Which of these test results would warrant withholding the drug and consulting with the prescriber?
    a. Erythrocyte sedimentation rate (ESR) 10 mm/hr
    b. Hematocrit (Hct) 38%
    c. Peak expiratory flow (PEF) 54% of best
    d. Platelets 180,000/mm³

27. When teaching a patient who is receiving mitomycin, the nurse explains that the greatest danger of contracting an infection caused by the effect of the drug on the immune system usually occurs
    a. 4 to 6 weeks after the infusion.
    b. 6 to 8 days after the infusion.
    c. 24 to 48 hours after the infusion.
    d. during the infusion.

28. A patient is scheduled to receive gemtuzumab ozogamicin (Mylotarg). Before administering the drug, the nurse should consult with the prescriber regarding premedication with
    a. aspirin.
    b. dexamethasone.
    c. diphenhydramine.
    d. leucovorin.

▶ 29. Which of the following assessments would warrant stopping the infusion of paclitaxel (Abraxane) and consulting the prescriber?
   a. Pulse 58 beats/min
   b. Pulse 98 beats/min
   c. Respirations 15 breaths per minute
   d. Respirations 24 breaths per minute

▶ 30. Which of these assessment findings would be most significant if a patient was receiving docetaxel (Taxotere)?
   a. Blood pressure 147/90 mm Hg
   b. Eight-hour output of 850 mL of very dark amber urine
   c. Three soft formed stool in 8 hours
   d. Two plus pitting edema of the ankles

▶ 31. The husband of a patient who received a treatment of irinotecan (Camptosar) 3 days ago calls the oncology clinic nurse to report that his wife has been up all night with diarrhea. She is currently in bed and is too weak to stand up. He asks the nurse what he should do. The nurse should advise the husband to
   a. administer 1 loperamide (Imodium AD) tablet to his wife after each unformed stool.
   b. allow his wife to rest.
   c. get his wife to take frequent sips of a sports drink with sugar and electrolytes.
   d. take his wife to the hospital for evaluation.

▶ 32. The oncology clinic nurse is administering chemotherapy to several patients. Which of the following would warrant closest monitoring?
   a. 37-year-old female receiving carboplatin (Paraplatin) for ovarian cancer
   b. 78-year-old male receiving cyclophosphamide for non-Hodgkin's lymphoma
   c. 64-year-old female receiving gemcitabine (Gemzar) for pancreatic adenoma
   d. 54-year-old male receiving pemetrexed (Alimta) for mesothelioma

CASE STUDIES AND PATIENT TEACHING

(Use a separate piece of paper for your responses.)

Case Study 1

A 41-year-old female is admitted to the outpatient area for her first course of adjuvant chemotherapy for metastatic breast cancer. Four weeks ago, she underwent a left modified radical mastectomy and axillary lymph node dissection for infiltrating ductal carcinoma of the breast. Two of 20 nodes sampled were positive for cancer. The patient will be receiving standard dosage therapy of Adriamycin, Cytoxan, and 5-FU (mg/m^2) IV bolus. Premedications include Zofran 32 mg as IV push bolus (IVPB) and Decadron 20 mg IV. In addition, she will receive filgrastim 300 mcg SQ daily for 10 days beginning 24 hours after chemotherapy completion.

1. What techniques should the nurse use when administering these cytotoxic chemotherapy agents to prevent personal harm?

2. What administrative techniques should the nurse use to prevent patient injury from a vesicant anticancer drug?

Case Study 2

Chemotherapy prescribed for a 53-year-old male for advanced non-Hodgkin's lymphoma includes vincristine. The nurse is preparing a plan of nursing care relating to probable adverse effects from this drug.

1. What nursing diagnoses should the nurse consider?

Case Study 3

The nurse is preparing to administer paclitaxel (Taxol) to a 38-year-old patient with ovarian cancer.

1. Developmentally, what effect of this drug would be a priority for the nurse to prepare this patient to experience?

2. What teaching should the nurse provide relating to the likelihood of the drug causing neutropenia?

3. Filgrastim (Neupogen) is prescribed 5 mcg/kg/day. The patient weighs 132 lb. What dose should be administered?

4. Dexamethasone, diphenhydramine, and cimetidine are prescribed "before treatment." What information can the nurse research to determine how soon after administering these drugs the chemotherapy infusion should be initiated?

5. What actions should the nurse take when administering paclitaxel to prevent harm to the patient relating to this specific drug?

6. The patient experiences a tingling sensation around her lips 10 minutes after the paclitaxel infusion is started. What action should the nurse take at this time?

7. The patient returns 3 weeks later. She is very concerned when the nurse informs her that prescribed therapy still includes paclitaxel (Abraxane). What explanation by the oncologist can the nurse reinforce?

102

Anticancer Drugs II: Hormonal Agents, Biologic Response Modifiers, and Targeted Drugs

Answers can be reviewed online at http://evolve.elsevier.com/Lehne/.

OBJECTIVES

See page 28 for the Objectives.

CRITICAL THINKING AND STUDY QUESTIONS

1. An important nursing concern for patients receiving drugs that deprive prostate tumors of testosterone involves the risk of
   a. constipation.
   b. impaired skin integrity.
   c. ineffective breathing pattern.
   d. sexual dysfunction.

2. The nurse is reinforcing the prescriber's teaching about the expected effects of leuprolide (Lupron), which has been prescribed for a 62-year-old male with advanced prostate cancer. Which of the following statements, if made by the patient, suggests a need for further teaching?
   a. "I might have more trouble passing my water for a short time after I start this drug."
   b. "I need to be careful to avoid going out in crowds while taking this drug."
   c. "I should pick up throw rugs in my house so I don't trip and fall."
   d. "It is important for me to try to walk regularly."

3. A patient with advanced prostate cancer treated with the GnRH analog triptorelin has been depressed and has a poor appetite. The nurse is sitting with the patient to encourage him to eat his lunch. Based on adverse effects of this drug therapy, which of the following foods on the patient's lunch tray would be most important for the patient to eat?
   a. Ham sandwich
   b. Orange
   c. Tossed salad
   d. Yogurt

4. Which of these laboratory tests would be most important for the nurse to assess when a patient with prostate cancer is receiving goserelin (Zoladex) and flutamide (Eulexin)?
   a. Alkaline phosphatase (ALP)
   b. Blood urea nitrogen (BUN)
   c. Platelets
   d. Neutrophils

5. An important teaching for a patient who has been prescribed nilutamide (Nilandron) is
   a. change positions slowly to prevent dizziness or fainting.
   b. limit your fluid intake in the evening so you do not need to get up to go to the bathroom.
   c. night driving may not be safe.
   d. use an electric razor to prevent cutting yourself.

6. Which of the following teachings would not be necessary when the nurse is teaching a patient regarding adverse effects of abarelix (Plenaxis)?
   a. Avoid stimulation for several hours before bedtime to improve sleep.
   b. Blood pressure monitoring for hypotension is important.
   c. Eating whole grains, fruits, and vegetables can prevent constipation.
   d. You must stay in the office for at least 30 minutes after the injection because this drug has been known to cause allergic reactions.

▶ 7. Because diethylstilbestrol diphosphate (Stilphostrol) can cause hypercalcemia, the nurse assesses patients receiving this drug for
   a. abdominal cramps and borborygmi.
   b. bleeding gums and bruising.
   c. muscle weakness and constipation.
   d. positive Chvostek's and Trousseau's signs.

✳ 8. A priority nursing concern for a patient who is receiving multiple drugs including ketoconazole (Nizoral) for prostate cancer is
   a. allergy.
   b. body image.
   c. fatigue.
   d. impairment in drug metabolism.

✳ 9. Which of the following assessment findings, if present in a patient who is receiving estramustine (Emcyt) for prostate cancer, would be of most concern to the nurse?
   a. Calf swelling—unilateral
   b. Headache
   c. Nausea
   d. Serum calcium 11 mg/dL

▶ 10. Which of the following nursing actions would be most likely to support patient adherence to taking antiestrogen drug therapy for breast cancer?
   a. Demonstrating administration techniques
   b. Emphasizing benefits of therapy

   c. Identifying patient concerns
   d. Teaching mechanism of action of the drugs

11. When taking a history from a 52-year-old woman with high risk for breast cancer for whom tamoxifen therapy is being considered, which of the following questions would be most important for the nurse to ask?
   a. "Has anyone in your family ever had breast cancer?"
   b. "Have you ever been told that your cholesterol is high?"
   c. "Have you had your bone density measured recently?"
   d. "Have you had any blood clots?"

12. Toremifene (Fareston) therapy is prescribed to prevent recurrence of breast cancer for a patient who takes carbamazepine (Tegretol) and phenytoin (Dilantin) for a seizure disorder. These drugs induce the CYP3A4 hepatic enzyme needed for metabolism of tamoxifen. The nurse is aware that dosage of tamoxifen for this patient will be
   a. the same as usual, but may be less effective.
   b. the same as usual, but may be more likely to produce adverse effects.
   c. higher than usual.
   d. lower than usual.

13. A patient who is receiving tamoxifen read in the newspaper that a STAR study is being conducted on a similar drug raloxifene (Evista). The patient asks the nurse why they are studying this drug if it is so similar to tamoxifen. The basis of the nurse's response is that research suggests that raloxifene
   a. does not cause hot flashes.
   b. does not increase the risk of uterine cancer.
   c. does not promote clot formation.
   d. improves bone density better than tamoxifen.

14. The nurse is preparing to administer fulvestrant (Faslodex). Based on current recommendations for intramuscular (IM) injections and the incidence of injection-site pain, the best site for this 5-mL IM injection would be
   a. one 5-mL injection in either dorsogluteal site.
   b. two 2.5-mL injections in bilateral dorsogluteal sites.
   c. one 5-mL injection in either ventrogluteal site.
   d. two 2.5-mL injections in bilateral ventrogluteal sites.

✳ 15. A priority teaching relating to expected adverse effects for a patient who is prescribed the aromatase inhibitor anastrozole (Arimidex) is
 a. eat small frequent meals to prevent nausea.
 b. hot flushes may wake you at night.
 c. safety precautions to prevent falls in the home.
 d. wear layers of clothing.

✳ 16. The nurse is reviewing laboratory test results for a 50-year-old woman with breast cancer. The oncologist is considering prescribing letrozole (Femara). Which of the following laboratory test results would be a priority to report to the prescriber?
 a. ALP 125 international units/L
 b. eGFR 98 mL/min
 c. Hematocrit 38%
 d. hCG 825 milli-international units/mL

▶ 17. Trastuzumab (Herceptin) is prescribed for a patient with a breast cancer tumor that produces excessive HER2. The nurse would notify the prescriber immediately if patient suddenly develops
 a. a headache.
 b. crackles throughout the lung fields.
 c. dizziness with sudden position changes.
 d. a temperature of 100.4°F (38°C).

18. A patient asks the nurse how interferon alfa-2a (Roferon-A) is fighting his cancer. The basis of the nurse's response is that this drug (Select all that apply.)
 a. alters DNA preventing cancer cell reproduction.
 b. blocks microtubule assembly.
 c. causes nonreproducing cancer cells to stay nonreproducing.
 d. deprives cancer cells of hormones needed for survival.
 e. disrupts cellular protein synthesis.
 f. improves the body's ability to fight cancer cells.
 g. promotes cancer cells' change into forms that do not reproduce.
 h. suppresses cancer genes.

19. To prevent some of the most common adverse effects of interferon alfa-2a (Roferon-A), the nurse teaches the patient about administering which of the following drugs?
 a. Acetaminophen (Tylenol)
 b. Dexamethasone (Decadron)

 c. Diphenhydramine (Benadryl)
 d. Ondansetron (Zofran)

20. The oncology nurse is infusing aldesleukin (Proleukin) when the patient suddenly becomes very short of breath. The first response by the nurse should be to
 a. assess the patient's vital signs.
 b. elevate the head of the bed.
 c. notify the oncologist.
 d. stop the drug infusion.

21. Nursing preparation for administration of BCG vaccine includes
 a. accessing a central venous line.
 b. assessing the intravenous site for patency.
 c. inserting a urethral catheter.
 d. identifying the appropriate landmarks for IM infusion.

22. The nurse teaches a patient who is receiving BCG vaccine to use precautions to protect from contamination with excreted urine for 6 hours after the end of therapy, including cleaning the toilet with
 a. alcohol.
 b. ammonia.
 c. bleach.
 d. peroxide.

23. The oncology clinic nurse is monitoring the chemotherapy infusions of the following patients. The patient receiving which of the following drugs would warrant close observation and access to epinephrine and cardiopulmonary resuscitation because of the known risk of an anaphylactic reaction? (Select all that apply.)
 a. Bevacizumab (Avastin)
 b. Bexxar (Tositumomab with I^{131} Tosituomab)
 c. Bortezomib (Velcade)
 d. Cetuximab (Erbitux)
 e. Denileukin diftitox (Ontak)
 f. Erlotinib (Tarceva)
 g. Gemtuzumab ozogamicin (Mylotarg)
 h. Rituximab (Rituxan)

24. The teaching plan for patients receiving EGFR-tyrosine kinase inhibitors should include the importance of reporting sudden onset of which of the following symptoms to the oncologist?
 a. Fever
 b. Irritability
 c. Nausea
 d. Shortness of breath

✳ 25. Because cetuximab (Erbitux) can lower serum magnesium levels, it is a priority for the nurse to monitor the patient receiving this drug for
   a. anorexia.
   b. 4+ DTR.
   c. fever.
   d. hypotension.

▸ 26. Which of the following symptoms, if occurring 12 to 24 hours after the first infusion of rituximab (Rituxan), suggests possible drug-induced tumor lysis syndrome (TLS)?
   a. Hypotension and cool, clammy skin
   b. Muscle spasms and tingling around the mouth
   c. Nausea and constipation
   d. Weakness and thirst

▸ 27. A patient is receiving rituximab (Rituxan). The nurse should teach the patient to observe for critical adverse effects that warrant immediate medical attention, including
   a. fever and chills.
   b. muscle aches and pains.
   c. stomatitis and widespread rash.
   d. vomiting and diarrhea.

28. Teaching should include prompt reporting of abdominal pain, chest pain, shortness of breath, change in mental status, and blood in sputum when a patient is receiving treatment with
   a. bevacizumab (Avastin).
   b. bortezomib (Velcade).
   c. gemtuzumab ozogamicin (Mylotarg).
   d. rituximab (Rituxan).

29. The priority nursing consideration for the visiting nurse when caring for a patient who has started therapy with bevacizumab (Avastin) after a colon resection and who spends long periods of the day in bed is the risk for
   a. altered nutrition related to loss of appetite and nausea.
   b. altered tissue perfusion, altered coagulation, and sluggish circulation.
   c. constipation related to decreased mobility and loss of appetite.
   d. fluid imbalance caused by decreased intake of fluids and possible diarrhea.

▸ 30. The nurse notes a 2-lb weight gain in 24 hours when assessing a hospitalized patient who has been receiving imatinib (Gleevec) for chronic myeloid leukemia (CML). It is a priority for the nurse to assess this patient's
   a. cardiopulmonary status.
   b. gastrointestinal status.
   c. musculoskeletal status.
   d. neurologic status.

31. Why have so many new drugs in the class BCR-ABL tyrosine kinase inhibitors been developed?

32. A patient diagnosed with multiple myeloma who has been receiving Bortezomib (Velcade) develops severe diarrhea. Which of the following symptoms suggest that the patient is experiencing the most likely electrolyte imbalance?
   a. Bruising with minimal trauma
   b. Confusion and thirst
   c. Hyperactive DTRs
   d. Weakness and lethargy

33. Which of the following assessment findings would be of greatest concern to the nurse caring for a male patient who is prescribed Sunitinib (Sutent) for advanced renal cell carcinoma?
   a. 10 mm Hg increase in BP over baseline
   b. Dizziness with position changes
   c. Gain of 2 pounds in 24 hours
   d. Hemoglobin 13.2 g/dL

▸ 34. Because gemtuzumab ozogamicin (Mylotarg) damages myeloid colony-forming cells, the nurse who is caring for a patient who is receiving this drug should monitor for the need to institute
   a. contact isolation precautions.
   b. neutropenic precautions.
   c. orthostatic hypotension precautions.
   d. respiratory droplet isolation precautions.

35. A patient who has been receiving arsenic tri-oxide (Trisenox) for promyelocytic leukemia is hospitalized with pleural and pericardial effusions. High-dose glucocorticoid therapy is initiated. When assessing the patient, the nurse notes that the patient is confused; his skin is hot and dry, and he is breathing rapidly. When reporting the patient's condition to the pre-scriber, it would be particularly important to also include results of
    a. BUN levels.
    b. deep tendon reflexes.
    c. metered blood glucose.
    d. urine output.

✳ 36. The nurse is caring for a patient who is receiv-ing denileukin diftitox (Ontak) for cutaneous T-cell lymphoma (CTCL). The drug book states that asthenia is a common adverse effect. A pri-ority nursing concern related to this potential adverse effect is
    a. hydration.
    b. infection.
    c. pain.
    d. safety.

CASE STUDIES AND PATIENT TEACHING

(Use a separate piece of paper for your responses.)

Case Study 1

The nurse works in a busy gynecologic practice. She is responsible for assisting the patients with completing an initial patient history and highlighting abnormali-ties to alert the primary care provider.

1. What information on the history would suggest an increased risk for breast cancer?

2. A 53-year-old patient has a sister who died at age 48 of metastatic breast cancer. The patient is 5 feet 4 inches and 187 lb. She asks the nurse how losing weight can decrease her risk of breast cancer. How should the nurse respond?

3. The patient has been advised to consider tamoxifen (Nolvadex) therapy because of her high risk for breast cancer. She asks the nurse how this drug will help prevent breast cancer. What explanation can the nurse provide?

4. Why is it important for the nurse to assess the patient's smoking status and recommend smoking cessation if the patient smokes and is considering tamoxifen therapy?

5. The patient has not had a menstrual period for 2 years. Why would the nurse advise this patient to come in to be seen if she experiences any vaginal bleeding?

6. What other symptoms or serious adverse effects of tamoxifen would the nurse teach the patient to report immediately?

7. Adherence to tamoxifen therapy is affected by the patient's ability to cope with adverse effects. What information can the nurse provide to this patient to assist her in dealing with the following adverse effects?
    a. Hot flushes
    b. Fluid retention
    c. Nausea and vomiting

Case Study 2

A 76-year-old male with a history of non-Hodgkin's lymphoma, chronic obstructive pulmonary disease (COPD), type 2 diabetes mellitus, atrial fibrillation, and hypothyroidism is admitted to the nursing unit with a diagnosis of community acquired pneumonia. He is pre-scribed intravenous tobramycin 120 mg 3 times a day, metformin 500 mg twice a day, diltiazem (Cardizem CD) 240 mg once a day, levothyroxine (Synthroid) 0.075 mg once a day, and tiotropium (Spiriva) inhalation once a day. Respiratory therapy is ordered every 4 hours and PRN. The patient's primary cancer site was in his lung 20 years ago, and he has experienced 7 relapses and/or metastases that have been treated with partial lung lobectomy, gastric and duodenal resection, and cyto-toxic chemotherapy. His most recent site of metastasis is the esophagus at which time he had pleural and peri-cardial effusions, requiring thoracotomy and chest tube insertion. He is currently being treated with rituximab (Rituxan). The patient's wife is very attentive, and the nurse believes that she has been a major factor in the patient's survival. The patient's wife tells the nurse that the patient's most recent prostate-specific antigen (PSA) was 8 (ng/mL). She is concerned because the oncolo-gist is not considering surgery and has not ordered any additional chemotherapy.

1. How should the nurse respond?

2. The oncologist discusses concerns that additional chemotherapy would not be effective and that the patient's overall condition makes surgery a greater risk than the cancer. He discusses therapy with tamsulosin (Flomax) for symptom relief. Why is androgen deprivation therapy not being offered in this case?

3. What nursing diagnoses should the nurse consider for this patient and his wife?

Case Study 3

A 43-year-old female with multiple myeloma has been prescribed prednisolone to decrease serum calcium and to relieve the pain of spinal cord compression.

1. What symptoms should the nurse be assessing when looking for hypercalcemia?

2. What are possible nursing issues relating to the hypercalcemia?

3. What are possible nursing issues relating to the adverse effects of high-dose glucocorticoids?

4. What are possible outcomes for glucocorticoid therapy?

Case Study 4

Cetuximab is prescribed for a patient with metastatic, EGFR-positive colorectal cancer. The chemotherapy nurse is precepting a student nurse. When reviewing drugs, the student asks why the following drugs are kept on hand in case of adverse effects.

1. What should be included in the explanation for these drugs?
   a. Epinephrine
   b. Glucocorticoids
   c. IV antihistamines
   d. Bronchodilators

2. The student asks the nurse why she is assessing the patient's lung sounds before starting the infusion. What should be included in the explanation?

3. The student nurse notes that the patient has severe acne-like lesions on most of his body. He asks the nurse why the patient is not in isolation. What would be included in the nurse's response?

Answers can be reviewed online at http://evolve.elsevier.com/Lehne/.

OBJECTIVES

See page 28 for the Objectives.

CRITICAL THINKING AND STUDY QUESTIONS

✳ 1. The most important thing that a nurse can do to prevent blindness from primary open-angle glaucoma (POAG) is
   a. administer eye medications as ordered.
   b. explain the importance of following recommendations for eye screening.
   c. identify individuals at high risk for glaucoma.
   d. teach the common symptoms of glaucoma.

✳ 2. The nurse is providing telephone guidance as a service of an insurance company. Which of the following calls most warrants referral for immediate care?
   a. Halos appearing around lights
   b. Itching and watering of eyes
   c. Sensitivity to light
   d. Severe eye pain that started 10 minutes ago

▶ 3. The nurse has performed a head-to-toe assessment on a patient who is receiving timolol optic drops (Timoptic) for POAG. Even though systemic effects of the drug are uncommon, which of the following findings would be a reason for the nurse to contact the prescriber before administering the drops? (Select all that apply.)
   a. Audible wheezing
   b. Blood pressure 170/100 mm Hg
   c. Clouding of lens of eye
   d. End inspiratory crackles
   e. Keyhole appearance to pupil
   f. Pulse 50 beats/min

▶ 4. If a brown discoloration of the iris of a patient with hazel eyes is noted on a patient receiving latanoprost (Xalatan), the nurse should
   a. administer the medication and note the finding.
   b. assess for symptoms of a migraine headache.

   c. teach the patient proper eye cleansing hygiene.
   d. withhold the medication and contact the prescriber.

✳ 5. It is important for the nurse to teach orthostatic blood pressure precautions when a patient is prescribed which of the following drugs for POAG?
   a. Apraclonidine (Iopidine)
   b. Bimatoprost (Lumigan)
   c. Brimonidine (Alphagan)
   d. Latanoprost (Xalatan)

✳ 6. The drug handbook lists retinal detachment as an uncommon, but serious adverse effect of pilocarpine used for glaucoma. The nurse determines that the patient needs more teaching if the patient includes which of the following in the list of things that he should report immediately to his ophthamologist?
   a. Floaters in the field of vision
   b. Halos around lights
   c. Light flashes
   d. Painless loss of part of his vision

✳ 7. Because of possible parasympathetic response if echothiophate (Phospholine Iodide) is absorbed into systemic circulation, it would be important to alert the prescriber if a patient who is receiving this drug develops which of the following types of infection?
   a. *Clostridium difficile*
   b. methicillin-resistant *Staphylococcus aureus* (MRSA)
   c. vancomycin-resistant enterococci (VRE)

8. A patient who has been prescribed oral acetazolamide (Diamox) for refractory POAG and experiences the adverse effects of severe vomiting and diarrhea should be monitored by the nurse for
   a. calcium greater than 11 mg/dL.
   b. capillary bloode glucose less than 70 mg/dL.
   c. potassium less than 3.5 mEq/L.
   d. sodium greater than 145 mEq/L.

9. Which of the following most likely suggests that a patient who has received mydriatic drugs is experiencing closed-angle glaucoma?
   a. Clouding of vision
   b. Headache
   c. Ocular discharge
   d. Severe sudden eye pain

10. A patient asks the nurse why his prescriber does not advise using the ocular decongestant tetrahydrozoline (Visine) for his allergic conjunctivitis. Which of the following would be included in the nurse's explanation?
    a. Benefits take several days to develop.
    b. Rebound congestion is likely.
    c. The drug can cause cataracts.
    d. The drug can elevate intraocular pressure.

11. The nurse can help decrease the progression of age-related macular degeneration (ARMD) by teaching patients at risk to
    a. have preventative laser surgery.
    b. have adequate light when reading.
    c. take specific supplements of vitamins C and E, beta carotene, zinc, and copper.
    d. wear sunscreen and sunglasses in bright light.

12. Patients with ARMD should be taught to protect their skin from light for 5 days after therapy that includes the drug
    a. brimonidine.
    b. pegaptanib.
    c. phenylephrine.
    d. verteporfin.

13. It is important for the nurse to teach a patient who had vitreous humor injection of pegaptanib (Macugen) to immediately seek medical care if which of the following occur?
    a. Blurred vision and halos
    b. Light sensitivity and pain
    c. Conjunctival redness and edema
    d. Floaters and decreased visual acuity

CASE STUDIES AND PATIENT TEACHING

(Use a separate piece of paper for your responses.)

Case Study 1

A 62-year-old female is seen by her ophthalmologist at the direction of her primary care physician (PCP). She has a history of chronic obstructive pulmonary disease (COPD), psoriasis, and breast cancer. She is accompanied by her daughter and is reluctant to seek care because her eyes are "fine." A topical anesthetic is placed in the eye, and the ophthalmologist measures her intraocular pressure (IOP) to be 23 mm Hg. Tropicamide (Tropicacyl) drops are applied, and the patient is sent to wait until mydriatic and cytoplegic effects occur.

1. What are mydriatic and cytoplegic effects, and what are their purposes in this situation?

2. After further examination, the patient is diagnosed with primary open-angle glaucoma (POAG). Her daughter asks how she could have this disease, glaucoma, and not be aware of it. How should the nurse respond?

3. The patient is prescribed latanoprost (Xalatan) 1 drop to each eye at bedtime. The prescription is denied by the patient's insurer. The prescriber changes the order to betaxolol (Betoptic) 1 drop in each eye twice a day. Why had the prescriber originally chosen latanoprost instead of betaxolol for this patient?

4. What teaching should the nurse provide the patient regarding the betaxolol prescription and her glaucoma?

5. The patient returns to the ophthalmologist to have her IOP checked. Her IOP measures at 25 mm Hg. The prescriber adds brimonidine (Alphagan) 1 drop instilled in each eye 3 times a day and dorzolamide (Trusopt) 1 drop 3 times a day. The patient asks why the prescriber did not just order the additional drops of latanoprost (Xalatan). How should the nurse respond?

6. What teaching should the nurse provide about therapy with brimonidine and dorzolamide ?

Answers can be reviewed online at http://evolve.elsevier.com/Lehne/.

OBJECTIVES

See page 28 for the Objectives.

CRITICAL THINKING AND STUDY QUESTIONS

1. The nurse is teaching the parents of a 2½-year-old child about administration of topical glucocorticoid therapy prescribed for their son's eczema. Which of the following statements, if made by a parent, would suggest a need for further teaching?
   a. "I should apply a thick film when using the cream on his chin."
   b. "I should not cover the area of the skin where the cream was applied with a bandage or any type of plastic item unless the doctor tells me to."
   c. "It is important that I only apply the cream to areas with the rash."
   d. "The cream can help stop itching so he won't scratch and get it infected."

✳ 2. A patient who was admitted for a knee replacement asks the nurse to get an order for "cortisone cream" because she has an irritated area of skin under her breast. It is most important for the nurse to
   a. explain that cortisone cream should not be used in moist areas.
   b. insist that the nurse apply the cream.
   c. keep the area covered with a dressing.
   d. assess the area and communicate findings to the prescriber.

✳ 3. The nurse is teaching an adolescent about expected and adverse effects of applying prescribed salicylic acid. A priority teaching would be instructing the patient to report
   a. feeling short of breath.
   b. flaking of skin.
   c. headache.
   d. itching in the area where the drug was applied.

4. The nurse is responsible for answering telephone questions in a dermatology practice. A patient who has recently been prescribed benzoyl peroxide calls because she has been experiencing scaling and swelling at the site of application. An expected protocol for the nurse's response normally would include
   a. continue to use the benzoyl peroxide and try an oil-based moisturizer to relieve the severe dryness.
   b. continue to use the benzoyl peroxide as prescribed because this is an expected therapeutic effect.
   c. continue to use the benzoyl peroxide, but use it less often.
   d. stop using the benzoyl peroxide.

▶ 5. A 24-year-old college student with acne asks the health center nurse if she can use her brother's unopened topical clindamycin because she does not have health insurance to pay for the clindamycin/benzoyl peroxide (BenzaClin) that has been prescribed. The basis of the nurse's response should be that the combination product
   a. causes less drying and peeling of the skin.
   b. decreases the chance that antibiotic resistance will occur.
   c. prevents allergic reactions.
   d. prevents systemic absorption of the drug components.

6. A 56-year-old patient asks the nurse what she can tell her about using tretinoin (Retin-A) to prevent wrinkles. The nurse could share the research that suggests that tretinoin
   a. causes the skin to feel softer.
   b. eliminates deep wrinkles.
   c. prevents sunburn.
   d. repairs sun-damaged skin.

7. A patient has been prescribed adapalene (Differin) for acne. Which of the following would the nurse include in teaching? (Select all that apply.)
   a. An increase in acne lesions is common early in therapy.
   b. Apply a sunscreen, such as zinc oxide, before applying the cream.
   c. Apply the cream twice a day, morning and bedtime.
   d. Expect a decrease in blackheads, whiteheads, and inflamed lesions.
   e. Stop the drug if a burning sensation or peeling of the skin occurs.
   f. Use a sunscreen every morning, even if you are not going to be outside.

8. It would be particularly important for the nurse to teach patients with a dark complexion who have been prescribed azelaic acid (Azelex) to apply the cream
   a. after washing and taking care to thoroughly dry the face.
   b. evenly but avoiding mucous membranes.
   c. only to active lesions.
   d. to every area that is red.

9. Which of the following should the nurse teach a patient to report to the prescriber when prescribed isotretinoin for severe acne? (Select all that apply.)
   a. Back pain and muscle stiffness
   b. Burns easily when out in sun
   c. Frequent nosebleeds
   d. Missed menstrual period
   e. No longer interested in normally pleasurable activities
   f. Peeling of skin from palms and soles
   g. Severe headache followed by transient blurred vision

▶ 10. The oral contraceptive, Estrostep, is prescribed for a 17-year-old female with acne who desires contraception. Developmentally, which of the following effects of the estrogen component of this drug is most likely to be a concern to this patient?
   a. Anorexia
   b. Nausea
   c. Swollen breasts
   d. Weight gain

▶ 11. A patient has been prescribed Ortho Tri-Cyclen and spironolactone (Aldactone) for contraception and treatment of acne that has been resistant to topical treatments. It is important for the patient to be instructed to report which of the following symptoms of the most likely electrolyte disturbance related to this therapy?
   a. Persistent abdominal cramps and diarrhea
   b. Persistent bone pain and constipation
   c. Persistent fatigue and cool, clammy skin
   d. Persistent thirst and flushed skin

12. The nurse teaches her family to use sunscreens that contain avobenzone because it is
   a. effective on prominent body parts such as the nose.
   b. the only ingredient that absorbs UVA1 rays.
   c. currently available in a clear formula.
   d. most efficient in reflecting the sun's rays.

13. Recent research suggests that psoriasis is caused by
   a. an inflammatory disorder.
   b. excessive production of sebum.
   c. excessive reproduction of keratinocytes.
   d. poor hygiene.

14. A patient asks the nurse why he should not use his high-potency glucocorticoid on his face. The basis of the nurse's response is that the face is especially prone to what effect of topical glucocorticoids?
   a. Acne-like eruptions
   b. Changes in pigmentation
   c. Sensitivity to sunlight
   d. Thinning of the skin

▶ 15. A patient is admitted with fatigue, nausea, vomiting, and constipation. Lab test results include Na^+ 136 mEq/L, K^+ 3.5 mEq/L, and Ca^{++} 12 mg/dL. The nurse notes red patches with silvery, flaking scales on a patient's knees, elbows, and scalp. It is important for the nurse to determine the dose and frequency of medication if this patient is being treated for psoriasis with
   a. anthralin.
   b. calcipotriene (Dovonex).
   c. tars.
   d. tazarotene (Tazorac).

▶ 16. A 28-year-old female patient is prescribed anthralin. Which of the following statements, if made by the patient, suggests a need for additional teaching?
   a. "I need to be especially careful to wash my hands after apply the cream."
   b. "It is best if I put the cream on at bedtime."
   c. "I need to cover the cream so that it does not stain my clothing."
   d. "I need to contact my prescriber if the area around my psoriasis becomes red."

▶ 17. Which of the following laboratory results for a 57-year-old female patient who is receiving methotrexate for psoriasis would be of most concern to the nurse?
   a. Alanine aminotransferase 35 international units/L
   b. Hemoglobin 12 gm/dL
   c. Platelet count 6000/mm³
   d. White blood cell (WBC) count 9000/mm³

▶ 18. The nurse would be especially vigilant with monitoring the cardiovascular system of an obese patient with severe psoriasis being treated with acitretin (Soriatane) who has a history of
   a. chronic obstructive pulmonary disease (COPD).
   b. diabetes mellitus (DM).
   c. gastroesophageal reflux disease (GERD).
   d. osteoarthritis (OA) degenerative joint disease (DJD).

19. Match the following drugs for psoriasis and their common adverse effects. (Some items have more than one answer.)

_____ a. Acitretin (Soriatane)   1. Alopecia
_____ b. Alefacept (Amevive)   2. Assess for bleeding
                                  3. Chills
_____ c. Efalizumab (Raptiva)   4. Damage to liver
                                  5. Decreased RBC count
_____ d. Etanercept (Enbrel)   6. Increased risk of cancer
                                  7. Increased risk of infection
_____ e. Methotrexate   8. Teratogenic

✳ ▶ 20. The most important intervention that a nurse can provide to prevent squamous cell carcinoma is teaching people to
   a. avoid chronic exposure of the skin to sunlight.
   b. examine moles for irregular borders.
   c. report rough scaly red-brown papules to your primary care provider.
   d. use sunscreen.

21. The nurse in a long-term care facility is administering topical fluorouracil (Carac) to an actinic keratosis lesion. Which of the following assessments suggests that therapy has achieved the desired effect and treatment can be stopped?
   a. Burning and vesicle formation
   b. Erosion, ulceration, and necrosis
   c. Mild inflammation with redness
   d. Severe inflammation and stinging

22. An important nursing teaching for patients using diclofenac gel (Solaraze) or imiquimod cream (Aldara) is to
   a. avoid sun exposure.
   b. cover the treated area with an occlusive dressing.
   c. discontinue treatment if redness or itching occurs.
   d. be aware that the medications may stain clothing.

23. Which of the following should be included in the teaching of a patient immediately after application of aminolevulinic acid for actinic keratosis areas of the face?
   a. Avoid exposing your face to sunlight.
   b. Report any burning or stinging.
   c. Use a sunscreen with SPF of at least 30 between application and blue light treatment.
   d. You need to return in 18 hours for the blue light treatment.

▶ 24. The nurse would consult with the pediatrician before administering which of the following immunizations if a child is prescribed topical tacrolimus (Protopic) for atopic dermatitis?
   a. Prevnar (pneumococcal)
   b. Recombivax HB (hepatitis B)
   c. Tripedia (DTaP)
   d. Varivax (varicella)

✳▶ 25. Which of the following laboratory results for a 27-year-old female patient who is receiving podophyllum (Podocon-25) for genital warts would be most important for the nurse to report to the gynecologist administering treatment?
   a. Alanine aminotransferase 35 international units/L
   b. hCG positive
   c. Hemoglobin 12 gm/dL
   d. White blood cell (WBC) count 5000/mm³

26. A patient is convinced that the aluminum in antiperspirants causes breast cancer and asks a nurse how deodorants work. The basis of the nurse's response is that deodorants
    a. cover odor with a pleasant fragrance.
    b. decrease flow of apocrine but not eccrine sweat glands.
    c. inhibit release of acetylcholine.
    d. slow growth of skin bacteria.

27. The principle of treatment for seborrheic dermatitis is suppression of
    a. cellular reproduction.
    b. growth of yeasts.
    c. histamine release.
    d. scalp oil production.

28. A 34-year-old male asks the nurse about finasteride (Propecia) used to prevent baldness. Which of the following best suggests an understanding of the drug's effects?
    a. "It doesn't work on everyone but it can't hurt to try."
    b. "It could help my wife's thinning hair also."
    c. "I need to think about the bad effects before deciding if this is for me."
    d. "It work great but you have to keep taking them."

29. The expected therapeutic effect of eflornithine (Vaniqua) is
    a. finer, lighter hair growth.
    b. removal of unwanted facial hair.
    c. halted growth of unwanted facial hair.

30. The nurse would expect an order for which of the following preparations for a patient who tests positive for methicillin-resistant *Staphylococcus aureus* (MRSA) on nasal swab?
    a. Mupirocin
    b. Neosporin
    c. Retapamulin
    d. Vancomycin

31. A patient asks the nurse why botulinum toxin (Botox) injections have to be repeated. The best answer to this question includes
    a. discussion of the half-life of the drug.
    b. enzyme degradation of the toxin.
    c. neurons grow new terminals.
    d. reactivation of vesicles.

▸ 32. The nurse is providing information to a patient who regularly takes aspirin and is considering botulinum toxin (Botox) injections. It is recommended that a patient avoid aspirin for a week preceding treatment. It would be important for the nurse to inform the patient not to discontinue taking aspirin without consulting the prescriber if the aspirin is being taken for
    a. analgesia.
    b. fever reduction.
    c. joint pain.
    d. platelet inhibition.

CASE STUDIES AND PATIENT TEACHING

(Use a separate piece of paper for your responses.)

Case Study 1

The nurse identifies that body image is a priority concern when collecting data from a 46-year-old patient who is being seen in the dermatology practice. The patient has heard of friends using tretinoin (Renova) to prevent aging of the skin. She asks if this drug really works.

1. What information can the nurse provide?

2. The patient is concerned about cost and asks if tretinoin is better than face creams that you can buy in the drugstore. What does research suggest on this topic?

3. The patient and prescriber agree that tretinoin (Renova) is appropriate for this patient. What information can the nurse provide when she asks how this differs from the tretinoin (Retin-A Micro) prescribed for her daughter's acne?

4. What teaching should the nurse provide about use of tretinoin products?

5. The patient reports that she has always used a sunscreen of at least SPF 30 and reapplies it regularly because she enjoys activities out in the sun. What teaching about skin protection should the nurse provide to this patient?

Case Study 2

An 18-year-old female high school senior is being seen at the dermatology office after treatment with antibiotics, benzoyl peroxide, tretinoin (Rein-A Micro), and adapalene (Differin) over the past 2 years have failed to provide acceptable results.

1. What data needs to be collected when the prescriber is considering treatment with isotretinoin (Accutane?)

2. The dermatologist has decided to prescribe isotretinoin (Accutane) and has asked the office nurse to reinforce teaching regarding this drug. What are some nursing diagnoses that should be included when planning teaching relating to this patient, this diagnosis, and this treatment?

3. How should the nurse respond to the patient's question of how isotretinoin therapy differs from tretinoin?

4. Because patients do not always remember what is explained to them, what teaching methods besides oral explanation should the nurse provide to this patient?

5. What teaching must the nurse provide this patient regarding the iPLEDGE program?

Case Study 3

When preparing a 3-year-old for a well child check, a nurse who works in a pediatric office learns that the family is leaving for a vacation to the beach.

1. What information should be included in teaching about protecting the skin from sun damage?

105

Drugs for the Ear

Answers can be reviewed online at http://evolve.elsevier.com/Lehne/.

OBJECTIVES

See page 28 for the Objectives.

CRITICAL THINKING AND STUDY QUESTIONS

1. Which of the following is true regarding acute otitis media (AOM)? (Select all that apply.)
   a. AOM can be caused by eustachian tube malfunction.
   b. Presence of otalgia suggests serious complications have occurred.
   c. In an otherwise healthy child with AOM, it is more important to treat the pain than the infecting microbe.
   d. AOM primarily occurs in children aged 5 to 12 years.
   e. Treatment of bacterial AOM should always include antibiotics.

2. The nurse is caring for a 2-year-old child. When bathing the child, the nurse notes sticky, crusting exudate filling the right external ear canal. The nurse would use which of the following terms when documenting this finding?
   a. Otalgia
   b. Otitis media
   c. Otorrhea
   d. Otosclerosis

✳ 3. A child who was a preemie and weighs 10 pounds at 3 months is prescribed amoxicillin 200 mg to be administered twice a day for AOM. The pharmacy supplies an oral suspension of 250 mg/mL. For each dose, the nurse administers
   a. 0.08 mL measured in a 1-mL syringe.
   b. 0.8 mL measured in either a needleless 1-mL or 3-mL syringe.
   c. 1.25 mL measured in a needleless 3-mL syringe.
   d. 1.25 mL measured in needleless 1-mL and 3-mL syringes.

4. Which of the following assessment findings in a child receiving amoxicillin would be a reason for the parent to contact the prescriber?
   a. Allergy to clarithromycin
   b. Diarrhea
   c. Facial rash that is maculopapular and does not itch
   d. Multiple intensely itchy and swollen raised areas on the skin of the chest and back

5. The most significant reason why prophylactic antibiotic therapy for recurrent otitis media is not currently recommended is because it
   a. increases the development of antibiotic resistance.
   b. involves the use of drugs that stain the teeth.
   c. frequently causes diarrhea.
   d. is too expensive.

6. Recommendations for acute otitis externa include instilling into the ear canal a 2% solution of the acid found in
   a. alcohol.
   b. oranges.
   c. peroxide.
   d. vinegar.

7. The nurse is doing telephone triage in a primary care office. A patient calls complaining of ear pain. Which of the following information would warrant the patient being seen immediately? (Select all that apply.)
   a. Child less than 12 years of age
   b. Elderly diabetic
   c. History of impacted cerumen
   d. Immunocompromised
   e. Pain when the outer ear is touched
   f. Purulent otic discharge
   g. Uses cotton swabs regularly to clean ear canal

8. Which of the following childhood vaccinations has been shown to decrease the need for tympanostomy tubes related to AOM?
   a. DTaP
   b. MMR
   c. OPV
   d. PVC

9. Amoxicillin-clavulanate is used for antibiotic-resistant acute otitis media because the clavulanate
   a. allows for a lower dose of amoxicillin.
   b. decreases incidence of adverse effects.
   c. increases antibacterial action against *Streptococcus pneumoniae*.
   d. prevents destruction of the antibiotic by bacterial enzymes.

CASE STUDIES AND PATIENT TEACHING

(Use a separate piece of paper for your responses.)

Case Study 1

A pregnant mother has brought her 2 ½-year-old child to the pediatrician because he was fussy all last night. The pediatric nurse practitioner (PNP) diagnoses acute otitis media (AOM), but does not prescribe an antibiotic.

1. What factors did the PNP consider when deciding whether or not to treat with an antibiotic?

2. The mother is upset and complains to the office nurse that she always received a prescription in the past when her older son had an ear infection. What should the nurse include in the explanation of why antibiotics are not being prescribed?

3. What drug treatment should be provided for this child?

4. What symptoms should the nurse teach the mother to report regarding the need for the child to be brought back for re-evaluation?

5. The nurse notes that this child has had multiple episodes of otitis media. What teaching can the nurse provide that may decrease the incidence of otitis media for this child and the new sibling when born?

Case Study 2

A patient has been prescribed Cipro HC drops for otitis externa.

1. What information should the nurse include when teaching about administration of these drops?

2. What technique should the nurse use to evaluate the learning if the child's mother does not appear to understand oral instruction?

3. The patient asks if she can use old drops from a previous infection. What should the nurse include in her response?

4. The nurse notes that the patient has had repeated episodes of otitis externa. What teaching can the nurse provide that might decrease the number of episodes?

106
Miscellaneous Noteworthy Drugs

Answers can be reviewed online at http://evolve.elsevier.com/Lehne/.

OBJECTIVES

See page 28 for the Objectives.

CRITICAL THINKING AND STUDY QUESTIONS

✱▶ 1. A priority nursing diagnosis for a patient with pulmonary hypertension is
   a. decreased cardiac output.
   b. fatigue.
   c. fluid volume deficit.
   d. ineffective airway clearance.

2. The nurse has been caring for a patient who is receiving an intravenous drip of epoprostenol (Flolan) for pulmonary hypertension. Which of the following symptoms suggest that the patient may be developing a septic state?
   a. Facial flushing
   b. Drop of 10 beats per minute in pulse from baseline
   c. Drop of 30 mm Hg in systolic BP from baseline
   d. Increase in temperature from 97.8°F at 0800 to 99°F at 1600

▶ 3. When administering bosentan (Tracleer) to a patient admitted with pulmonary arterial hypertension (PAH), which of the following nursing assessments would indicate that therapy is achieving the desired effect?
   a. Blood pressure 110/70 mm Hg
   b. Jugular venous pulsation 2.5 cm above sternal angle
   c. Lower extremity peripheral edema decreased from 3+ to 2+ bilaterally
   d. Peak expiratory volume (PEV) 75% of best

✱▶ 4. A priority nursing instruction to a patient with PAH who is receiving iloprost (Ventavis) is
   a. change positions slowly.
   b. cough and deep breathe.
   c. do not cross your legs.
   d. use pursed-lip breathing.

✱▶ 5. Which of these laboratory test results, if identified for a patient who is receiving bosentan (Tracleer), should the nurse report to the prescriber immediately?
   a. BNP 87 pg/mL
   b. Creatinine 1.4 mg/dL
   c. hCG positive
   d. Urine leukocyte esterase positive

▶ 6. The most recent ALT result for a patient receiving bosentan (Tracleer) is 85 international units/L. The nurse should
   a. administer the drug as prescribed.
   b. withhold the drug and consult with the prescriber regarding a dose decrease or interruption.
   c. withhold the drug and consult with the prescriber regarding discontinuing the drug.

7. Which of the following statements, if made by a patient who has just been prescribed sildenafil (Revatio) for PAH, would warrant teaching to prevent a possible fatal reaction?
   a. "I know I should exercise more but I often do not have enough energy."
   b. "I use aspirin when I get a headache because I also heard that it is good fro my heart."
   c. "I use the little tablets that dissolve under the tongue that the doctor prescribed for my wife when I get chest pain."
   d. "My hearing is not as good as it used to be."

∗▸ 8. The nurse is performing an abdominal assessment on a septic patient who is receiving drug therapy with drotrecogin alfa activated (DrotAA, Xigris). Which of the following assessment findings suggests a critical complication of therapy with this drug warranting immediate consultation with the prescriber?
   a. Distended abdomen
   b. Hyperactive bowel sounds
   c. Hypoactive bowel sounds
   d. Rigid abdomen

9. The recommended dose of drotrecogin alfa activated (DrotAA, Xigris) is 24 mcg/kg/hr. What is the recommended hourly dose for a patient who weighs 137.5 lb?

▸ 10. A patient is prescribed 1.5 mg/hr of drotrecogin alfa activated (DrotAA, Xigris). The drug is reconstituted in normal saline solution (NSS) at a concentration of 100 mcg/mL. The infusion pump is calibrated in mL/hr. What rate of infusion should be programmed into the pump?

▸ 11. Which of the following laboratory results would warrant consulting the prescriber of drotrecogin alfa activated (DrotAA, Xigris)?
   a. ALT 400 international units/L
   b. INR 3
   c. Platelet count 40,000,000/mL
   d. RBC 4.5 10^6/mcL

∗▸ 12. The nurse is administering intramuscular (IM) dexamethasone to a pregnant woman who is at risk for premature delivery of the fetus. The patient's skin is hot and dry, and the patient is voiding 200 to 250 mL every hour. Which diagnostic test results should the nurse check at this time?
   a. BUN
   b. Creatinine
   c. SMBG
   d. Urine specific gravity

∗▸ 13. A priority nursing diagnosis relating to administration of beractant (Survanta) to a premature neonate is related to the risk of
   a. airway clearance impairment.
   b. deficient fluid volume.
   c. hypothermia.
   d. ineffective breast-feeding.

▸ 14. For maximal therapeutic results, dornase alfa (Pulmozyme) should be administered to patients with cystic fibrosis
   a. after chest physiotherapy.
   b. after meals.
   c. before chest physiotherapy.
   d. before meals.

▸ 15. The nurse is caring for a 15-year-old girl who has been admitted in a sickle cell crisis. The patient complains of severe joint pain (10 of 10). The nurse notes that the child is sitting quietly in bed conversing with her parents. Intravenous morphine 0.5 mg and oral ibuprofen 200 mg are ordered every 3 hours as needed. The patient has not had any analgesic medication in the past 3 hours. The nurse should
   a. administer the ibuprofen.
   b. administer the morphine.
   c. assess for other physiologic indicators of pain.
   d. provide nonpharmacologic pain relief measures.

16. A 16-year-old with sickle cell anemia has been prescribed hydroxyurea (Droxia). Developmentally, which nursing problems would be of most concern relating to this drug therapy?
    a. Adherence to prescribed regimen
    b. Body image
    c. Infection
    d. Tissue perfusion

17. A toddler has come to the outpatient oncology clinic for an infusion of rasburicase (Elitek) to be administered daily for 5 days before the start of chemotherapy. The nursing plan of care should address prevention and relief of the most common adverse effect of this therapy, including the possible need for an
    a. analgesic.
    b. antidiarrheal.
    c. antiemetic.
    d. antihistamine.

18. When a patient is receiving riluzole (Rilutek) for amyotrophic lateral sclerosis (ALS), it is most important for the nurse to assess for which of the following symptoms of the underlying condition?
    a. Dizziness
    b. Nausea and vomiting
    c. Respiratory distress
    d. Weakness

19. A patient with end-stage renal disease (ESRD) who receives hemodialysis is prescribed calcium carbonate (PhosLo) to lower blood phosphate. In order to achieve maximum binding of phosphate and minimal absorption of the calcium, the drug should be administered
    a. first thing in the morning.
    b. at least 1 hour before meals.
    c. at least 2 hours after meals.
    d. with meals.

20. The nurse is caring for a patient who is prescribed sevelamer HCl (Renagel) to prevent hyperphosphatemia of ESRD. Which of the following respiratory changes suggests that the patient may be experiencing metabolic acidosis?
    a. Deep exhalations
    b. Diminished lung sounds
    c. Lower lobe crackles (rales)
    d. Sonorous gurgles (rhonchi)

CASE STUDIES AND PATIENT TEACHING

(Use a separate piece of paper for your responses.)

Case Study 1

A 14-year-old female with cystic fibrosis has come to the emergency department because of sudden onset of shaking chills, fever 102.5°F, and greenish-colored sputum. She tells the nurse that she is worse than she was 6 months ago. Her last airway studies show a decreased vital capacity and increased residual volume. She appears very depressed. The patient is 5 feet tall and weighs 80 pounds. She is being admitted to the adult unit since the adolescent unit has no beds. This upsets the patient because she is a frequent patient and knows the adolescent unit staff well. The nurse begins planning care.

1. What are some possible nursing diagnoses for this patient?

2. The nurse is having difficulty reaching the patient's primary care provider to obtain orders for the patient's routine enzymes. Why is it so important to promptly obtain these orders?

3. The patient snaps at the nurse when she brings the enzymes one-half hour after lunch was served. How should the nurse respond?

Case Study 2

A 22-month-old African-American child is admitted to a pediatric hospital because of fever, irritability, jaundice, and unremitting malaise. Laboratory test results reveal anemia and presence of hemoglobin S, confirming the diagnosis of sickle cell disease. The boy's mother asks the nurse why his eyes are so yellow.

1. What would be the logical explanation for jaundice in sickle cell disease?

2. The mother has heard of a new drug, hydroxyurea, and asks why it has not been prescribed for her child. The best explanation is that the drug
    a. has adverse effects.
    b. has only been approved for patients who are ages 18 and older.
    c. is an orphan drug.
    d. is only used as a last resort.

3. The mother asks the nurse if there is anything that she can do to prevent her child from experiencing sickle cell crises. How should the nurse respond?

Case Study 3

A 38-year-old female patient who is prescribed thalidomide (Thalomid) for multiple myeloma complains to the nurse of the need to obtain a pregnancy test within

24 hours before the first dose, every 2 weeks for a month, then once a menstrual cycle. She states that she has had regular periods and has been using the same oral contraceptives without problems for many years.

1. What information should the nurse provide to this patient'?

107
Dietary Supplements

Answers can be reviewed online at http://evolve.elsevier.com/Lehne/.

OBJECTIVES

See page 28 for the Objectives.

CRITICAL THINKING AND STUDY QUESTIONS

1. Match the dietary products to their primary use.

_____ a. Black cohosh
_____ b. Echinacea
_____ c. Feverfew
_____ d. Garlic
_____ e. Ginger root
_____ f. *Ginkgo biloba*
_____ g. Flaxseed
_____ h. Ma Huang (ephedra)
_____ i. St John's wort
_____ j. Saw palmetto
_____ k. Valerian

1. Benign prostatic hyperplasia
2. Decrease triglycerides
3. Depression
4. Improve memory
5. Migraine headache prophylaxis
6. Morning sickness of pregnancy
7. PMS and menopause symptoms
8. Prevent colds
9. Promote sleep
10. Constipation
11. Weight loss

2. Health concerns about the use of herbal products include which of the following statements? (Select all that apply.)
   a. Products marketed as dietary supplements did not require rigorous evaluation before marketing.
   b. The FDA could not remove the product from the market even if there is evidence that it causes harm.

c. The product may have contained harmful ingredients such as arsenic, mercury, and lead.
   d. The product may not have contained the stated ingredients in the amount listed on the label.
   e. Their labels could claim to treat disease without adequate research supporting the claim.
   f. There was no evidence that any of these products are effective or safe.

3. Lack of oversight of the accuracy of an herbal product's label can be particularly dangerous for patients who are
   a. allergic to inert ingredients often found in pills.
   b. in lower socioeconomic groups.
   c. using a generic brand of a product.
   d. using the product to promote health.

4. The 2007 ruling on Current Good Manufacturing Practices (CGMPs) of dietary supplements seeks to (Select all that apply.)
   a. eliminate contaminants in herbal products.
   b. ensure accuracy of labels on herbal products.
   c. ensure the herb produces the effect that it claims to produce.
   d. ensure potency of the herbal product.
   e. ensure the herbal product is safe.
   f. protect small companies by phasing in regulations with small companies affected last.

5. The nurse should teach a patient who chooses to use an herbal product that it is best to
   a. always buy the more expensive brand.
   b. take the herb with at least 8 ounces of water.
   c. use products that have the seal of approval from the USP.
   d. use the lowest dose possible.

✳ 6. The priority nursing action when a nurse discovers that a patient self-prescribes herbal products is to
   a. assess for adverse effects of the product.
   b. be an advocate for the patient's right to make choices.
   c. convince the patient to stop taking the products.
   d. teach the patient the importance of informing all healthcare providers of all products being used.

7. A patient who is taking metronidazole is at risk for a drug interaction if also taking an herbal product in which of the following forms?
   a. Decoctions, teas, and infusions
   b. Fluid extracts and tinctures
   c. Glycerites
   d. Solid extracts

8. Which of the following laboratory tests would be important for the nurse to monitor if a patient with heart failure was prescribed warfarin and self-prescribes coenzyme Q-10?
   a. ALT
   b. CBC
   c. INR
   d. Sodium

9. Research suggests that possible effects of cranberry juice include
   a. increasing excretion of bacteria.
   b. making urine acidic, which kills bacteria.
   c. preventing bacteria from adhering to the bladder wall.
   d. preventing kidney stones.

10. Based on German studies, it is important for the nurse to teach postmenopausal women who are taking black cohosh for hot flashes and insomnia to
   a. avoid prolonged exposure to the sun.
   b. change positions slowly.
   c. drink adequate amounts of fluids.
   d. stop taking the herb if you experience a headache.

11. Pregnant nurses should wear gloves if they are administering which of the following herbal supplements?
   a. Aloe
   b. Feverfew
   c. Ginger
   d. Saw palmetto

12. Echinacea (Select all that apply.)
   a. can aggravate autoimmune disorders.
   b. can produce an allergic reaction the first time taken in patients allergic to ragweed.
   c. can stimulate the immune system.
   d. can suppress the immune system.
   e. decreases the severity of the common cold.
   f. prevents symptoms of the common cold.
   g. should be avoided by people with immune suppression.

▶ 13. The nurse is assessing a new admission. The patient lists echinacea, garlic, and kava among the products that she uses regularly. On first observation, the nurse notes that the patient's skin has a yellowish color. The most appropriate action for the nurse to take next is to
   a. continue to assess the patient.
   b. document jaundice in the nursing note.
   c. notify the healthcare provider of the findings stat.
   d. tell the patient to stop taking the herbal products.

14. A patient who regularly takes feverfew to prevent migraine headaches stopped taking the herb before elective surgery. The nurse should assess the patient for possible adverse effects of discontinuation of this therapy, including
   a. bleeding.
   b. flatulence.
   c. insomnia.
   d. nausea.

15. A patient who is prescribed glipizide (Glucatrol) for type 2 diabetes mellitus and celecoxib (Celebrex) for inflamed joints informs the nurse that she has started taking ginger because she read in a magazine that it helps arthritis. It would be most important for the nurse to teach this patient what to do if she experiences which of the following adverse effects?
   a. Bruising with minor injuries
   b. Headache
   c. Loss of appetite
   d. Palpitations and sweating

16. Patients who are at risk for seizures should be cautioned about taking ginkgo, especially in combination with
    a. analgesics.
    b. antihistamines.
    c. antipyretics.
    d. laxatives.

17. An appropriate outcome for a 6-month-old infant relating to Culturelle prescribed during a rotavirus infection is
    a. soft, formed stool.
    b. no bacterial growth in urine.
    c. temperature 98°F to 99°F.
    d. no adventitious lung sounds.

18. A priority concern for the nurse when a patient with multiple medical disorders self-prescribes St John's wort is
    a. affect on other prescribed drugs.
    b. constipation.
    c. photosensitivity.
    d. potency of the preparation.

19. The nurse is aware that which of the following herbal supplements has been associated with liver failure?
    a. Black cohosh
    b. Ginger
    c. Kava
    d. Valerian

▶ 20. The nurse is caring for a patient who regularly uses Ma Huang (ephedra) for weight loss. It is important for the nurse to
    a. assess mental status.
    b. monitor vital signs.
    c. not administer any other sedatives.
    d. weigh the patient daily.

21. The nurse should monitor the patient for bleeding if the patient uses which of the following herbal products? (Select all that apply.)
    a. Aloe
    b. Black cohosh
    c. Echinacea
    d. Feverfew
    e. Garlic
    f. Ginger

g. *Ginkgo biloba*
h. Goldenseal
i. Kava
j. Ma Huang (ephedra)
k. St John's wort
l. Saw palmetto
m. Valerian

CASE STUDIES AND PATIENT TEACHING

(Use a separate piece of paper for your responses.)

Case Study 1

A 52-year-old man is admitted with chest pain. Assessment findings include height 5 feet, 8 inches, weight 220 lb, waist circumference 42 inches, BP 145/86 mm Hg, and pulse 78 beats/min. Lab results include triglycerides 380 mg/dL, LDL 240 mg/dL, and HDL 34 mg/dL. He is diagnosed with gastroesophageal reflux disease (GERD) and metabolic syndrome. He informs his healthcare provider that he wants to try natural therapy and has heard that garlic can help many things. The healthcare provider asks the nurse to discuss therapy with garlic with this patient.

1. What are possible positive effects of garlic supplementation for this patient?

2. The healthcare provider recommends enteric-coated garlic supplement. What can the nurse teach the patient to ensure that the product that he purchases contains effective amounts of allicin?

3. The patient insists on using raw garlic. What information should the nurse provide about raw garlic therapy?

4. Why is it important for the patient to inform all healthcare providers and his pharmacist that he is using garlic therapy?

Case Study 2

An 85-year-old with atrial fibrillation is being treated with digoxin (Lanoxin) and warfarin (Coumadin). At times, she is fatigued and forgetful. Her friend suggests that she take ginkgo to give her more energy.

1. What possible complications can occur with this combination of drugs and herbs?

2. What teaching should the nurse provide this patient regarding the use of herbal products?

3. The patient informs the nurse that she is not going to get her annual flu shot because she has purchased a bottle of echinacea. How would the nurse respond?

108
Management of Poisoning

Answers can be reviewed online at http://evolve.elsevier.com/Lehne/.

OBJECTIVES

See page 28 for the Objectives.

CRITICAL THINKING AND STUDY QUESTIONS

✻ 1. The initial priority of nursing care of a patient with a suspected poisoning is
   a. administering an antidote.
   b. identifying the poison.
   c. preventing absorption of poison that has not been absorbed.
   d. removing residual poison that has not been absorbed.

▶ 2. A person with an unknown medical history arrives at the emergency department (ED) after ingesting an unidentified poison. The patient is comatose when arriving at the ED. An intravenous (IV) line of normal saline is infusing, respirations are unlabored at 17 breaths per minute, and BP is 118/72 mm Hg. Which of the following assessment findings suggest hypoglycemia? (Select all that apply)
   a. Capillary refill 2-3 seconds
   b. Diaphoresis
   c. DTR 2+
   d. Dry mucous membranes
   e. Pulse 108 beats/min

3. The nurse knows that the most accurate and efficient method of identifying the poison and the dose is
   a. analysis of body fluids by a laboratory.
   b. evaluation of patient symptoms.
   c. examining the container.
   d. interviewing the caregiver.

4. The purpose of an antidote to a poison is to
   a. increase renal excretion of the poison.
   b. prevent absorption of the poison.
   c. remove residual poison from the gastrointestinal (GI) tract.
   d. reverse the effects of the poison.

5. Household stocking of over-the-counter sale of syrup of ipecac, an emetic, was promoted in the past for noncaustic poisoning. This is no longer routinely recommended primarily because it
   a. causes electrolyte imbalances.
   b. does not work.
   c. involves complicated directions.
   d. may delay seeking time-sensitive professional care.

6. Charcoal is most effective in binding with poisons in the GI tract and preventing absorption if administered
   a. after syrup of ipecac.
   b. after the patient has vomited.
   c. within 30 minutes of poison ingestion.
   d. for fat soluble poisons.

▸ 7. The nurse assessing a 3-year-old patient who is receiving 0.5 L/hr of polyethylene glycol (GoLYTELY) via nasogastric (NG) tube after the child ingested 60 tablets of adult iron supplement. Which of the following assessment findings would be of most concern to the nurse?
   a. BP 80/52 mm Hg
   b. Hyperactive bowel sound in right upper quadrant (RUQ) and absent in left lower quadrant (LLQ)
   c. Pulse 120 beats/min
   d. 475 mL of yellow-tinged liquid stool in past hour

8. A child has ingested several bottles of children's chewable aspirin (acetylsalicylic acid). The ED resident informs the nurse that treatment will include enhancing renal excretion of the drug. The nurse would question orders for all of the following substances except
   a. acetic acid.
   b. ammonium chloride.
   c. citric acid.
   d. sodium bicarbonate.

9. A patient has been treated for poisoning by hemoperfusion, which passes blood over an absorbent resin. The nurse should monitor the patient for
   a. bleeding.
   b. dehydration.
   c. hyperglycemia.
   d. seizures.

10. Match the following chelating agents and the metal(s) they bind with.

   _____ a. Deferoxamine (Desferal)
   _____ b. Dimercaprol (BAL in oil)
   _____ c. Edetate calcium disodium (Calcium EDTA)
   _____ d. Fomepizole (Antizole)
   _____ e. Penicillamine (Depen)
   _____ f. Succimer (Chemet)

   1. Arsenic
   2. Copper
   3. Ethylene glycol (antifreeze)
   4. Gold
   5. Iron
   6. Lead
   7. Mercury

11. A patient is being treated for acute ferric iron poisoning with deferoxamine (Desferal). The nurse knows that this drug works by
   a. binding with iron in the blood, causing excretion in the urine.
   b. binding with iron in the GI tract, preventing absorption.
   c. flushing the GI tract.
   d. inducing vomiting.

▸ 12. A nurse assesses the vital signs of a patient who is being treated for ferric iron poisoning with IV deferoxamine (Desferal). Which of the following findings suggests that the administration rate of the drug might be too rapid?
   a. Blood pressure 150/85 mm Hg
   b. Pulse 105 beats/min
   c. Respirations 15 breaths per minute
   d. Temperature 100.4 °F (38 °C)

13. The nurse is teaching a patient who has been prescribed deferasirox (Exjade) for iron overload associated with beta-thalassemia. Which of the following statements, if made by the patient, suggests a need for additional instruction?
   a. "I need to have bloodwork done as directed to make sure that the drug dose and my kidneys are okay."
   b. "I need to crush the tablet and mix it with a full glass of juice."
   c. "I should stop taking this drug if I have a fever higher than 100.4 °F."
   d. "If I take this with a drug for heartburn, it won't be absorbed."

▸ 14. Which of the following would be an appropriate technique when the nurse is administering dimercaprol (BAL in oil)?
   a. Deep injection into the dorsogluteal muscle
   b. Subcutaneous injection into abdominal fat
   c. Subcutaneous injection above the vastus lateralis
   d. Z-track injection into the ventrogluteal muscle

15. The nurse is caring for a 3-year-old who weighs 15 kg and is scheduled to receive an intramuscular dose of edetate calcium EDTA for lead poisoning. The child's urinary output has averaged 15 mL/hr for the last 4 hours. The nurse should
    a. administer the drug and continue nursing care.
    b. consult the prescriber regarding the need for additional fluids.
    c. withhold the medication and consult the prescriber.
    d. withhold the medication and assess for renal failure.

16. To detect serious adverse effects, it is most important for the nurse to monitor the results of which laboratory test when caring for a patient with Wilson's disease who is receiving penicillamine (Depen)?
    a. Alanine aminotransferase
    b. Blood urea nitrogen
    c. Complete blood count and differential (CBC and diff)
    d. Creatinine

17. The nurse would withhold calcium EDTA and contact the prescriber if which of the following laboratory test results occur?
    a. Albumin 5 g/dL.
    b. Amylase 190 international units/L
    c. Protein total 8.3 g/dL
    d. Protein in urine 287 mg/dL

18. A child who was admitted after ingesting antifreeze is treated with fomepizole (Antizole). The prescriber orders a loading dose followed by doses every 12 hours. The child's kidneys are failing and hemodialysis is ordered. The nurse should consult the prescriber regarding
    a. extending the time between doses.
    b. shortening the time between doses.
    c. lowering the dose of fomepizole (Antizole).
    d. raising the dose of fomepizole (Antizole).

19. The nurse teaches parents that dialing 1-800-222-1222 will connect them with
    a. the national poison center.
    b. a pharmacist.
    c. a local certified poison center.
    d. a specially trained nurse.

CASE STUDIES AND PATIENT TEACHING

(Use a separate piece of paper for your responses.)

Case Study 1

A 4-year-old, who has been playing outside in her yard, comes in the house and says she doesn't feel well. Her mother notices a purple stain on the child's face. Knowing that they do not have any grape juice in the house, the mother asks her daughter what she has eaten. The child tells her about some berries she found in the yard. The mother calls the poison control center and the child is rushed to the ED of the hospital.

1. Why didn't the poison control center recommend syrup of ipecac?

2. When the nurse questions the mother, she describes "weeds" growing at the back of the yard with blueberry-size purple berries that her daughter may have ingested. What should be done to identify the ingested substance?

3. The stomach contents contain a noncaustic neurotoxin. What data can the nurse collect to assist the emergency physician with deciding if charcoal, gastric lavage, or whole bowel irrigation is the best approach for this poisoning?

4. The mother is sure that the ingestion of the poison occurred less than 30 minutes ago. Gastric lavage and aspiration is ordered. What is the nurse's role?

5. The child is stabilized and observed overnight. What instruction should the nurse provide this family before discharge?

Case Study 2

A patient has been admitted after being accidentally sprayed with a toxic liquid.

1. What procedure should the nursing staff take to decontaminate the patient while protecting themselves?

Answers can be reviewed online at http://evolve.elsevier.com/Lehne/.

OBJECTIVES

See page 28 for the Objectives.

CRITICAL THINKING AND STUDY QUESTIONS

1. Which of the following symptoms suggest a smallpox infection?
   a. Headache, high fever, chills, and rigors
   b. Multiple red spots on the tongue and buccal mucosa
   c. Painless ulcers with a necrotic core that develop black eschar
   d. Tender, enlarged, inflamed lymph nodes

2. The basis of nursing actions to prevent transmission when *Bacillus anthracis* presence is suspected is based on the knowledge that
   a. dividing bacteria produces spores when adequate nutrition is present.
   b. mature bacteria can survive for long periods in a moist, dark environment.
   c. spores can survive for long periods in many environmental conditions.
   d. the bacteria is easily transmitted from person to person.

3. Which of the following statements, if made by a patient receiving ciprofloxacin for cutaneous anthrax, would indicate understanding of drug therapy teaching?
   a. "I must take all of the prescription as directed because if I do not serious illness and death could occur."
   b. "I should take the antibiotic until the scabs fall off."
   c. "If I start the antibiotic immediately, there is a chance that I will not experience itchy vesicles."
   d. "My prescription needs to be changed if I get pregnant."

4. The community health nurse, who works in areas known to have the presence of *B. anthracis*, promotes routine vaccination with anthrax vaccine (BioThrax) for
   a. police.
   b. postal workers.
   c. receptionists.
   d. sheep farmers.

5. Intramuscular streptomycin 0.5 gm twice a day is prescribed for a 150-lb adult male who has been diagnosed with tularemia. The drug is provided in a solution of 100 mg/mL. Nursing assessments before administration of the drug include BP 140/72 mm Hg, pulse 88 beats/min, respirations 24 breaths per minute, moist cough, and end inspiratory crackles in upper lobes. The nurse should
   a. administer the drug and consult the prescriber regarding the dose.
   b. administer the drug as one injection in the dorsogluteal site.
   c. wear a high-efficiency particulate mask when administering the drug.
   d. withhold the drug and consult the prescriber.

6. A patient is admitted with a diagnosis of pneumonic plague. Which of the following precautions would be needed to prevent spread of this infection?
   a. Airborne precautions
   b. Contact precautions
   c. Droplet precautions
   d. Prophylactic vaccination of staff

7. The public health nurse is administering smallpox vaccine (Dryvax) to police officers. Which of the following statements, if made by a vaccination recipient, would indicate a need for further teaching?
   a. "I should keep the site covered to avoid spreading the live vaccine."
   b. "I should report any drainage that occurs from the vaccination site."

c. "It is important that I not get pregnant for at least 4 weeks after receiving this vaccination."

d. "This vaccination should be effective even if I was exposed to smallpox yesterday."

8. The Department of Health and Human Services has contracted to buy the modified vaccinia virus Ankara (MVA) instead of vaccinia virus (Dryvax) in case of a terrorist attack with smallpox because MVA
   a. is safe for immunocompromised people.
   b. does not have a risk of postvaccinal encephalitis or cardiac problems.
   c. is the only drug approved by the FDA.
   d. is less expensive and more effective than Dryvax.

▶ 9. The nurse is preparing to vaccinate a person who has been exposed to the smallpox virus. The patient states that she is pregnant. The nurse should
   a. administer the vaccine.
   b. administer cidofovir before administering the smallpox vaccine.
   c. assess if the patient has been informed of benefits and risks of vaccination.
   d. withhold the vaccine.

✳▶10. The most important nursing priority for a patient with botulism poisoning is
   a. effective breathing.
   b. impaired mobility.
   c. swallowing ability.
   d. visual acuity.

▶ 11. The nurse is providing emergency care after a disaster at a nuclear power plant that caused the release of radioactive material. Which of the following doses of potassium iodide should be administered to a 16-year-old pregnant female?
   a. None
   b. 65 mg daily
   c. 130 mg daily
   d. 195 mg daily

▶ 12. To prevent magnesium deficiency when receiving zinc trisodium (Zn-DTPA), the nurse teaches a patient to include adequate amounts of which of the following foods?
   a. Eggs
   b. Liver
   c. Red meat
   d. Whole grains

13. Which of the following statements, if made by a patient who has been prescribed Ca-DPTA therapy for americium poisoning, would suggest understanding of teaching?
   a. "I cannot receive these drugs if my kidneys are not functioning properly."
   b. "I need to take a pill every day for at least 2 months."
   c. "I should drink 100 ounces of fluid, especially water, each day."
   d. "I should try to empty my bladder at least once every 8 hours."

14. The nurse knows that adverse effects of ferric hexacyanoferrate (Prussian blue) used to increase excretion of nonradiaoctive thallium can increase the risk of toxicity of which of the following medications?
   a. Acetaminophen
   b. Atenolol
   c. Digoxin
   d. Furosemide

CASE STUDIES AND PATIENT TEACHING

(Use a separate piece of paper for your responses.)

Case Study 1

People died from inhalation of anthrax spores in the United States in October 2001. The nation was on alert for terrorist attacks.

1. What are possible reasons for the infections not being promptly diagnosed and treated in time to prevent all deaths?

2. How can the nurse contribute to early recognition of infections caused by biologic agents?

3. People who were possibly exposed to the *B. anthracis* were offered prophylactic drug therapy. What teaching should be provided by the community health nurses assisting with this mass prophylaxis?

Case Study 2

A patient has come to the emergency department because of exposure to an unknown powder.

1. If this person was exposed to anthrax bacilli, how can the infection spread to other people?

2. What precautions should the nurse take to prevent the spread of anthrax infection?

Case Study 3

The military nurse is participating in a mock drill imitating exposure of soldiers to mustard gas.

1. What would be the first action that the nurse should take?

2. How can the nurse prevent additional exposure to the agent for the soldiers and healthcare providers?

3. What questions about the episode would the nurse ask to determine which persons probably received the most exposure to the gas?

4. What symptoms would the nurse expect to occur first?

5. What should the nurse assess to determine if the most serious consequences could be occurring?

Case Study 4

Reports of ricin being used by terrorists cause a great deal of fear.

1. Why is ricin a logical weapon of bioterrorism?

2. What treatment would the nurse anticipate if a patient is admitted with inhalation of ricin?

3. What test would detect the early effects of ricin on the GI tract?